Monoclonal Antibodies against Bacteria

Volume III

Monoclonal Antibodies against Bacteria

Volume III

Edited by

Alberto J. L. Macario
Everly Conway de Macario

Wadsworth Center for Laboratories and Research
New York State Department of Health
Albany, New York

1986

ACADEMIC PRESS, INC.
Harcourt Brace Jovanovich, Publishers
Orlando   San Diego   New York   Austin
Boston   London   Sydney   Tokyo   Toronto

ACADEMIC PRESS, INC.
Orlando, Florida 32887

United Kingdom Edition published by
ACADEMIC PRESS INC. (LONDON) LTD.
24–28 Oval Road, London NW1 7DX

Library of Congress Cataloging in Publication Data
(Revised for vol. 3)

Monoclonal antibodies against bacteria.

Includes bibliographies and indexes.
 1. Bacterial antigens—Analysis—Collected works.
2. Antibodies, Monoclonal—Collected works. I. Macario,
Alberto J. L. II. Conway de Macario, Everly. [DNLM:
1. Antibodies, Monoclonal. 2. Bacteria. QW 575 M7472]
QR186.6.B33M66 1985   616.9'20793   84-24455
ISBN 0-12-463003-0 (v. 3 : alk. paper)

PRINTED IN THE UNITED STATES OF AMERICA

86 87 88 89   9 8 7 6 5 4 3 2 1

To our parents.
They built a present for themselves
and the future for us.

Contents

1 Identification and Characterization of *Treponema pallidum* Antigens by Monoclonal Antibodies

Sheila A. Lukehart

2 Diagnostic Uses of Monoclonal Antibodies to *Salmonella*

Pak Leong Lim

3 Monoclonal Antibodies and Immunodetection Methods for *Vibrio cholerae* and *Escherichia coli* Enterotoxins

Ann-Mari Svennerholm, Marianne Wikström, Leif Lindholm, and Jan Holmgren

4 Monoclonal Antibodies against *Campylobacter* Strains

Timo U. Kosunen and Mikko Hurme

5 Monoclonal Antibodies to the Lipopolysaccharide and Capsular Polysaccharide of *Bacteroides fragilis*

Matti K. Viljanen, Linnéa Linko, Pertti Arstila, Olli-Pekka Lehtonen, and Andrej Weintraub

6 Monoclonal Antibodies against Surface Components of *Streptococcus pneumoniae*

Larry S. McDaniel and David E. Briles

7 Monoclonal Antibodies to *Bordetella pertussis*

Charlotte D. Parker

8 Molecular Structures of Bacteria Elucidated by Monoclonal Antibodies with Special Reference to Antigenic Determinants of the Methanogens' Envelopes

Everly Conway de Macario and Alberto J. L. Macario

9 Monoclonal Antibodies against *Clostridium perfringens* θ Toxin (Perfringolysin O)

Hiroko Sato

10 Monoclonal Antibodies against Diphtheria Toxin: Their Use in Analysis of the Function and Structure of the Toxin and Their Application to Cell Biology

T. Yoshimori and T. Uchida

11 Application of Monoclonal Antibodies to the Study of Oral Bacteria and Their Virulence Factors

Joseph M. DiRienzo

12 Current and Future Applications of Monoclonal Antibodies against Bacteria in Veterinary Medicine

David M. Sherman and R. J. F. Markham

Contributors

Numbers in parentheses indicate the pages on which the authors' contributions begin.

Pertti Arstila (119), Department of Virology, University of Turku, SF-20520 Turku, Finland

David E. Briles (143), The Cellular Immunobiology Unit of the Tumor Institute, Departments of Microbiology and Pediatrics, and The Comprehensive Cancer Center, University of Alabama at Birmingham, Birmingham, Alabama 35294

Everly Conway de Macario (181), Wadsworth Center for Laboratories and Research, New York State Department of Health, Albany, New York 12201

Joseph M. DiRienzo (249), Department of Microbiology, School of Dental Medicine, University of Pennsylvania, Philadelphia, Pennsylvania 19104

Jan Holmgren (77), Department of Medical Microbiology, University of Göteborg, S-413 46 Göteborg, Sweden

Mikko Hurme (99), Department of Bacteriology and Immunology, University of Helsinki, 00290 Helsinki, Finland

Timo U. Kosunen (99), Department of Bacteriology and Immunology, University of Helsinki, 00290 Helsinki, Finland

Olli-Pekka Lehtonen (119), Department of Medical Microbiology, University of Turku, SF-20520 Turku, Finland

Pak Leong Lim (29), Department of Microbiology, University of Hong Kong, Hong Kong

Leif Lindholm (77), Department of Medical Microbiology, University of Göteborg, S-413 46 Göteborg, Sweden

Linnéa Linko (119), Department of Medical Microbiology, University of Turku, SF-20520 Turku, Finland

Sheila A. Lukehart (1), Department of Medicine, University of Washington School of Medicine, Seattle, Washington 98195

Alberto J. L. Macario (181), Wadsworth Center for Laboratories and Research, New York State Department of Health, Albany, New York 12201

R. J. F. Markham[1] (295), Department of Large Animal Clinical Sciences, College of Veterinary Medicine, University of Minnesota, St. Paul, Minnesota 55108

Larry S. McDaniel (143), The Cellular Immunobiology Unit of the Tumor Institute, Departments of Microbiology and Pediatrics, and The Comprehensive Cancer Center, University of Alabama at Birmingham, Birmingham, Alabama 35294

Charlotte D. Parker (165), Department of Microbiology, School of Medicine, University of Missouri, Columbia, Missouri 65212

Hiroko Sato (203), Department of Applied Immunology, National Institute of Health, Shinagawa-ku, Kamiosaki, Tokyo 141, Japan

David M. Sherman (295), Department of Large Animal Clinical Sciences, College of Veterinary Medicine, University of Minnesota, St. Paul, Minnesota 55108

Ann-Mari Svennerholm (77), Department of Medical Microbiology, University of Göteborg, S-413 46 Göteborg, Sweden

T. Uchida (229), Institute for Molecular and Cellular Biology, Osaka University, Suita, Osaka 565, Japan

Matti K. Viljanen (119), Department of Medical Microbiology, University of Turku, SF-20520 Turku, Finland

Andrej Weintraub (119), Karolinska Institute, Department of Clinical Bacteriology, Huddinge University Hospital, Huddinge, Sweden

Marianne Wikström (77), Department of Medical Microbiology, University of Göteborg, S-413 46 Göteborg, Sweden

T. Yoshimori (229), Department of Physiology, Kansai Medical University, Moriguchi-shi, Osaka 570, Japan

[1]Present address: Department of Pathology and Microbiology, Faculty of Veterinary Medicine, University of Prince Edward Island, Charlottetown, Prince Edward Island, Canada C1A 4P3.

Preface

This volume was conceived following the same principles that guided the production of the earlier ones. A variety of topics is encompassed by the twelve chapters. They are linked by the basic principles of hybridoma technology, which are similar, if not identical, no matter which bacterial species is studied. While these basic principles ensure unity, the special features of each chapter endow this volume with a wealth of knowledge. A broad range of biologic, medical, and biotechnologic themes is covered. A representative cross-section of contemporary developments involving monoclonal antibodies against bacteria is presented.

The format of the chapters is the same as that of those in Volumes I and II. Introductory material helps to explain the novel data presented in the Results and Discussion sections. Anticipated developments are included near the end of each contribution. (These extrapolations are as inspiring as the data presented.) Each chapter closes with a comprehensive bibliography.

A call has recently been made to "revive systematics" [E. O. Wilson (1985). *Science* **230,** 1227]. Systematics is much more than classification of organisms. It is a source of knowledge, a springboard for launching research aimed at understanding biologic diversity at all levels. From this vantage point, monoclonal antibodies emerge as essential instruments, particularly in bacteriology, as illustrated by the contents of this treatise. For example, discovering better ways to extract energy from biomass depends to a significant extent on taxonomic exploration (see E. O. Wilson, cited above). Paradigmatic in this respect are monoclonal antibodies against bacteria that produce methane gas from organic wastes.

Another important field of biotechnology in which monoclonal antibodies against bacteria are playing a momentous role is vaccine design and production.

The antibodies are useful for identifying antigens which elicit protective immunity and which should be part of a vaccine. The same antibodies aid in preparing the vaccine, in the quality control of its production, and in monitoring the response it elicits in vaccinated individuals.

What next? Research aimed at improving hybridoma technology and monoclonal antibody generation goes on. Major efforts are devoted toward optimizing *in vitro* procedures to immunize lymphocytes before fusion and toward producing large amounts of antibodies (thus avoiding the use of animals for this purpose). Techniques to obtain human monoclonal antibodies are also being actively tested. Especially interesting is work concerned with designing antibody molecules, in the laboratory, according to specifications. This work draws on hybridoma and recombinant DNA technologies and on genetic and chemical strategies. Manipulations of the components of the antibody molecule (fragments, chains) and of their DNA and RNA counterparts are employed. The ideal of constructing antibody molecules with all the necessary attributes to meet certain demands, but lacking unwanted properties, is approaching its realization. Undoubtedly these advances will greatly benefit bacterial immunology.

Recent work with bacteria found in plants [S. H. DeBoer and A. Wieczorek (1984). *Phytopathology* **74,** 1431] adds still another facet to the theme of monoclonal antibodies against bacteria. The same could be said about studies using monoclonal antibodies for the investigation of cell differentiation and the formation of supracellular structures in fruiting bacteria [J. Gill, E. Stellwag, and M. Dworkin (1985). *Ann. Inst. Pasteur/Microbiol.* **136A,** 11]. These two examples from very different disciplines, with the variety of topics dealt with in this treatise, demonstrate that monoclonal antibodies against bacteria have become an essential component of bacteriology in various areas of scientific endeavor. Consequently, Volume III aims to provide, as does the treatise as a whole, a forum in which medicine, dentistry, and veterinary science cross-fertilize with one another and with other disciplines such as engineering. Interaction of scientists across traditional borders that divide science into compartments may quicken the progress of research toward achievements of practical interest. This is, at least, our hope.

The chapters in this volume are concerned with important topics: treponemal antigens of significance for understanding syphilis, yaws, and pinta (Chapter 1): salmonellosis (Chapter 2) and other gastroenteropathies (Chapters 3–5); pediatric infections (Chapters 6 and 7); strategies for molecular analyses of bacterial antigens, focusing on cell walls, S layers, and sheaths (Chapter 8); bacterial toxins involved in gaseous gangrene (Chapter 9) and other forms of cell damage, as in diphtheria (Chapter 10); caries and periodontal disease (Chapter 11); and bacteria relevant to animal sciences (Chapter 12).

Alberto J. L. Macario
Everly Conway de Macario

Contents of Previous Volumes

Monoclonal Antibodies against Bacteria

Volume III

1

Identification and Characterization of *Treponema pallidum* Antigens by Monoclonal Antibodies

SHEILA A. LUKEHART
Department of Medicine
University of Washington School of Medicine
Seattle, Washington

I. INTRODUCTION

Treponemal infections in humans are complex, chronic, systemic diseases with protean clinical manifestations and the risk of serious late sequelae. Syph-

1

ilis, which is the most widely known, is a sexually transmitted disease with worldwide distribution, while the nonvenereal treponematoses (yaws, bejel, and pinta) occur primarily in tropical or semiarid regions of the developing world, particularly in Africa and Southeast Asia. These diseases progress from an initial, primary skin or mucous membrane lesion to the secondary disseminated and destructive tertiary stages, interrupted by long periods of latency. The numerous and varied clinical manifestations of syphilis have been recognized for centuries, but little real progress has been made in understanding the pathogenesis of the disease or the role of the host's immune response in modifying disease progression. The definition of the antigenic structure of pathogenic treponemes has been limited by the inability to cultivate the organisms continuously *in vitro,* and consequently, much of our knowledge of the antigenic structure of members of the genus *Treponema* is based on studies of cultivable nonpathogenic treponemes and cumbersome absorption of polyvalent antisera. Major advances have been made since 1980 in the identification of the major antigens of *Treponema pallidum* and in the definition of the host's immune response to those molecules. This chapter briefly reviews the current knowledge of treponemal biology and antigenic structure, and will detail the recent production of monoclonal antibodies to *T. pallidum* as well as the potential contributions of monoclonal antibodies to the study of treponemal infections.

II. BACKGROUND

A. Taxonomy

The genus *Treponema* includes the etiologic agents of venereal and endemic syphilis, yaws, and pinta, as well as numerous nonpathogenic commensal species which are found on the mucosal surfaces of the mouth, genitalia, and gastrointestinal tract (73). The pathogenic treponemes are distinguishable from the nonpathogens by their morphology, motility, and inability to be cultured *in vitro.* Although a considerable degree of antigenic relatedness exists between the pathogenic and nonpathogenic treponemes, no DNA homology has been reported between virulent *T. pallidum* (Nichols strain) and the nonpathogenic *Treponema phagedenis* or *Treponema refringens* (50).

The four human pathogens are morphologically identical and, to date, are indistinguishable serologically. Historically, they have been classified as separate species on the basis of the characteristic diseases they cause and, to some degree, their animal host ranges. Recent DNA sequence homology studies revealed 100% reassociation of DNA from *T. pallidum* Nichols strain (venereal syphilis) with that of *Treponema pertenue,* the causative agent of yaws (51). Based on these studies, the pathogenic treponemes were recently reclassified

(73): *T. pallidum* subsp. *pallidum* (venereal syphilis), *T. pallidum* subsp. *pertenue* (yaws), *T. pallidum* subsp. *endemicum* (endemic syphilis or bejel), and *T. carateum* (pinta). With rare exceptions, the discussion below concerning pathogenesis, host response, and antigenic structure will be based on studies involving the Nichols strain of *T. pallidum* subsp. *pallidum*.

B. Growth and Morphology

Treponemes are motile, helical bacteria, 5–20 μm in length, with multiple periplasmic flagella (axial filaments) lying within the outer membrane. Beneath the flagella is a layer of peptidoglycan and a trilaminar cytoplasmic membrane. The existence of a distinct mucopolysaccharide coating or outer envelope remains controversial (36), although freshly isolated *T. pallidum* are coated with host-derived proteins (1,39) and/or mucopolysaccharides (18, 24, 27, 77, 78, 85, 90, 91).

Limited multiplication of *T. pallidum* has been achieved in a tissue culture system (21,59) under microaerophilic conditions, although continuous passage has not been achieved and organisms must be propagated by serial passage in susceptible mammals, usually rabbits. Because the organisms must be extracted from infected tissue, large numbers of bacteria are expensive and cumbersome to obtain, with additional difficulties encountered in purification of the organisms from host tissue.

C. Clinical Course of Treponemal Infections

Treponemal infections are transmitted by direct contact with an infectious lesion. Because the organisms do not survive for long periods outside of an animal host, fomite transmission is very rare. Venereal syphilis is acquired by sexual contact, while the nonvenereal treponemal infections are usually acquired in childhood under conditions of crowding and poor hygiene. The organisms penetrate abraded skin or intact mucous membranes and begin to multiply at the site of inoculation. Within minutes or hours, the bacteria gain access to the circulatory and lymphatic systems, and disseminate to the spleen, liver, lymph nodes, and other tissues. Invasion of the central nervous system in venereal syphilis, when it occurs, is thought to take place within the first days or weeks of infection.

The organisms remaining at the site of inoculation multiply with a generation time of approximately 33 hr (19) resulting, after an average incubation period of 3 weeks, in the appearance of a firm, indurated primary lesion or chancre. Initially a painless papule, the chancre quickly enlarges and ulcerates. Because of the sexual nature of syphilis transmission, primary lesions occur most frequently in the genital, perianal, and oral areas, although any part of the body may be involved. Histologic examination reveals a pronounced perivascular mononuclear infiltrate, with lymphocytes and macrophages predominating. Plasma cells are frequently present and endothelial proliferation is characteristic. Because treponemes are not known to elaborate any toxin or to have clear cytopathic activity, the pathogenesis of treponemal disease is thought to be due to the host's immune response to bacterial antigens. Treponemes may be found in abundance early in the course of lesion development and are frequently found in perivascular areas.

The primary lesion heals spontaneously within 1 to 2 months and the disseminated rash of secondary syphilis then appears as macular, papular, or (more rarely) pustular lesions, located on the trunk, extremities, palms, and soles. Other evidence of systemic infection (lymphadenopathy, pharyngitis, malaise, headache, fever, and liver or kidney involvement) frequently accompanies or precedes the development of dermatologic manifestations. Histologically, secondary lesions are very similar to primary chancres, with lymphocytes, plasma cells, and macrophages being the prominent cell types.

Again, the lesions heal spontaneously and the patient enters a period of latency which extends for variable times from several months to decades. Although the patient has no clinical manifestations, persistent organisms may be identified in various tissues including spleen, lymph nodes, and liver. The precise location (intracellular versus extracellular) and metabolic status of *T. pallidum* during latency is unknown; however, no inflammatory response is apparent in infected tissues.

Approximately 30% of patients with untreated syphilis develop tertiary disease involving (a) gummatous destruction of the skin, bone, mucous membranes, or other internal organs; (b) symptomatic or asymptomatic central nervous system involvement; and (c) cardiovascular involvement, primarily aortitis. The remaining patients are latently infected for the remainder of their lives, with no further clinical evidence of disease. There is no firm evidence for spontaneous cure.

Infection of the fetus via the transplacental route can occur during any stage of syphilis, however, women with early active disease are more likely to have affected fetuses. Congenital infection can result in stillbirth, spontaneous abortion, perinatal death, or birth of a live infant with active or latent syphilis. Untreated congenital syphilis can progress to the tertiary stage.

The nonvenereal treponemal infections (yaws, pinta, endemic syphilis) follow the same basic clinical course as venereal syphilis except that cardiovascular or central nervous system involvement and congenital infection have not been documented in any of the nonvenereal treponematoses.

D. Pathogenesis and the Immune Response

The pathogenic mechanisms of treponemal infections are not well defined. It has been hypothesized that one of the first steps in infection is the attachment of the treponeme to the mammalian cell by specific receptor sites on the tip of the bacterium (22,23,34). Recent evidence indicates that fibronectin may be an important component in the attachment of *T. pallidum* to host tissues (25,26,64,79,80); laminin and collagen have also been implicated as mediators of attachment (25).

Dissemination of the infection from the site of inoculation occurs very early, by an unknown mechanism(s), through the walls of capillaries and lymphatic vessels and across the blood–brain and placental barriers. Fitzgerald (24) has suggested that hyaluronidase (or other mucopolysaccharidase) of treponemal origin may serve as a "spreading factor" which destroys the mucopolysaccharide ground substance of capillary and lymphatic vessels, thus allowing the dissemination of the organism to other tissues. This hypothesis is speculative at this point and there is no firm evidence that *T. pallidum* produces a mucopolysaccharidase or that the enzyme is required for pathogenesis.

During active infection, most treponemes are found in the extracellular spaces; however, they have also been detected by electron microscopy within cells. The intracellular location of treponemes may contribute to their ability to evade the host's immune response and persist during the latent stage. The passive or active acquisition of proteins or mucopolysaccharides of host origin may also serve to protect the organisms from the effects of antibody, complement, or phagocytic cells and thus permit persistence.

The host responds to treponemal infection by the production of antibodies, sensitization of T lymphocytes, and activation of macrophages. In experimental infection of rabbits, antitreponemal antibodies can be detected by immunofluorescence and Western blotting within 1 week following intratesticular infection (31,48), and neutralizing or immobilizing activity is first detectable at 1 month (15). The role of antibody in protection against treponemal infection has been examined extensively using polyvalent antisera. These studies have shown that antibody, with complement, can immobilize *T. pallidum in vitro* (57) and render the organism noninfectious (15,16). Passive administration of rabbits with antiserum to *T. pallidum* delays and alters lesion development (14,28,63,72,83, 84,88) but does not eliminate the challenge organisms. Passively administered antiserum completely protects hamsters from endemic syphilis infection (4) but does not confer complete protection against yaws infection (68).

There are several mechanisms by which antibody can contribute to protection against treponemal infection, including complement-dependent immobilization (57) or neutralization (15,16), opsonization (40), and inhibition of bacterial attachment to mammalian cells (23,34,89) or extracellular matrix (25). The observation that humans develop the rash of secondary syphilis, with a very large number of detectable treponemes, in the presence of high-titered, antitreponemal antibodies indicates that the antibody which is produced is not effective alone.

Histologic studies have strongly implicated the T lymphocyte and macrophage as the major infiltrating cells in healing primary lesions in rabbits (5,41,70), and treponemes have been identified within macrophages *in vivo* (5,42,71). Numerous investigators have examined the cellular arm of the immune response *in vitro* using lymphocyte blast transformation and lymphokine release assays, and adoptive transfer. These studies (reviewed in 45) have shown that T lymphocytes are sensitized to treponemal antigens early in infection and that these lymphocytes release soluble macrophage-activating factors (43). The phagocytosis of *T. pallidum* by macrophages has been demonstrated (40) and is significantly enhanced by immune serum.

E. Identification and Characterization of *Treponema pallidum* Antigens Using Polyvalent Antisera

Historically, the analysis of the antigenic structure of *T. pallidum* has been limited because of the inability to grow the organism *in vitro*. Although Fieldsteel and others (21,59) have reported the multiplication of *T. pallidum in vitro,* continuous culture has not yet been achieved. The organisms must therefore be propagated by intratesticular passage in rabbits and extracted from minced rabbit tissue. In addition to treponemes, these suspensions contain varying amounts of host tissue including erythrocytes, lymphocytes, serum proteins, spermatozoa, and noncellular tissue debris. Although gross cellular debris can be removed by low-speed centrifugation, the removal of serum proteins and noncellular tissue components has proved difficult.

Because of the inability to obtain large quantities of purified *T. pallidum,* much of the early knowledge of treponemal antigenic structure was derived from studies on nonpathogenic, cultivable treponemes such as *T. phagedenis,* biotype Reiter. The Reiter organism contains a protein antigen which is shared with other treponemes, including *T. pallidum* (17,20). This protein, determined by Hardy *et al.* (33) to be located primarily in the axial filaments, has served as the basis for a serologic test for syphilis. In an examination of *T. pallidum* antigens, Miller *et al.* (52) described both heat-labile and heat-stable antigens which were specific for *T. pallidum* (Nichols and other human strains). In addition, protein and lipopolysaccharide antigens related to Reiter antigens were described. In a later report, Miller *et al.* (53) described a heat-stable, radiation-resistant, noncardiolipin antigen which was specific for the Nichols strain of *T. pallidum.*

1. Identification of Antigenic Molecules

Since 1980, technical advances, including immunoblotting, have resulted in a rapid increase in our knowledge of the major antigenic molecules of *T. pallidum.* Using polyvalent antisera with sodium dodecyl sulfate–polyacrylamide gel electrophoresis (SDS–PAGE) and immunoblotting (6–9,12,29–31,44,48,62,86) or radioimmunoprecipitation (2,3,11,37,54,55,74,81) techniques, a fairly clear profile of the antigens of *T. pallidum* has emerged, consisting of approximately 23 molecules ranging in molecular weight from 115,000 to 12,000 (Fig. 1). The major antigens are molecules of 69, 47–48, 40, 37, 35, 33, 30, 14, and 12 kDa. Thornburg and Baseman (81) and Norris and Sell (60) examined *T. pallidum* using two-dimensional electrophoresis and identified many more treponemal proteins, 67 of which reacted with antibody from syphilitic rabbits (60).

The reported molecular weights of *T. pallidum* molecules vary by 3000 to 5000 Da between laboratories, and no standardized nomenclature has yet been devised. Although this fact makes it difficult to compare the results from different laboratories, similar antigenic profiles have been proposed by investigators using similar techniques.

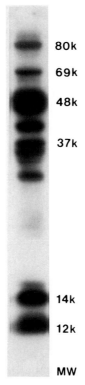

80k

69k

48k

37k

14k

12k

MW

Fig. 1.   Antigenic profile of *Treponema pallidum* Nichols strain, as revealed by autoradiography with pooled human syphilitic sera and ^{125}I-labeled protein A. Treponemes were disrupted by sonication, solubilized in SDS, and electrophoresed on 12.5% polyacrylamide gels prior to electrophoretic transfer onto nitrocellulose paper for reaction with antibody and ^{125}I-labeled protein A. Twenty-two antigenic molecules were identified; approximate molecular weights are shown. Reproduced with permission from Lukehart (47).

2. Biochemical Characterization of Antigenic Molecules

Because of the electrophoretic mobility of the identified molecules and their ability to be stained by Coomassie Blue, the antigenic molecules are assumed to be polypeptides; however, the precise chemical nature of the antigenic determinants has not been defined.

Two laboratories have examined *T. pallidum* antigens for the presence of carbohydrate moieties. Using [^{14}C]glucosamine incorporation *in vitro,* Moskophidis and Muller (55) identified four surface glycoproteins, with molecular weights of 59,000, 35,000, 33,000, and 30,500. Using a modification of the immunoblotting technique, Baker-Zander and Lukehart (10) have identified 14 antigenic molecules which bind ^{125}I-labeled lectins. These lectins also agglutinate washed *T. pallidum,* indicating that at least some of the carbohydrate is located on the outer membrane. Periodate oxidation of the molecules prior to reaction destroys the ability of the [^{125}I]concanavalin A to bind, and competition by specific sugars blocks lectin binding, thus confirming the carbohydrate nature of the lectin-binding moiety.

3. Identification of Molecules Containing Common and Pathogen-Specific Determinants

Antigenic cross-reactivity between *T. pallidum* and the nonpathogenic treponemes has been recognized for many years, however the molecules responsible for this cross-reactivity have been identified only recently. Five cross-reactive molecules of the Reiter treponeme were identified by Strandberg-Pedersen *et al.* (76) by reaction with sera from patients with secondary syphilis; one of these antigens was thought to represent the axial filament. Bharier and Allis (13) reported earlier that the axial filaments, which contain common antigens, are composed of three molecules between 33,000 and 36,500 Da. A recent study by Limberger and Charon (38) identified two molecules from purified *T. phagedenis* axial filaments with molecular weights of 39,800 and 33,000. Antiserum raised against the 33-kDa molecule cross-reacted with *T. pallidum.* Studies of purified axial filaments of *T. pallidum* (62) revealed the presence of three molecules with reported molecular weights ranging from 33,500 to 37,000.

Lukehart *et al.* (44), Hanff *et al.* (30), Moskophidis and Muller (54), and Baughn *et al.* (12) investigated the molecules containing antigens common to *T. pallidum* and the Reiter treponeme, and identified 4–15 molecules containing common antigens. Molecules of approximately 80, 69, 47, 37, 35, 33, and 30 kDa were identified by at least three of the four laboratories. Hanff *et al.* (30) and Lukehart *et al.* (44) speculated that the 30- and 33-kDa or 35- and 33-kDa molecules, respectively, represent axial filament components.

Pathogen-specific determinants were hypothesized by Lukehart *et al.* (44) to be located on molecules of 48, 14, and 12 kDa. Although reactivity of syphilitic rabbit serum to a 37-kDa molecule was not completely removed by absorption with the Reiter treponeme, a 37-kDa molecule of *T. pallidum* was identified with anti-Reiter antiserum. It is possible that the 37- and 48-kDa molecules each contain common and pathogen-specific determinants. Jones *et al.* (37) detected pathogen-specific determinants on the 47–48 kDa molecule using polyvalent antisera; however, they could not detect common determinants with their methodologies. Hanff *et al.* (30) report the identification of 14 pathogen-specific molecules; however, molecular weights are not given.

Baker-Zander and Lukehart (7) examined the molecular basis for cross-reactivity of *T. pallidum* with related spirochetes including the rabbit pathogen *Treponema paraluiscuniculi,* the swine pathogen *Treponema hyodysenteriae, Borrelia hermsii,* and *Leptospira interrogans.* The *T. pallidum* antigens recognized by immunoblotting with antiserum to *T. paraluiscuniculi* were virtually identical to those recognized by human or rabbit syphilitic sera, while the number of molecules identified by antiserum to more distantly related species was substantially lower. This study provided evidence, however, for the existence of one or more common spirochete antigens; the *T. pallidum* molecules most frequently recognized by heterologous antisera were 80, 69, 47, 37, 35, 33, and 30 kDa. These are the same molecules identified as containing antigens cross-reactive with the Reiter treponeme.

4. Comparison of Strains and Subspecies of Treponema pallidum

Baker-Zander and Lukehart (6), Thornburg and Baseman (81), and Stamm and Bassford (74) compared the major protein antigens of *T. pallidum* subsp. *pallidum* and *pertenue* using one- or two-dimensional gel electrophoresis and immunoblotting or radioimmunoprecipitation. Only minor molecular weight differences of several molecules were noted. Stamm and Bassford (74) also compared the antigenic profiles of the Nichols strain of *T. pallidum* with a more recent isolate, Street 14, and detected only minor differences.

5. Location and Function of Antigenic Molecules

The surface location of *T. pallidum* antigens has been examined by several laboratories (2,37,55,60,74,81) using ^{125}I-labeling of intact organisms. The number of putative outer membrane proteins varies from 9 to 20, depending on the report, but there appears to be consensus that the immunodominant 46–48 kDa molecule is surface exposed, as well as a molecule of approximately 39–40 kDa.

Baseman and co-workers have identified three outer membrane molecules which serve as receptor ligands for *T. pallidum* binding to fibronectin and cell surfaces (11,64,79,80). Although the reported molecular weights of these receptors has varied in each of their publications, Thomas *et al.* (80) recently reported corrected values of 89,500, 37,000, and 32,000. These molecules were recently demonstrated by proteolytic digestion and peptide mapping to have a common functional domain of 12,000 Da (80).

F. Unanswered Questions

Syphilis has been a well-described clinical entity for centuries, but our knowledge of the mechanisms of pathogenesis and bacterial persistence is very limited. Although we know that immobilizing, neutralizing, and opsonizing antibodies are produced in response to infection, the precise antigens to which these antibody activities are directed are not known. Sensitized T lymphocytes proliferate and produce macrophage-activating factors in the presence of sonicated *T. pallidum,* yet the specific antigens responsible for T-cell stimulation have not been defined.

The technical difficulties associated with the study of a bacterium which must be cultivated *in vivo* have resulted in a relative dearth of knowledge of the antigenic structure of *T. pallidum.* The recent development of hybridoma technology and gene cloning will finally permit the examination of purified antigenic determinants of *T. pallidum* in order to unravel the complex host–parasite relationship of syphilis. Monoclonal antibodies to *T. pallidum* have recently been produced and their use in antigenic analysis of the organism is just beginning. The discussion below addresses the production and characterization of these antibodies and their respective contributions, current and future, to the definition of treponemal antigens, examination of the host immune response, and the improved diagnosis of the disease.

III. RESULTS AND DISCUSSION

A. Production of Monoclonal Antibodies

Six laboratories have reported the production of monoclonal antibodies with specificity for *T. pallidum.* The immunizing preparations, schedules, and doses differed between laboratories (Table I).

1. Immunizing Preparation

The primary goal in the development of monoclonal antibodies to *T. pallidum* is to aid in the examination of the antigens of the bacterium which are expressed during infection of an animal or human host. The optimal method for immunizing mice for production of such antibodies, then, is actively to infect them with *T. pallidum.* Unfortunately, infection of mice with *T. pallidum* results in a self-limited asymptomatic condition in which the organisms are rapidly cleared and only low levels of antibody are produced. For that reason, one cannot depend on

TABLE I

Production of Monoclonal Antibodies to *Treponema pallidum*

Reference	Immunizing preparation	Duration	Route[a]	Total dose	Adjuvant	Myeloma cell line
Robertson et al. (65)	Freshly isolated *T. pallidum*	87 days	ip, iv	2.7×10^8	CFA	SP2/0
Saunders and Folds (67)	Virulent *T. pallidum*	6 weeks	id, ip	Not specified	CFA	P3 × 63-Ag8.653 or SP2/0
Van Embden et al. (87)	Viable, urografin-purified *T. pallidum*	1, 3, 5 months	ip, iv	7×10^7	None	Not specified
Thornburg et al. (81, 82)	Freshly extracted Methocel–Hypaque purified *T. pallidum*	24 days	im, sc, ip	1.2×10^9	CFA	SP2/0
Lukehart et al. (46)	CPE-purified *T. pallidum*[a]	37 days	sc, ip, iv	9×10^7	CFA	NS1/1
Moskophidis and Muller (56)	Freshly extracted, urografin-purified *T. pallidum*	63 days	ip	2.8×10^8	CFA	SP2/0

[a] CPE, Continuous-particle electrophoresis; CFA, Freund's complete adjuvant; id, intradermal; ip, intraperitoneal; im, intramuscular; iv, intravenous; sc, subcutaneous.

the infectious process to stimulate appropriate antibody production (as with rabbits or humans), and *T. pallidum* must be treated simply as an inert antigen to be administered using a standard immunization protocol.

T. pallidum must be obtained from infected rabbit tissue and a major consideration in the immunization of mice is the presence of contaminating rabbit testicular tissue in the treponemal preparations. Because the organisms used for screening the hybridoma cells have also been derived from infected rabbit testes, the possibility exists for misidentification of some antirabbit antibodies as antitreponemal. Two laboratories attempted to remove gross rabbit cellular debris from the immunizing preparation by differential centifugation, three laboratories purified the bacteria by density gradient centrifugation, and one laboratory used commercially available continuous-particle electrophoresis (CPE)-purified *T. pallidum*. The use by Robertson et al. (65) and Saunders and Folds (67) of intact, freshly isolated, virulent organisms was an attempt to preserve, in the immunizing preparation, any loosely associated antigens of *T. pallidum,* so that, theoretically, all relevant antigens might be recognized. It would be anticipated that immunization with this suspension would result in the production of many anti-rabbit monoclonal antibodies. Both laboratories reported that several of their clones produced antibodies which reacted by enzyme-linked immunosorbent assay (ELISA) or radioimmunoassay (RIA) with normal rabbit tissue (NRT) as well as *T. pallidum* preparations. Saunders and Folds (67) used Percoll density gradient-purified organisms in their screening tests to minimize possible errors in interpretation, whereas Robertson *et al.* (65) used a *T. pallidum* preparation for screening which had been subjected only to differential centrifugation.

The remaining laboratories immunized mice with treponemal preparations that had been purified by density gradient centrifugation or CPE. These methods significantly reduce the amount of contaminating rabbit tissue in the treponemal suspension. The number of antirabbit antibodies reported by these investigators was variable. Lukehart *et al.* (46) and Van Embden *et al.* (87) found no NRT-reactive antibodies among 13 and 3 characterized antibodies, respectively. The use by Lukehart *et al.* of indirect immunofluorescence (IIF) of CPE-purified *T. pallidum* as a secondary screen of primary fusion wells reduced the possibility of propagating ''false-positive'' cell lines early in the procedure. Similarly, Moskophidis and Muller (56) performed NRT ELISA screening on primary wells and eliminated 34 fusion wells which contained anti-NRT activity. Thornburg *et al.* (82) do not report that their antibodies were tested for reactivity with rabbit tissue. Because the number of anti-NRT antibodies reported by the various laboratories is dependent on the screening strategy, as well as the purity of the immunizing preparation, one cannot conclude from these results that the purity of the immunizing preparation is really critical to the success of the fusion. Theoretically, less antigenic competition would occur during the immunization step if rabbit tissue were removed from the immunizing preparation; however, this point has not been examined directly by any investigator. A more important consideration may be the choice of screening strategies (Section III,A,3).

2. Immunization Protocol

The routes of immunization varied between laboratories, but always included at least one intraperitoneal injection. There was no clear advantage to any partic-ular route or protocol. The duration of immunization varied from 24 days to 5 months, with a median of 6 to 8 weeks. There was no obvious advantage, in terms of numbers of clones or in subclass of immunoglobulins produced, to a longer immunization schedule.

The total number of *T. pallidum* organisms used for immunization ranged from 7×10^7 to 1.2×10^9. Again, no obvious benefit was obtained by increas-ing the total dose above 3×10^8. All immunization protocols resulted in the production of numerous antibody-producing clones, except for that used by Van Embden *et al.* (87), who reported the production of only three anti-*T. pallidum* antibodies from three separate fusions. Several technical points should be considered in this regard. Van Embden *et al.* immunized with the lowest number of treponemes (7×10^7), using only an initial injection followed by three daily injections immediately prior to fusion. In addition, this laboratory was the only one which did not employ Freund's complete adjuvant (CFA). Lukehart *et al.* (46) also used a low total dose of organisms (9×10^7) in CFA, with a booster injection 1 week before the final injection. Although the total dose and schedule of injections are not significantly different between the two laboratories, the relative yield of the fusions was vastly different, and that difference may be due, in part, to the use of CFA. The theoretical concern of concurrent immunization with mycobacterial antigens by use of CFA appears to be unimportant in this setting.

3. Screening Strategies

Methods which employ a 96-well configuration are clearly the most practical for screening the large number of wells required for monoclonal antibody production. Two approaches have been used for *T. pallidum:* ELISA and solid-phase RIA. Although most laboratories found that sonicated *T. pallidum* was a better preparation for use in these assays, Thornburg *et al.* (82) used whole fixed *T. pallidum.* Most laboratories used a single method for the entire screening process, and then used multiple methodologies (immunofluorescence, immunoblot, hemagglutination, immobilization, competition assays) for later characterization. Lukehart *et al.* (46) used a double-screening method at each step of the cloning process: after initially identifying positive wells in an ELISA assay, each positive well was reevaluated by an IIF assay in which morphologic criteria and antigen purity were also used as a measure of specificity. Clearly the screening strategy is dependent on the intended uses of the monoclonal antibodies. Because Lukehart *et al.* were interested only in antibodies which reacted by IF, an early IF screen was necessary. Similarly, if one is interested in antibodies which react only with pathogenic treponemes, screening against one of the nonpathogenic treponemes is preferable during the cloning and selection process, in order to avoid propagation of clones reacting with common treponemal antigens.

It is apparent that all antitreponemal antibodies must be screened ultimately for anti-NRT reactivity. The stage at which this screening occurs, however, may affect the ultimate yield of the fusion. Because primary wells frequently contain multiple fusion products, the elimination of the primary wells containing anti-NRT reactivity may result in the inadvertent elimination of other valuable anti-*T. pallidum* clones. A preferable method in the initial screening may be the use of a positive-selection method (e.g., IIF of purified *T. pallidum*). This confirms the presence of specific anti-*T. pallidum* activity initially and defers the elimination of antirabbit clones to a later stage in which fewer clones are represented in a single well.

B. Characterization of Monoclonal Antibody Reactivity to *Treponema pallidum* and Related Organisms

1. Reactivity with Other Treponema pallidum *Strains*

All treponemal monoclonal antibodies reported to date have been produced using the Nichols strain of *T. pallidum* subsp. *pallidum* as the immunizing strain. This strain was isolated in 1915 and has been maintained by rabbit passage since that time. Because cross-protection studies have demonstrated antigenic differences between strains, the utility (for diagnostic purposes or identification of protective antigens) of information derived from *T. pallidum* monoclonal antibodies is dependent on the relevance of those antibodies to antigens expressed on modern "street strains" of *T. pallidum*. Only two laboratories have examined the reactivity of their antibodies with strains other than the immunizing strain. Lukehart *et al.* (46) measured the reactivity of 13 antibodies against four recently isolated (fewer than five passages in rabbits) *T. pallidum* strains by IIF and found that the degree of reactivity in each case was comparable to that seen with the Nichols strain. The eight antibodies described by Saunders and Folds (67) reacted by ELISA and RIA equally well with the Street 14 and Nichols strains.

Only the H9-1 antibody produced by Lukehart *et al.* (46) has been examined for reactivity with *T. pallidum* that have not been passaged in rabbits; this antibody has demonstrated high sensitivity and specificity for detection of *T. pallidum* in lesion exudates from patients with syphilis (35,66; see also Section III,D), indicating the conservation of the H9-1-defined epitope of *T. pallidum* from 1915 to the present.

2. Antigens Common to Nonpathogenic Treponemes

The antigenic cross-reactivity of the pathogenic and nonpathogenic treponemes is well established, and numerous investigators have identified distinct molecules which contain common and pathogen-specific antigenic determinants (Section II,E,3). Monoclonal antibodies provide a means for examining these treponemal antigens without tedious absorption of polyvalent antisera. All investigators reporting the production of *T. pallidum* monoclonal antibodies tested their antibodies for reactivity with the nonpathogenic Reiter treponeme. Although Saunders and Folds (67) report that some of their antibodies reacted with the Reiter treponeme, no data are shown and the molecular specificity of these antibodies was not explored. Thornburg *et al.* (82) report the result of one monoclonal antibody which did not react with the Reiter treponeme; the other antibodies were reportedly tested but no results were given. None of three antibodies reported by Van Embden *et al.* (87) reacted with the Reiter treponeme. Ten of 45 antibodies reported by Moskophidis and Muller (56), 3 of 39 reported by Robertson *et al.* (65), and 2 of 13 reported by Lukehart *et al.* (46) reacted by ELISA, IIF, and/or RIA with *T. pallidum* and the Reiter treponeme, but not with

NRT. The molecular specificities of such antibodies were examined only by Lukehart *et al.* (46). Antibody C2-1, which reacts with *T. pallidum* and the Reiter treponeme by ELISA and IIF, was shown by the immunoblotting technique to bind a determinant located on a molecule of approximately 48,000 Da. A molecule with an identical apparent molecular weight was also determined (Section II,E,3) to have pathogen-specific antigenic determinants. The binding of both pathogen-specific (Section III,B,3) and common treponemal monoclonal antibodies with a molecule of the same apparent molecular weight confirms the hypothesis of Lukehart *et al.* (44), based on studies with extensively absorbed polyvalent antisera, that both common and specific determinants reside on the 48-kDa molecule. Until two-dimensional electrophoresis is performed, however, one cannot state definitively that the determinants are on the same molecule, rather than on separate, comigrating molecules.

Thornburg *et al.* (82) examined the reactivity of antibody $13F_3$, which identifies an epitope on a 45-kDa molecule, against the swine pathogen, *T. hyodysenteriae* and found no binding. Lukehart *et al.* (46) tested all 13 of their monoclonal antibodies against a panel of pathogenic and nonpathogenic spirochetes, including *Treponema denticola* (strains 11 and W), *Treponema refringens* (Noguchi), *Treponema vincentii* (N-9), *T. hyodysenteriae* (B204), *Leptospira interrogans* (Canicola), and *Borrelia recurrentis*. Antibodies C2-1 and G2-1, which had been shown to react with an antigen on the Reiter treponeme, also reacted with each of the organisms listed above, confirming the presence of a common spirochetal antigen as suggested by Baker-Zander and Lukehart (7). In order to eliminate the possibility that these two IgM antibodies reacted with an antigen common to all bacteria or to mammalian cells, they were also tested by immunofluorescence against *Chlamydia trachomatis*-infected HeLa cells (75), with no reaction. The remaining 11 antibodies, which reacted with *T. pallidum* but not with the Reiter treponeme, also failed to react with any of the panel of spirochetes, confirming their specificity for human pathogens of the genus *Treponema*.

3. Identification of Pathogen-Specific Antigens

Most investigators have concentrated their efforts on the characterization of pathogen-specific antigens, and consequently those antibodies which react with *T. pallidum,* but not with the Reiter treponeme, are the best characterized. Although the production of many such antibodies has been reported, the molecular specificities of relatively few have been determined (Table II). The immunodominant molecule of *T. pallidum* has a reported molecular weight of 45,000 to 48,000 depending on the laboratory. All investigators (except Saunders and Folds, who did not examine molecular specificities) reported antibodies which reacted with this immunodominant molecule. In addition, the 44, 37, 33, 15.5, and 12 kDa molecules were shown to contain pathogen-specific determi-

TABLE II

Characterization of *Treponema pallidum* Antigens by Monoclonal Antibodies

Molecular weight	Common determinant	Pathogen-specific determinant	Surface location	Immobilization
48,000[a]	+(46)[c]	+(46)	+[d]	
47,000[a]		+(37)	+(37,49)	+(37)
46,000[a]		+(56,87)	+(56)	+(56)
45,000[a]		+(82)	+(82)	
44,000		+(56,87)	+(56)	+(56)
37,000		+(46)		
33,000		+(56)		+(56)
15,500[b]		+(56)		+(56)
12,000[b]		+(46)		

[a] Probably the same molecule.
[b] May be the same molecule.
[c] Reference numbers are in parentheses.
[d] E. M. Walker, N. H. Bishop, and S. A. Lukehart (unpublished observations).

nants by immunoblotting using characterized monoclonal antibodies. Each of these molecules had previously been identified in *T. pallidum* using polyvalent antisera and, except for the 33- and 44-kDa molecules, all had been hypothesized to contain pathogen-specific determinants.

4. Subspecies Differentiation Using Monoclonal Antibodies

Because antigenic differences between subspecies of *T. pallidum* are expected to be minor, the exquisite specificity of monoclonal antibodies holds the promise for serologic classification of these organisms. Although no laboratory has reported the production of subspecies-specific monoclonal antibodies, three laboratories have examined the reactivity of their antibodies with other *T. pallidum* subspecies. Marchitto *et al.* (49) evaluated two anti-47-kDa antibodies for reactivity with *T. pallidum* subsp. *pertenue* and *endemicum* by RIA, immunoblotting, and surface-binding assays. Although both antibodies bound to all organisms, the degree of binding varied. Marchitto and co-workers concluded that, although the 47-kDa antigen was present on all subspecies, its orientation or expression differed between organisms, making it more, or less, available for binding by antibody.

Preliminary studies by S. A. Lukehart and S. A. Baker-Zander (unpublished observations) also indicate differential reactivity of five to nine monoclonal antibodies with *T. pallidum* subsp. *pallidum* and *pertenue* by IIF assays. There was not a clear absence of reactivity with *T. pallidum* subsp. *pertenue;* rather the degree of fluorescence was significantly lower, suggesting reduced availability of the determinant for binding. Titration of the antibodies resulted in disappearance of reactivity to *T. pallidum* subsp. *pertenue,* while reactivity with *T. pallidum* subsp. *pallidum* persisted. Interestingly, differential binding of these same monoclonal antibodies was not observed in ELISA or RIA using sonicated organisms. This finding supports the hypothesis that certain determinants, while present in both organisms, may be oriented or exposed differently in the two organisms, as suggested by Marchitto *et al.* (49).

C. Location and Function of Antigens Defined by Monoclonal Antibodies

1. Surface Location

As discussed earlier (Section II,E,5), surface radioiodination studies, immunoprecipitation with polyvalent antisera, and SDS–PAGE have identified 9–20 outer membrane proteins of *T. pallidum,* including the immunodominant 46–48 kDa molecule. The use of monoclonal antibodies to determine the location of antigenic molecules on *T. pallidum* has been very limited to date. Reactivity of these antibodies with treponemal antigens is commonly measured by ELISA or RIA using sonicated organisms or by IIF using fixed bacteria. Under these conditions, the precise location of the binding cannot be determined. Marchitto *et al.* (49), using a surface-binding assay with two ^{125}I-labeled monoclonal antibodies (specific for the 47-kDa molecule) demonstrated binding to intact whole *T. pallidum* subsp. *pallidum* and *pertenue,* suggesting a surface location for this molecule. Electron micrographic studies confirmed, by staphylococcal protein A–colloidal gold visualization of monoclonal antibody binding, that the 47-kDa molecule is located on the surface of the bacterium. Electron micrographic studies using monoclonal antibodies A8-1 and IIG10-1 of Lukehart *et al.* (46) also confirm the binding of anti-48-kDa antibodies to the outer membrane of *T. pallidum* (Fig. 2; E. M. Walker, N. H. Bishop, and S. A. Lukehart, unpublished observations).

2. Attachment to Mammalian Cells

Although the 47-kDa molecule has not been implicated by others in the attachment of *T. pallidum* to mammalian cells, a monoclonal antibody specific for this molecule reportedly blocks the attachment of *T. pallidum* to host cells by 50% (37). Although the significance of this finding is unclear, it provides further evidence for the surface location of the 47-kDa molecule. The ability of other *T. pallidum* monoclonal antibodies to block attachment to mammalian cells has not been reported.

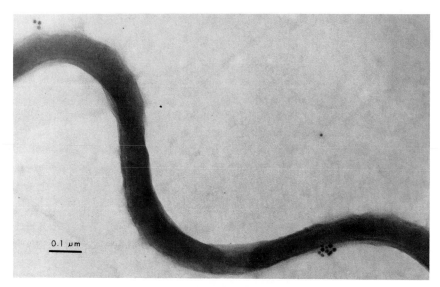

Fig. 2. The surface location of the 48,000-Da molecule of *Treponema pallidum* Nichols strain is confirmed by the binding of monoclonal antibody IIG10-1 to the outer membrane of the intact, unwashed bacterium. Bound antibody, detected by clusters of colloidal gold-labeled goat anti-mouse IgG, is probably localized to areas in which the outer membrane is exposed by disruption of surface-associated rabbit molecules. No colloidal gold particles are associated with the organism in the absence of antibody IIG10-1 or in the presence of an unrelated (anti-*Neisseria gonorrhoeae*) monoclonal antibody. Magnification × 50,000.

3. Immobilizing Activity

Reactivity of monoclonal antibodies in the *Treponema pallidum* immobilization (TPI) test has been used by some investigators to suggest the surface location of the target antigen (37). Jones *et al.* (37) showed that antibody to the 47-kDa molecule immobilized *T. pallidum* in the TPI test; Moskophidis and Muller (56) reported that two of two antibodies reacting with the 46-kDa molecule had immobilizing activity. Similarly, TPI reactivity was found in monoclonal antibodies with specificity for the 44, 33, and 15.5 kDa molecules; each of these molecules had been shown in previous studies from that laboratory to be located on the bacterial surface.

D. Diagnostic Applications of Monoclonal Antibodies

Diagnosis of syphilis infection is based on the identification of *T. pallidum* in exudate from skin or mucous membrane lesions and/or reactivity in various serologic tests. Culture diagnosis, which is used for most infectious diseases, is not possible for syphilis. In primary syphilis, the serologic screening tests are nonreactive in 30% of patients, and diagnosis must be based in these cases on microscopic identification of *T. pallidum* in lesion material by darkfield examination. Although darkfield microscopy is a valuable diagnostic tool in specialty clinics, microscopes with darkfield condensers are not available in most physicians' offices. The accuracy of the darkfield examination is dependent solely on the ability of the microscopist to differentiate *T. pallidum* from numerous commensal spirochetes on the basis of characteristic motility and morphology. In addition, darkfield microscopy is not reliable for persons with oral lesions because of the inability to distinguish *T. pallidum* from certain oral spirochetes.

Monoclonal antibodies with inherent specificity for the pathogenic treponemes provide the basis for the development of specific and sensitive methods for detection of *T. pallidum* in lesion exudate, tissue biopsy material, or other body fluids. Two laboratories have investigated the use of *T. pallidum* monoclonal antibodies for diagnosis of syphilis.

Norgard *et al.* (58) developed a solid-phase immunoblot assay to detect *T. pallidum* which had been air-dried onto nitrocellulose, using ^{125}I-labeled rabbit anti-mouse IgG and autoradiography. Three monoclonal antibodies were able to detect 10^3 treponemes, and one antibody could detect as few as 500 organisms, with a 2- to 4-day autoradiography period. Antibodies with the highest sensitivity were directed against the 47-kDa molecule. The specificity of this method was tested by a similar examination of the Reiter treponeme, *Haemophilus ducreyi, Neisseria gonorrhoeae,* herpes simplex virus type 2, and NRT. The test was developed using rabbit-derived *T. pallidum,* and the sensitivity and specificity of the method for detection of *T. pallidum* in clinical specimens has not been examined.

Direct immunofluorescence staining for detection of *T. pallidum* was described by Lukehart *et al.* (46) and has been evaluated in two reported clinical trials. This test has the advantage for the clinician of rapid results (<1 hr) and inherent specificity. Antibody H9-1, which has specificity for the immunodominant 48-kDa molecule, was purified and conjugated with fluorescein isothiocyanate for direct immunofluorescence (35). Exudate from lesions of patients attending sexually transmitted diseases clinics for evaluation of genital or cutaneous ulcers was collected on microscope slides and allowed to air-dry before acetone fixation and immunofluorescent staining. Hook *et al.* (35) evaluated 61 patients (30 with syphilis, 31 without syphilis) using the direct monoclonal antibody test, as well as microscopic, culture, and serologic testing routinely used for evaluation of genital ulcer disease. Compared to diagnosis based on standard diagnostic methods, the monoclonal antibody test was 100% sensitive and specific. Further, it detected *T. pallidum* in one syphilis patient for whom darkfield microscopic examination was negative, and identified two nonsyphilitic patients in whom microscopists incorrectly identified commensal spirochetes as *T. pallidum.*

This same antibody was used by Romanowski *et al.* (66) to evaluate 128 patients presenting to a sexually transmitted disease clinic in Canada. In this study the monoclonal antibody test was 89% sensitive compared to darkfield microscopic examination and was 100% specific for patients with syphilis.

IV. CONCLUSIONS

Monoclonal antibodies to *T. pallidum* have recently been developed and characterized in terms of their reactivity with various pathogenic and nonpathogenic spirochetes, molecular specificity, and functional activity (Table II). The exploitation of these antibodies, however, has only begun, and their early uses have been limited to confirmation of information obtained using polyvalent antisera and other techniques. The immunodominant 45–48 kDa molecule of *T. pallidum* has been the subject of the most intensive investigation using monoclonal antibodies. This molecule, which contains both common treponemal and pathogen-specific antigenic determinants, is located in the outer membrane of the bacterium. Antibodies directed against determinants found on this molecule are able to immobilize the organism in the presence of complement.

Based on studies with polyvalent antisera, the 37,000- and 33,000-Da molecules were hypothesized to contain common treponemal antigens. Monoclonal antibody reactivity has shown that they also appear to contain pathogen-specific determinants. Although molecules with similar molecular weights have been localized to the surface of the organism, detailed studies with monoclonal antibodies have not been completed. Molecules of 37,000 and 32,000 Da are reported by Thomas *et al.* (79) to be cytoadhesins; however the ability of monoclonal antibodies with these specificities to block binding of *T. pallidum* to fibronectin or mammalian cells has not been reported. Antibodies directed against the 33,000-Da molecule have immobilizing activity.

The low molecular weight pathogen-specific molecule(s) detected by monoclonal antibodies is poorly characterized. The reported molecular weights for this antigen vary from 12,000 to 16,000 and it is quite likely that the 15,500-Da molecule recognized by Moskophidis and Muller's monoclonal antibody (56) is the same as the 12,000-Da molecule recognized by antibody F5-1 of Lukehart *et al.* (46).

Monoclonal antibodies to *T. pallidum* have proved, and will continue, to be useful in the characterization of treponemal antigens. They also have permitted the development of specific and sensitive diagnostic tests for syphilis. Because these tests are sensitive in early disease, when serologic diagnosis is difficult or impossible, they fill a void in the methodologies available to most physicians for the differential diagnosis of genital ulcer disease. The inherent specificity of the monoclonal antibody test broadens the utility of the test beyond that of darkfield microscopy.

V. PROSPECTS FOR THE FUTURE

Because most investigators have only recently produced and characterized *T. pallidum* monoclonal antibodies, the actual application of those antibodies to antigenic analysis and purification has only begun. The potential applications are far ranging, from the clarification of taxonomic and evolutionary relatedness of spirochetes to epitope mapping of individual molecules and improved diagnosis of syphilis. The antibodies will be invaluable in determining, by immunoelectron microscopy, the location of specific antigenic molecules, including those located on the periplasmic flagella. Although surface location can be inferred from surface-labeling and surface-binding experiments, the integrity of the outer membrane in those experiments is not discernible and the results are therefore not definitive. The precise antibody-binding site can be visualized by immunoelectron microscopy.

Monoclonal antibodies will be useful in examining the pathogenesis of treponemal infections in terms of cell attachment and localization of organisms during the various stages of syphilis. Antigenic modulation has been hypothesized to explain the reappearance of bacteria during the secondary stage and their persistence during latency despite the presence of immobilizing antibody. Monoclonal antibodies might permit the examination of the expression and disappearance of specific antigens during the course of infection.

Purification of individual *T. pallidum* antigens is problematic because of the contaminating host material which is present in suspensions of the organisms. One of the major future applications of monoclonal antibodies will be the purification of antigenic molecules by affinity chromatography or large-scale immunoprecipitation. In this way, purified molecules can be obtained for biochemical analysis, and immunologic and vaccine studies. Epitope mapping of antigenic molecules using monoclonal antibodies will define shared domains of molecules within the same organism, as well as determinants shared by different species.

The production of *T. pallidum* antigens by recombinant *Escherichia coli* is being investigated in several laboratories. Monoclonal antibodies with known specificities would be invaluable in screening clones in order to select the specific antigen of interest. Van Embden and co-workers (32,87) have isolated a recombinant clone which expresses a determinant of the 44-kDa molecule of *T. pallidum,* as determined by monoclonal antibody reactivity.

In addition to the research applications of *T. pallidum* monoclonal antibodies, new diagnostic tests will result directly from the use of the antibodies to detect *T. pallidum* in lesions, tissues, or body fluids. Antigens, native or cloned, which are identified and characterized by monoclonal antibodies may serve as the basis for new serodiagnostic tests.

VI. SUMMARY

Monoclonal antibodies of *T. pallidum* Nichols strain have been produced and characterized in terms of their reactivity with various pathogenic and non-pathogenic treponemes and related spirochetes. These antibodies have defined an immunodominant surface molecule of 45–48 kDa which contains both common treponemal and pathogen-specific determinants. Other molecules recognized by pathogen-specific monoclonal antibodies have molecular weights of 44,000, 37,000, 33,000 and 12,000–15,500. Complement-dependent immobilization of *T. pallidum* is mediated by monoclonal antibodies with specificity for the 45–48, 44, and 33 kDa surface antigens and the 15.5-kDa molecule. Diagnostic applications of monoclonal antibodies have been explored, and clinical studies reveal high sensitivity and specificity of direct immunofluorescence staining for identification of *T. pallidum* in lesion material.

ACKNOWLEDGMENTS

The author thanks Sharon Baker-Zander for helpful discussions, Ferdinand Muller for providing a copy of his manuscript prior to publication, Barbara Romanowski for unpublished data, Eldon Walker and Nancy Bishop for providing the immunoelectron micrograph, and Ferne Beier and Mark Todd for manuscript preparation. This work was supported by Public Health Service Grant AI 18988 from the National Institutes of Health.

REFERENCES

1. Alderete, J. F., and Baseman, J. B. (1979). Surface-associated host proteins on virulent *Treponema pallidum*. *Infect. Immun.* **26,** 1048–1056.
2. Alderete, J. F., and Baseman, J. B. (1980). Surface characterization of virulent *Treponema pallidum*. *Infect. Immun.* **30,** 814–823.
3. Alderete, J. F., and Baseman, J. B. (1981). Analysis of serum IgG against *Treponema pallidum* protein antigens in experimentally infected rabbits. *Br. J. Vener. Dis.* **57,** 302–308.
4. Azadegan, A. A., Schell, R. F., and LeFrock, J. L. (1983). Immune serum confers protection against syphilitic infection on hamsters. *Infect. Immun.* **42,** 42–47.
5. Baker-Zander, S. A., and Sell, S. (1980). A histopathologic and immunologic study of the course of syphilis in the experimentally infected rabbit. Demonstration of long-lasting cellular immunity. *Am. J. Pathol.* **101,** 387–414.

6. Baker-Zander, S. A., and Lukehart, S. A. (1983). Molecular basis of immunological cross-reactivity between *Treponema pallidum* and *Treponema pertenue*. *Infect. Immun.* **42,** 634–638.
7. Baker-Zander, S. A., and Lukehart, S. A. (1984). Antigenic cross-reactivity between *Treponema pallidum* and other pathogenic members of the family Spirochaetaceae. *Infect. Immun.* **46,** 116–121.
8. Baker-Zander, S. A., Hook, E. W., III, Bonin, P., Handsfield, H. H., and Lukehart, S. A. (1985). Antigens of *Treponema pallidum* recognized by IgG and IgM antibodies during syphilis in humans. *J. Infect. Dis.* **151,** 264–272.
9. Baker-Zander, S. A., Roddy, R. E., Handsfield, H. H., and Lukehart, S. A. (1986). IgG and IgM antibody reactivity to antigens of *Treponema pallidum* following treatment of syphilis. *Sex. Transm. Dis.* **13,** (in press).
10. Baker-Zander, S. A., and Lukehart, S. A. (1985). Detection of glycoproteins of *Treponema pallidum* by lectin binding. Meet., Int. Soc. STD Res., *6th,* Brighton, Engl. Abstr. No. 177.
11. Baseman, J. E., and Hayes, E. C. (1980). Molecular characterization of receptor binding proteins and immunogens of virulent *Treponema pallidum*. *J. Exp. Med.* **151,** 573–586.
12. Baughn, R. E., Adams, C. B., and Musher, D. M. (1983). Circulating immune complexes in experimental syphilis: Identification of treponemal antigens in isolated complexes. *Infect. Immun.* **42,** 585–593.
13. Bharier, M., and Allis, D. (1974). Purification and characterization of axial filaments from *Treponema phagedenis* biotype *reiterii* (the Reiter treponeme). *J. Bacteriol.* **120,** 1434–1442.
14. Bishop, N. H., and Miller, J. N. (1976). Humoral immunity in experimental syphilis. I. The demonstration of resistance conferred by passive immunization. *J. Immunol.* **117,** 191–196.
15. Bishop, N. H., and Miller, J. N. (1976). Humoral immunity in experimental syphilis. II. The relationship of neutralizing factors in immune serum to acquired resistance. *J. Immunol.* **117,** 197–207.
16. Blanco, D. R., Miller, J. N., and Hanff, P. A. (1984). Humoral immunity in experimental syphilis: The demonstration of IgG as a treponemicidal factor in immune rabbit serum. *J. Immunol.* **133,** 2693–2697.
17. Cannefax, G. R., and Garson, W. (1959). The demonstration of a common antigen in Reiter's treponeme and virulent *Treponema pallidum*. *J. Immunol.* **82,** 198–200.
18. Christiansen, S. (1963). Protective layer covering pathogenic Treponemata. *Lancet* **1,** 423–425.
19. Cumberland, M. C., and Turner, T. B. (1949). The rate of multiplication of *Treponema pallidum* in normal and immune rabbits. *Am. J. Syph., Gonorrhea, Vener. Dis.* **33,** 201–212.
20. D'Allesandro, G., and Dardanoni, L. (1953). Isolation and purification of the protein antigen of the Reiter treponeme. A study of its serologic reactions. *Am. J. Syph., Gonorrhea, Vener. Dis.* **37,** 137–150.
21. Fieldsteel, A. H., Cox, D. L., and Moeckli, R. A. (1981). Cultivation of virulent *Treponema pallidum* in tissue culture. *Infect. Immun.* **32,** 908–915.
22. Fitzgerald, T. J., Miller, J. N., and Sykes, J. A. (1975). *Treponema pallidum* (Nichols strain) in tissue culture: Cellular attachment, entry, and survival. *Infect. Immun.* **11,** 1133–1140.
23. Fitzgerald, T. J., Johnson, R. C., Miller, J. N., and Sykes, J. A. (1977). Characterization of the attachment of *Treponema pallidum* (Nichols strain) to cultured mammalian cells and the potential relationship of attachment to pathogenicity. *Infect. Immun.* **18,** 467–478.
24. Fitzgerald, T. J. (1983). Attachment of treponemes to cell surfaces. *In* "Pathogenesis and Immunology of Treponemal Infection" (R. F. Schell and D. M. Musher, eds.), pp. 195–228. Dekker, New York.
25. Fitzgerald, T. J., Repesh, L. A., Blanco, D. R., and Miller, J. N. (1984). Attachment of *Treponema pallidum* to fibronectin, laminin, collagen IV, and collagen I, and blockage of attachment by immune rabbit IgG. *Br. J. Vener. Dis.* **60,** 357–363.

26. Fitzgerald, T. J., and Repesh, L. A. (1985). Interactions of fibronectin with *Treponema pallidum. Genitourin. Med.* **61,** 147–155.

27. Fitzgerald, T. J., Miller, J. N., Repesh, L. A., Rice, M., and Urquhart, A. (1985). Binding of glycosaminoglycans to the surface of *Treponema pallidum* and subsequent effects on complement interactions between antigen and antibody. *Genitourin. Med.* **61,** 13–20.

28. Graves, S., and Alden J. (1979). Limited protection of rabbits against infection with *Treponema pallidum* by immune rabbit sera. *Br. J. Vener. Dis.* **55,** 399–403.

29. Hanff, P. A., Fehniger, T. E., Miller, J. N., and Lovett, M. A. (1982). Humoral immune response in human syphilis to polypeptides of *Treponema pallidum. J. Immunol.* **129,** 1287–1291.

30. Hanff, P. A., Miller, J. N., and Lovett, M. A. (1983). Molecular characterization of common treponemal antigens. *Infect. Immun.* **40,** 825–828.

31. Hanff, P. A., Bishop, N. H., Miller, J. N., and Lovett, M. A. (1983). Humoral immune response in experimental syphilis to polypeptides of *Treponema pallidum. J. Immunol.* **131,** 1973–1977.

32. Hansen, E. B., Pedersen, P. E., Schouls, L. M., Severin, E., and Van Embden, J. D. A. (1985). Genetic characterization and partial sequence determination of a *Treponema pallidum* operon expressing two immunogenic membrane proteins in *Escherichia coli. J. Bacteriol.* **162,** 1227–1237.

33. Hardy, P. H., Jr., Fredericks, W. R., and Nell, E. E. (1975). Isolation and antigenic characteristics of axial filaments from the Reiter treponeme. *Infect. Immun.* **11,** 380–386.

34. Hayes, N. S., Muse, K. E., Collier, A. M., and Baseman, J. B. (1977). Parasitism by virulent *Treponema pallidum* of host cell surfaces. *Infect. Immun.* **17,** 174–186.

35. Hook, E. W., III, Roddy, R. E., Lukehart, S. A., Hom, J., Holmes, K. K., and Tam, M. R. (1985). Detection of *Treponema pallidum* in lesion exudate with a pathogen-specific monoclonal antibody. *J. Clin Microbiol.* **22,** 241–244.

36. Hovind-Hougen, K. (1983). Morphology. *In* "Pathogenesis and Immunology of Treponemal Infection" (R. F. Schell and D. M. Musher, eds.), pp. 3–28. Dekker, New York.

37. Jones, S. A., Marchitto, K. S., Miller, J. N., and Norgard, M. V. (1984). Monoclonal antibody with hemagglutination, immobilization, and neutralization activities defines an immunodominant, 47,000 mol wt, surface-exposed immunogen of *Treponema pallidum* (Nichols). *J. Exp. Med.* **160,** 1404–1420.

38. Limberger, R. J., and Charon, N. W. (1985). Periplasmic flagellar proteins of *Treponema phagedenis. Annu. Meet., Am. Soc. Microbiol. 85th,* Las Vegas, Nevada, *Abstr.* D99.

39. Logan, L. C. (1974). Rabbit globulin and antiglobulin factors associated with *Treponema pallidum* grown in rabbits. *Br. J. Vener. Dis.* **50,** 421–427.

40. Lukehart, S. A., and Miller, J. N. (1978). Demonstration of the in vitro phagocytosis of *Treponema pallidum* by rabbit peritoneal macrophages. *J. Immunol.* **121,** 2014–2024.

41. Lukehart, S. A., Baker-Zander, S. A., Lloyd, R. M. C., and Sell, S. (1980). Characterization of lymphocyte responsiveness in early experimental syphilis. II. Nature of cellular infiltration and *Treponema pallidum* distribution in testicular lesions. *J. Immunol.* **124,** 461–467.

42. Lukehart, S. A., Baker-Zander, S. A., Lloyd, R. M. C., and Sell, S. (1981). Effect of cortisone administration on host-parasite relationships in early experimental syphilis. *J. Immunol.* **127,** 1361–1368.

43. Lukehart, S. A. (1982). Activation of macrophages by products of lymphocytes from normal and syphilitic rabbits. *Infect. Immun.* **37,** 64–69.

44. Lukehart, S. A., Baker-Zander, S. A., and Gubish, E. R., Jr. (1982). Identification of *Treponema pallidum* antigens: Comparison with a nonpathogenic treponeme. *J. Immunol.* **129,** 833–838.

45. Lukehart, S. A. (1983). Macrophages and host resistance. *In* "Pathogenesis and Immunology of

Treponemal Infection'' (R. F. Schell and D. M. Musher, eds.), pp. 349–364. Dekker, New York.

46. Lukehart, S. A., Tam, M. R., Hom, J., Baker-Zander, S. A., Holmes, K. K., and Nowinski, R. C. (1985). Characterization of monoclonal antibodies to *Treponema pallidum*. *J. Immunol.* **134,** 585–592.

47. Lukehart, S. A. (1985). Prospects for development of a treponemal vaccine. *Rev. Infect. Dis.* **7**(Suppl.), S305–S313.

48. Lukehart, S. A., Baker-Zander, S. A., and Sell, S. (1986). Characterization of the humoral immune response to antigens of *Treponema pallidum* following experimental infection and therapy in rabbits. *Sex. Transm. Dis.* **13,** 9–15.

49. Marchitto, K. S., Jones, S. A., Schell R. F., Holmans, P. L., and Norgard, M. V. (1984). Monoclonal antibody analysis of specific antigenic similarities among pathogenic *Treponema pallidum* subspecies. *Infect. Immun.* **45,** 660–666.

50. Miao, R., and Fieldsteel, A. H. (1978). Genetics of *Treponema*: Relationship between *Treponema pallidum* and five cultivable treponemes. *J. Bacteriol.* **133,** 101–107.

51. Miao, R. M., and Fieldsteel, A. H. (1980). Genetic relationship between *Treponema pallidum* and *Treponema pertenue,* two noncultivable human pathogens. *J. Bacteriol.* **141,** 427–429.

52. Miller, J. N., De Bruijn, J. H., Bekker, J. H., and Onvlee, P. C. (1966). The antigenic structure of *Treponema pallidum*, Nichols strain: I. The demonstration, nature and location of specific and shared antigens. *J. Immunol.* **96,** 450–456.

53. Miller, J. N., De Bruijn, J. H., Bekker, J. H., and Onvlee, P. C. (1969). The antigenic structure of *Treponema pallidum*, Nichols strain: II. Extraction of a polysaccharide antigen with ''strain-specific'' serologic activity. *J. Bacteriol.* **99,** 132–135.

54. Moskophidis, M., and Muller, F. (1984). Molecular analysis of immunoglobulins M and G immune response to protein antigens of *Treponema pallidum* in human syphilis. *Infect. Immun.* **43,** 127–132.

55. Moskophidis, M., and Muller, F. (1984). Molecular characterization of glycoprotein antigens on surface of *Treponema pallidum*: Comparison with nonpathogenic *Treponema phagedenis* biotype Reiter. *Infect. Immun.* **46,** 867–869.

56. Moskophidis, M., and Muller, F. (1985). Monoclonal antibodies to immunodominant surface-exposed protein antigens of *Treponema pallidum*. *Eur. J. Clin. Microbiol.* **4,** 473–477.

57. Nelson, R. A., Jr., and Mayer, M. M. (1949). Immobilization of *Treponema pallidum* in vitro by antibody produced in syphilitic infection. *J. Exp. Med.* **89,** 369–393.

58. Norgard, M. V., Selland, C. K., Kettman, J. R., and Miller, J. N. (1984). Sensitivity and specificity of monoclonal antibodies directed against antigenic determinants of *Treponema pallidum* Nichols in the diagnosis of syphilis. *J. Clin. Microbiol.,* **20,** 711–717.

59. Norris, S. J. (1982). *In vitro* cultivation of *Treponema pallidum*: Independent confirmation. *Infect. Immun.* **36,** 437–439.

60. Norris, S. J., and Sell, S. (1984). Antigenic complexity of *Treponema pallidum*: Antigenicity and surface localization of major polypeptides. *J. Immunol.* **133,** 2686–2692.

61. Penn, C. W., Bailey, M. J., and Cockayne, A. (1985). The axial filament antigen of *Treponema pallidum*. *Immunology* **54,** 635–641.

62. Penn, C. W., Bailey, M. J., and Cockayne, A. (1986). Molecular and immunochemical analysis of *Treponema pallidum*. *FEMS Microbiol. Rev.* **32,** 139–148.

63. Perine, P. L., Weiser, R. S., and Klebanoff, S. J. (1973). Immunity to syphilis. I. Passive transfer in rabbits with hyperimmune serum. *Infect. Immun.* **8,** 787–790.

64. Peterson, K. M., Baseman, J. B., and Alderete, J. F. (1983). *Treponema pallidum* receptor binding proteins interact with fibronectin. *J. Exp. Med.* **157,** 1958–1970.

65. Robertson, S. M., Kettman, J. R., Miller, J. N., and Norgard, M. V. (1982). Murine mono-

clonal antibodies specific for virulent *Treponema pallidum* (Nichols). *Infect. Immun.* **36,** 1076–1085.

66. Romanowski, B., Forsey, E., Prasad, E., Lukehart, S. A., Tam, M. R., and Hook, E. W., III. Fluorescent monoclonal antibody detection of *Treponema pallidum.* Submitted.

67. Saunders, J. M., and Folds, J. D. (1983). Development of monoclonal antibodies that recognize *Treponema pallidum. Infect. Immun.* **41,** 844–847.

68. Schell, R. F., LeFrock, J. L., and Babu, J. P. (1978). Passive transfer of resistance to frambesial infection in hamsters. *Infect. Immun.* **21,** 430–435.

69. Schell, R. F., Azadegan, A. A., Nitskansky, S. G., and LeFrock, J. L. (1982). Acquired resistance of hamsters to challenge with homologous and heterologous virulent treponemes. *Infect. Immun.* **37,** 617–621.

70. Sell, S., Gamboa, D., Baker-Zander, S. A., Lukehart, S. A., and Miller, J. N. (1980). Host response to *Treponema pallidum* in intradermally-infected rabbits: Evidence for persistence of infection at local and distant sites. *J. Invest. Dermatol.* **75,** 470–475.

71. Sell, S., Baker-Zander, S. A., and Powell, H. C. (1982). Experimental syphilitic orchitis in rabbits. Ultrastructural appearance of *Treponema pallidum* during phagocytosis and dissolution by macrophages *in vivo. Lab. Invest.* **46,** 355–364.

72. Sepetjian, M., Salussola, D., and Thivolet, J. (1973). Attempt to protect rabbits against experimental syphilis by passive immunization. *Br. J. Vener. Dis.* **49,** 335–337.

73. Smibert, R. M. (1984). Genus III. Treponema. *In* "Bergey's Manual of Systematic Bacteriology" (N. R. Krieg and J. G. Holt, eds.), Vol. 1, pp. 49–57. Williams & Wilkins, Baltimore, Maryland.

74. Stamm, L. V., and Bassford, P. J., Jr. (1985). Cellular and extracellular protein antigens of *Treponema pallidum* synthesized during *in vitro* incubation of freshly extracted organisms. *Infect. Immun.* **47,** 799–807.

75. Stephens, R. S., Tam, M. R., Kuo, C., and Nowinski, R. C. (1982). Monoclonal antibodies to *Chlamydia trachomatis:* Antibody specificities and antigen characterization. *J. Immunol.* **128,** 1083–1089.

76. Strandberg-Pedersen, N., Axelsen, N. H., Jorgensen, B. B., and Sand-Petersen, C. (1980). Antibodies in secondary syphilis against five of forty Reiter treponeme antigens. *Scand. J. Immunol.* **11,** 629–633.

77. Strugnell, R. A., Handley, C. J., Lowther, D. A., Faine, S., and Graves, S. R. (1984). *Treponema pallidum* does not synthesize *in vitro* a capsule containing glycosaminoglycans or proteoglycans. *Br. J. Vener. Dis.* **60,** 8–13.

78. Strugnell, R. A., Handley, C. J., Drummond, L., Faine, S., Lowther, D. A., and Graves, S. R. (1984). Polyanions in syphilis: Evidence that glycoproteins and macromolecules resembling glycosaminoglycans are synthesized by host tissues in response to infection with *Treponema pallidum. Br. J. Vener. Dis.* **60,** 75–82.

79. Thomas, D. D., Baseman, J. B., and Alderete, J. F. (1985). Fibronectin mediates *Treponema pallidum* cytadherence through recognition of fibronectin cell-binding domain. *J. Exp. Med.* **161,** 514–525.

80. Thomas, D. D., Baseman, J. B., and Alderete, J. F. (1985). Putative *Treponema pallidum* cytadhesins share a common functional domain. *Infect. Immun.* **49,** 833–835.

81. Thornburg, R. W., and Baseman, J. B. (1983). Comparison of major protein antigens and protein profiles of *Treponema pallidum* and *Treponema pertenue. Infect. Immun.* **42,** 623–627.

82. Thornburg, R. W., Morrison-Plummer, J., and Baseman, J. B. (1985). Monoclonal antibodies to *Treponema pallidum*: Recognition of a major polypeptide antigen. *Genitourin. Med.* **61,** 1–6.

83. Titus, R. G., and Weiser, R. S. (1979). Experimental syphilis in the rabbit: Passive transfer of immunity with immunoglobulin G from immune serum. *J. Infect. Dis.* **140,** 904–913.

84. Turner, T. B., Hardy, P. H., Jr., Newman, B., and Nell, E. E. (1973). Effects of passive immunization on experimental syphilis in the rabbit. *Johns Hopkins Med. J.* **133,** 241–251.
85. Van Der Sluis, J. J., Van Dijk, G., Boer, M., Stolz, E., and Van Joost, T. (1985). Mucopolysaccharides in suspensions of *Treponema pallidum* extracted from infected rabbit testes. *Genitourin. Med.* **61,** 7–12.
86. Van Eijk, R. V. W., and Van Embden, J. D. A. (1982). Molecular characterization of *Treponema pallidum* proteins responsible for the human immune response to syphilis. *Antonie van Leeuwenhoek* **48,** 486–487.
87. Van Embden, J. D., Van Der Donk, H. J., Van Eijk, R. V., Van Der Heide, H. G., De Jong, J. A., Van Olderen, M. F., Osterhaus, A. D., and Schouls, L. M. (1983). Molecular cloning and expression of *Treponema pallidum* DNA in *Escherichia coli* K-12. *Infect. Immun.* **42,** 187–196.
88. Weiser, R. S., Erickson, D., Perine, P. L., and Pearsall, N. N. (1976). Immunity to syphilis: Passive transfer in rabbits using serial doses of immune serum. *Infect. Immun.* **131,** 1402–1407.
89. Wong, G. H. W., Steiner, B., and Graves, S. (1983). Effect of syphilitic rabbit sera taken at different periods after infection on treponemal motility, treponemal attachment to mammalian cells in vitro, and treponemal infection in rabbits. *Br. J. Vener. Dis.* **59,** 220–224.
90. Wos, S. M., and Wicher, K. (1985). Antigenic evidence for host origin of exudative fluids in lesions of *Treponema pallidum*-infected rabbits. *Infect. Immun.* **47,** 228–233.
91. Zeigler, J. A., Jones, A. M., Jones, R. H., and Kubica, K. M. (1976). Demonstration of extracellular material at the surface of pathogenic *T. pallidum* cells. *Br. J. Vener. Dis.* **52,** 1–8.

2

Diagnostic Uses of Monoclonal Antibodies to *Salmonella*

PAK LEONG LIM

Department of Microbiology
University of Hong Kong
Hong Kong

I. INTRODUCTION

Salmonella organisms cause two major diseases, salmonellosis (acute gastroenteritis) and enteric fever. Both diseases are foodborne and require differential diagnosis to identify their cause. Salmonellosis is a common global problem recurring frequently as outbreaks of food poisoning. Enteric fever, which includes typhoid and paratyphoid, causes more serious illness and is endemic in certain geographical regions, including all the Southeast Asian countries, and

29

India, Egypt, and Chile. In Hong Kong, for example, 369 cases of enteric fever (6.9 cases per 100,000 inhabitants) were reported in 1983 (57). In Santiago, Chile, the annual incidence of typhoid fever is about 90 cases per 100,000 inhabitants (83), probably the highest in the world. More importantly, in these areas the number of typhoid carriers may be manyfold higher; these are the asymptomatic disseminators of the disease. Indeed, in Santiago, Levine *et al.* (55) estimated the number to be 694 per 100,000 population. In salmonellosis, on the other hand, animals are important reservoirs of the etiological agents.

Control of these diseases depends largely on public health measures, surveillance programs such as those which currently exist in the United States, the United Kingdom, and Australia, and, in the case of typhoid, on immunization as well (116). A key element in these measures is the proper identification of infected cases and the sources of infection. Rapid identification is essential to prevent spread of the disease epidemiologically, and also for patient management, since infantile salmonellosis and enteric fever can be fatal. Moreover, in the food industry, where screening of foods and feeds for presence of *Salmonella* has become more routine, rapid analysis could mean savings in cost due to storage. The most definitive diagnosis of *Salmonella* infections is by culture of the organism; however, this conventionally requires at least 3 days and is not always successful. Immunological diagnosis is also used for the enteric fevers. In this regard, the Widal test has remained the classical assay, although numerous investigators have denounced its usefulness and have devised better systems. Yet none of these developments have gained wide acceptance and, consequently, can only be regarded as experimental. Thus there is a dire need to improve both culture and immunological techniques. It would be desirable, for instance, to have an immunodiagnostic assay for typhoid that is simple, reliable, and easy to standardize for use in all laboratories. With the advent of monoclonal antibodies (MAbs) that are homogeneous and available in unlimited supplies, it may be possible to achieve such a goal. However, how can these antibodies be best utilized for diagnosis? Further, what kinds of antibodies should be used to achieve high specificities in assays? Can such antibodies be "tailor-made?"

These questions will be examined both from theoretical and practical standpoints in this review. To date, there are only two diagnostic systems described for *Salmonella* that utilize MAbs; the experience gained in these studies will be discussed in Section III. In view of the dearth, to date, of hybridoma-derived MAbs to *Salmonella,* the antigenic complexity of these organisms as revealed by conventional antisera and the progress made in the detection of these bacteria and their infections in the prehybridoma era will be extensively reviewed in Section II. The myeloma proteins that bind to *Salmonella* (81) will be included in the discussion since they are the forerunners of MAbs.

II. BACKGROUND

A. The *Salmonella* Bacteria

Salmonella is one of 21 genera of the Enterobacteriaceae ("the enterobacteria") (68), while classification of the *Salmonella* organisms themselves has been controversial over the years (29). The three-species (*S. choleraesuis, S. typhi, S. enteritidis*) concept of Edwards and Ewing (24), based on biochemical and serological differentiation, has been adopted widely; in this scheme, other antigenically distinct salmonellae are considered serotypes of *S. enteritidis*, rather than as separate species. However, recent DNA hybridization studies (54) suggested that there is only one species (*S. choleraesuis*) of *Salmonella* with six subspecies, of which subspecies I contains more than 99% of the *Salmonella* cultures derived from human disease.

In this review, as a matter of convenience, the serotypes will be referred to by their Linnaean names, as if they were species. A serotype of *Salmonella* is traditionally named after the place it was first isolated from, or the form of disease caused, and is distinguished from other serotypes by its antigenic structure, based on the O (somatic), H (flagellar), and Vi (capsular) antigens. These antigens, detected by specific antisera (Section II,D), will be discussed later. Based on these antigens, the salmonellae can be classified according to the Kauffmann–White scheme [see (24)], part of which is shown in Table I. Thus, serotypes with common O antigens are grouped together. For example, group D salmonellae have a common O antigen (O-9) that is absent in other groups. These organisms also share another O antigen (O-12) that is present in groups A and B as well. Hence, this antigen is not unique to group D salmonellae.

The organisms in groups A, B, and D cause 70% of the *Salmonella* infections in humans. The enteric fevers account for less than 10% of these (78), involving only a few serotypes (e.g., *S. typhi, S. paratyphi A, B,* and *C,* and *S. sendai*). These organisms are invasive and cause systemic rather than intestinal disease. *Salmonella typhi* organisms, for example, enter the body orally, invade the intestinal epithelium, enter the circulation, and then colonize the reticuloendothelial organs. After proliferation at these sites, after a week or so, they invade the bloodstream causing septicemia, and seed the intestine via the gallbladder and bile duct, causing hemorrhage and perforation of the Peyer's patches in severe cases. Thus, the organisms are usually recoverable from the blood (and urine) early in the disease, and from the stool probably between the third and fifth week of illness. Some convalescents may continue to excrete the organisms in the stool—sometimes in the urine too—but 2–5% of typhoid patients, especially those elderly or female, become chronic gallbladder carriers. In these carriers, it is often difficult to isolate the organism.

Some salmonellae (e.g., *S. choleraesuis* and *S. enteritidis*) can sometimes

TABLE I

Illustration of the Kauffmann–White Scheme of Serological Classification[a,b]

Group	*Salmonella* serotype	O Antigen	H antigen Phase 1	H antigen Phase 2
A	*S. paratyphi* A	*1*,2,12	a	—
B	*S. abortusequi*	4,12	—	e,n,x
	S. paratyphi B	*1*,4,(5),12	b	1,2
	S. limete	*1*,4,12,27	b	1,5
	S. abony	*1*,4,(5),12	b	e,n,x
	S. abortusbovis	*1*,4,12,27	b	e,n,x
	S. schleissheim	4,12,27	b,z_{12}	—
	S. wien	*1*,4,12,(*12*)	b	1,w
	S. abortusovis	4,12	c	1,6
	S. stanley	*1*,4,(5),12,27	d	1,2
	S. chester	4,(5),12	c,h	e,n,x
	S. derby	*1*,4,(5),12	(f),g	—
	S. typhimurium	*1*,4,(5),12	i	1,2
	S. agama	4,12	i	1,6
	S. gloucester	*1*,4,12,(*27*)	i	1.w
	S. bredeney	*1*,4,12,27	l,v	1,7
	S. heidelberg	*1*,4,(5),12	r	1,2
C1	*S. paratyphi* C	6,7,(Vi)	c	1.5
	S. choleraesuis	6,7	c	1,5
	S. montevideo	6.7	g,m,s	—
	S. oranienburg	6,7	m,t	—
	S. thompson	6,7	k	1,5
	S. bareilly	6,7	y	1,5
	S. tennessee	6,7	z_{29}	—
C2	*S. manhattan*	6,8	d	1,5
	S. Newport	6.8	e,h	1,2
	S. bovismorbificans	6,8	r	1,5
	S. kentucky	8,20	i	z_6
D	*S. sendai*	*1*,9,12	a	1,5
	S. typhi	9,12,Vi	d	—
	S. dublin	*1*,9,12,(Vi)	g,p	—
	S. panama	*1*,9,12	l,v	1,5
	S. gallinarum	*1*,9,12	—	—
E1	*S. anatum*	3,10	e,h	1,6
	S. meleagridis	3,10	e,h	1,w
	S. london	3,10	l,v	1,6
E2	*S. newington*	3,15	e,h	1,6
E3	*S. minneapolis*	(3),*15*,34	e,h	1,6
E4	*S. senftenberg*	1,3,19	g,s,t	—

[a] Reproduced with permission from Parker, M. T. (1984). The Salmonella. *In* "Topley and Wilson's Principles of Bacteriology, Virology and Immunity" (G. Wilson, A. Miles, and M. T. Parker, eds.), 7th Ed., p. 339. Arnold, London.

[b] Numbers in italics represent phage-determined antigenic factors. Numbers in parentheses represent antigens present only in some strains of the serotype.

cause localized infections in the abdominal aorta, meninges, bones, and other tissues, but the majority cause a self-limiting gastroenteritis confined to the intestine only. These organisms—unlike *S. typhi,* which inhabits humans only— can be found in a wide range of hosts, both warm and cold blooded; consequently, salmonellosis is often zoonotically acquired.

B. The Antigens of *Salmonella*

In this section, the antigenic composition of *Salmonella* will be discussed to indicate the diagnostic potential of some of the antigens. Like other gram-negative bacteria, *Salmonella* organisms have a surface envelope as depicted in Fig. 1. Two membranes that sandwich the peptidoglycan layer, composed of a

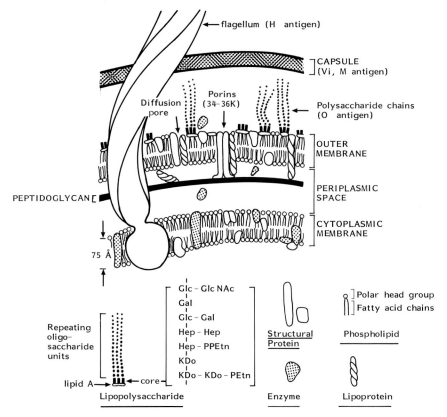

Fig. 1. Schematic cross section of the surface envelope of *Salmonella* bacteria. Glc, Glucose; NAc, *N*-acetyl; Gal, galactose; Hep, heptose; KDo, 2-keto-3-deoxyoctonic acid; PEtn and PPEtn, phospho- and diphosphoethanolamine. Adapted from DiRienzo *et al.* (22), p. 525, with permission from the *Annual Review of Biochemistry,* **47,** © 1978 by Annual Reviews, Inc.; and from Smit *et al.* (92), with permission. Also based on information in (1,42).

phospholipid bilayer but of different densities, are present. These are the inner cytoplasmic membrane and the outer membrane. The latter is diagnostically important, since it is exposed to the outside and contains the unique lipopolysaccharides (LPS), which bear the O antigens and cover 45% of the surface. In addition, the outer membrane embeds a number of important proteins namely, the porins and lipoproteins. Few salmonellae, notably, *S. typhi* and *S. paratyphi C,* also possess an outermost capsule that bears the Vi antigen. The majority of salmonellae are motile due to presence of flagellae (H antigens). There is, however, considerable variation in the expression of the O, Vi (including other capsular antigens), and H antigens in *Salmonella* cultures [see (24)].

The antigenic complexity of *Salmonella* is evidenced by the existence of some 60 O antigens (24). The isoelectric-focusing studies of DiPauli (21) confirmed the heterogeneity of the polysaccharides (>30 bands) in *S. typhimurium*, while more than 20 outer membrane proteins could also be identified in this serotype by sodium dodecyl sulfate–polyacrylamide gel electrophoresis (SDS–PAGE) analysis (2). Using crossed immunoelectrophoresis (XIE), Espersen *et al.* (28) observed 86 immunoprecipitates (antigens) in a cell lysate of *S. typhi,* developed with rabbit antisera. Only five antigens were specific for *Salmonella,* and two for *S. typhi,* of which one was LPS. A common antigen shared with *Pseudomonas aeruginosa,* but no *S. typhi*-specific protein antigen, was found. Fewer ($n = 19$) antigens were revealed with human sera (27), but LPS and the common antigen were again seen. More recently, Chau *et al.* (17), using a veronal buffer extract (VBE) of *S. typhi* in a similar approach, observed 27 antigens with rabbit antisera and 4 with human sera (Fig. 2). Again, LPS (antigen no. 7) and a common antigen (no. 19) were observed.

1. Lipopolysaccharide (LPS)

The serological analysis of the O antigens of *Salmonella* and the subsequent elucidation of their chemical basis have been extensively reviewed (42,60,61). Only pertinent conclusions will be summarized here.

LPS, prepared by the hot phenol–water method (42), is protein-free, unlike other preparations ["endotoxins" (71)] of the outer membrane. It consists of three structural parts (Fig. 1). Embedded in the membrane is lipid A, a lipoidal, acylated glycosamine disaccharide, which is the endotoxic principle of LPS, and is common (antigenically) to many gram-negative bacteria (31). Attached to it, in biosynthetic order, are KDo (2-keto-3-deoxyoctonic acid), heptose, and various other sugars (Fig. 1), forming what is commonly known as the core. Mutants ("rough") are known in each step. Though structurally very similar in all entero-

---

Fig. 2. XIE of *S. typhi* VBE developed with rabbit anti-VBE serum. Intermediate gel contained saline (A), or serum from typhoid patient/carrier (B). Immunoprecipitates formed from latter are numbered. Stained with Coomassie Brilliant Blue. Reprinted with permission from Chau *et al.* (17).

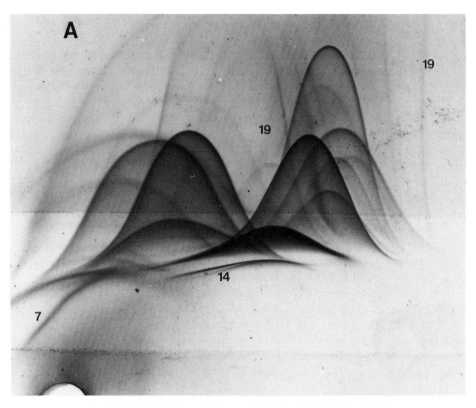

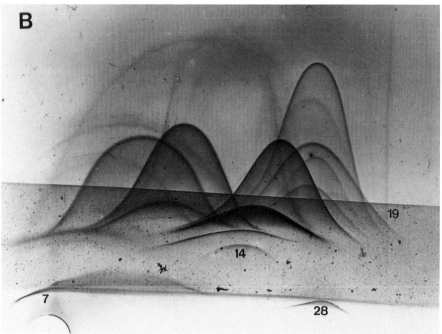

bacteria, the core may not be as antigenically common as once believed (66). However, Brade and Galanos (10) recently described an antigen residing in the KDo region, which was found expressed in many gram-negative bacteria belonging to six different families. In smooth strains of *Salmonella,* another structure is present that adjoins the core and extends outward from the cell. This is the O-polysaccharide chain, consisting of repeating oligosaccharide units. There is great variability in this region which accounts for the diversity of O antigens (and serotypes). Variability is due to the diverse combinations of different sugar residues. Figure 3 illustrates the following.

1. Elucidation of the chemical basis of an antigen is based on the inhibition of reaction between the antigen and its antiserum by different oligosaccharides. Usually, one constituent sugar gives the best inhibition, and this is termed the immunodominant sugar. (The term antigen is used broadly in this chapter to cover more specific terms such as factor, determinant, epitope, and antigenic site.)

2. Groups A, B, D, and E have a common repeating unit, -mannose-rhamnose-galactose-, although the glycosidic linkages involved may be different. In groups A, B, and D, the common antigen 12_2 is defined by the α-glycosyl group attached (1,4) to galactose in the main chain, while the group-specific antigens are specified by the respective α-3,6-dideoxyhexoses that join (1,3) to mannose: paratose for O-2 (group A), abequose for antigen O-4 (group B), and tyvelose for antigen O-9 (group D). The dideoxyhexoses, which are rarely found in nature outside the *Salmonella* group, except in *Yersinia pseudotuberculosis,* thus play an immunodominant role in specificity as terminal nonreducing sugars. However, they alone do not exhibit full specificity, but require for this at least the adjoining sugar and the linkages of this sugar in the main chain. This is seen, for instance, in the derivation of $O-27_D$ from O-9 by phage conversion. The only difference between these antigens is the galactosyl–mannose linkage (1,6 versus 1,2) in the main chain preceding the tyvelose side chain. O-9, however, is partly conserved in the converted strains (hence, termed partial or incomplete antigen); consequently, Staub and Bagdian (96) believed O-9 to be made up of two components $(9_1, 9_2)$ present on different sides of tyvelose, so that one (9_1) was independent of the galactosyl–mannose linkage. A further variation of O-9 is seen in group D_2 salmonellae in which a new antigen (O-46) is expressed; here, both linkages of mannose in the main chain are different from those in O-9.

3. Another evidence that antigenic specificity encompasses at least two sugar residues is the immunodominant role played by α-glucose in at least seven different antigens: O-1, $O-12_2$, O-19, O-34, O-6, O-7, and O-14. A common disaccharide, α-glycosyl–galactose, is involved in the first four, and the different specificities here are due to the different ways galactose is linked. For instance, O-1 (groups A,B) differs from $O-12_2$ (groups B,D) only in the glycosyl–galactose linkage (1,6 versus 1,4), and from O-19 (group E_4) only in the galactosyl–mannose linkage (1,2 versus 1,6). O-34 (group E_3) is similar to

O-12_2 in the α-glycosyl–galactose structure, but differs in the other linkages of galactose; despite their similarities, these two antigens showed very little cross-reactivity with one another.

4. A further example that an immunodominant sugar may exist on two non-cross-reacting antigens is abequose, present in O-4 (α-linked to D-mannose) and O-8 (α-linked to L-rhamnose).

5. If abequose in O-4 is substituted with an *O*-acetyl group, a new non-cross-reacting antigen (O-5) is generated; both forms are usually expressed in *S. typhimurium* strains.

6. Besides the spatially exposed terminal sugars, any sugar within a straight polysaccharide chain can express immunodominance. This is best seen in group E salmonellae. Thus, mannose is the immunodominant sugar for O-3, and its substitution by tyvelose in *S. strassbourg* (group D_2) probably accounts for the diminished expression of the antigen in this serotype; consequently, a division of O-3 [3a, (3)] has been suggested.

Although many of the O antigens are unique to *Salmonella,* present only in some serotypes, there are at least 14 antigens that are present also in *E. coli* [e.g., O-11, O-17, O-40, and O-50 (79)].

2. Vi Antigen

This "virulence" antigen (of uncertain pathogenic significance really) of *S. typhi* has been purified (115). Composed of repeating units of O- and N-acetylated galactosaminouronic acid, it is less O-acetylated than, but otherwise serologically identical to, the Vi antigen found in *Citrobacter ballerup* and *Escherichia freundii*. It has two main determinants: the *O*-acetyl moiety and another comprising the carboxyl and *N*-acetyl groups (102). Diagnostically it is important, since it (a) is readily accessible to antibodies (and often masks the O antigens), (b) serves as phage receptors, and (c) is present in very few other salmonellae or other bacteria (74). However, it may be less specific than believed, since it was found to cross-react with an acidic polysaccharide of *E. coli* B, which was not due to the *O*-acetyl group or other known reasons (103).

3. Flagellar (H) Antigens

These heat-labile antigens are detected by agglutination or immobilization and are important for bacterial identification. They are specified by amino acid sequences in the flagellins (monomers of flagella). A unique feature of these antigens is their expression in two alternative phases in most salmonellae (Table I). Phase 1 antigens are generally more specific than those in phase 2, but even these are widely distributed in *Salmonella*. *Salmonella adelaide* flagellins (MW 40,000) were found to stimulate good responses in rats (76), and the antigenic activities in these proteins seemed to be confined solely to a fragment (MW 18,000) obtained by cyanogen bromide cleavage or enzymatic digest (39).

SEROGROUP	SEROTYPE O-antigens	REPEATING OLIGOSACCHARIDE UNITS

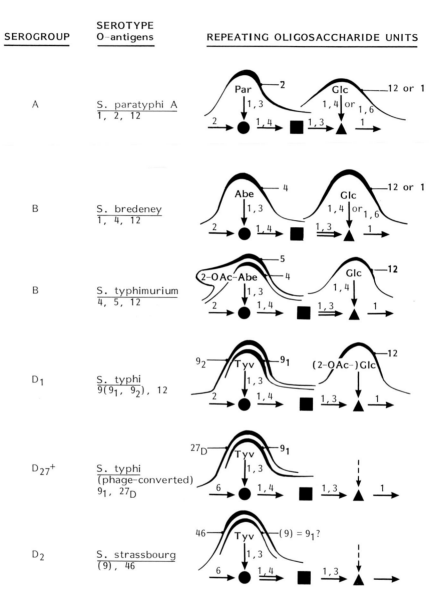

Fig. 3. Illustration of the biological repeating units of *Salmonella* LPS. The putative O antigens (numbered) are indicated by lines that are thickest over the immunodominant sugars. ●, Mannose; ■, rhamnose; ▲, galactose; —, α linkage; ＝, β linkage; ≡, linkage unknown; Par, paratose; Abe, abequose; Tyv, tyvelose; OAc, *O*-acetyl. Adapted with permission from Jann, K., and Westphal, O. (1975). Microbial Polysaccharides. *In* "The Antigens" (M. Sela, ed.), Vol. 3, p. 17. Academic Press, New York. Also based on information in (61,73,96).

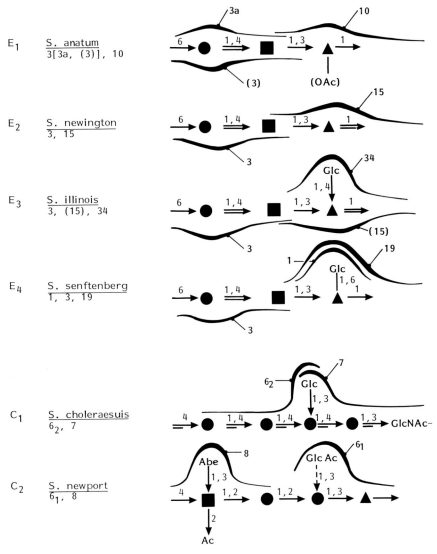

Fig. 3. *(Continued)*.

4. Porins

SDS–PAGE analysis of the *S. typhimurium* outer membrane revealed more than 20 proteins (2). Three major proteins, designated 34K, 35K, and 36K according to their molecular weights, form transmembrane pores for the diffusion of small hydrophilic compounds and hence are called "porins." These trypsin-resistant proteins are chemically related to, but distinct from, one another (109). A fourth major protein, 33K, is present, whose function is unknown. The porins are presumably exposed on the surface membrane, since they (a) also serve as phage receptors, (b) became coupled to activated dextran when this was applied to intact cells (46), and (c) stimulated protective antibodies in animals (51). The purified porins, however, were not immunogenic but required reconstitution with rough LPS for such activity (52).

It is not known whether analogous proteins present in *E. coli* [see (22)] and other bacteria (or salmonellae) are antigenically related to the *S. typhimurium* porins.

5. Lipoprotein

Present abundantly in *E. coli* is a 7000-Da lipoprotein, first isolated by Braun using boiling SDS [reviewed in (11) and (22)]. The protein shows highly repetitive sequences; its C-terminal lysine is either bound covalently to the peptidoglycan, or left free, while the N-terminal end contains fatty acids similar to those in phospholipids but different from lipid A. Much of the lipoprotein is buried in the outer membrane, and only part of it may be detected by specific antibodies in rough (LPS) mutants. A chemically and serologically similar protein was also found in many gram-negative bacilli, including *Salmonella, Arizona, Shigella,* and *Citrobacter* but not in *Proteus* or *Pseudomonas.*

6. Common and Cross-Reactive Antigens

In addition to the ones already mentioned, a number of antigens common to the enterobacteria exist, including a polysaccharide antigen (42% hexose, no KDo or heptose) isolated from *S. typhi* (43), and another first described by Kunin which is composed largely of D-glucosamine and D-mannosaminouronic acid (63). Both these antigens are associated with LPS in the native state and, like the porins (52), required this association for immunogenicity. Sompolinsky *et al.* (94) described a protein antigen (with two components) isolated from *P. aeruginosa* which is also present in *S. typhi* and at least 16 other bacteria.

Although common antigens probably represent phylogenetically conserved products, there are other cross-reactive antigens due to small determinant groups present, perhaps fortuitously, among the enterobacteria and in tissues. Thus, common determinants exist between some *Salmonella* O antigens and human blood group substances (e.g., *N*-acetylgalactosamine and L-fucose) (60) and between the O antigens of *Salmonella* and *E. coli* (79). However, there are other cross-reactions among bacteria that remain unexplained. Besides that of Vi and *E. coli* polysaccharide (103), there is the finding that an antiserum made against a parasite, *Trichinella spiralis,* agglutinated *S. typhi* and a few other *Salmonella* serotypes (112); O-12 was implicated, but this is not convincing. We have, in fact, obtained MAbs against *T. spiralis* that apparently bind to *S. typhi* LPS (W. T. Wong and P. L. Lim, unpublished observations).

C. Laboratory Detection of *Salmonella* and Its Infections

The presence of *Salmonella* bacteria in clinical specimens, foods, and feeds is usually detected by culture. However, this takes time and, although the salmonellae grow easily in culture, they can escape detection if they are present in scanty numbers in the samples or have been killed by antibiotics administered to the patient. Further, differentiation of these organisms from other enterobacteria is a major, time-consuming task of routine microbiology laboratories, and misidentification is not uncommon. Not all laboratories, especially those in developing countries, have the facilities or can afford the cost to implement this method properly. With the enteric fevers, there are immunological methods of diagnosis as well, although here again, these are not without problems. Both the cultural and immunodiagnostic approaches will be discussed below to indicate the problems and progress seen and the areas in which antibodies, notably monoclonal, can be used to advantage.

1. Culture

Since culturing is described in laboratory manuals [e.g., (24)], only an outline will be given. As indicated in Fig. 4, broth culture is usually used at the start. Thus, blood and blood clots are inoculated into nonselective broths, such as trypticase soy broth or ox bile, and growth is observed periodically, for up to 7 days in most cases. For stool, which contains a normal flora, a selective enrichment broth, such as selenite F or tetrathionate, is used which allows the salmonellae to proliferate preferentially over other enterobacteria. (Sometimes enrichment broth is not used and stool is inoculated directly onto solid media.) A nonselective medium (e.g., lactose broth) is normally used in food analysis prior to the selective enrichment. After overnight incubation, subcultures of the broth are transferred to a number of solid media. Many of these media are selective and differential. For example, the MacConkey and deoxycholate citrate agars contain bile salts that inhibit growth of many nonenterobacteria, and also contain lactose and a pH indicator which separate the enterobacteria into two types: the lactose fermenter (pink colonies) and the non-lactose fermenter (colorless). *Salmonella* colonies belong to the latter, and are further differentiated from other non-lactose fermenters by biochemical means, utilizing a minimal set of biochemical media ("screening tests") or a whole range. Based on the pattern of reactions in these media, usually obtained 3 days after the start of the investigation, suspect isolates are further characterized biochemically (if necessary) and are confirmed serologically in agglutination tests using specific antisera. Both polyvalent and appropriate monospecific antisera (see Section II,D) are used for identification according to the Kauffmann–White scheme. *Salmonella* isolates are further characterized by their sensitivities to antibiotics, and for epidemiological purposes by phage typing (82) or plasmid profile analysis (35).

There have been numerous attempts to simplify the conventional meth-

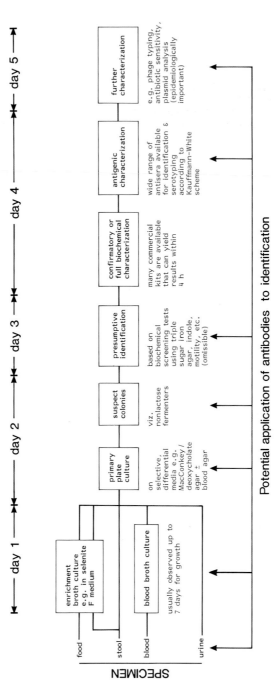

Fig. 4. General protocol for the bacteriological examination of clinical specimens, foods, and feeds for the presence of *Salmonella* organisms. Potential areas for the direct application of antibodies, notably monoclonal, for identification are indicated.

odology. For example, many simple (but expensive) kits are available in the market which permit accurate differentiation of the enterobacteria in as little as 4 hr (41). Specific antibodies have been used in different ways to identify *Salmonella* organisms directly at different stages of the protocol; some examples are discussed below; the potential areas for such applications are indicated in Fig. 4.

In food bacteriology, variable but encouraging results were obtained in attempts to detect salmonellae in food or feed samples in enrichment broth cultures, using polyvalent *Salmonella* antisera and the fluorescent-antibody or enrichment serology (agglutination) method. Based on results obtained by culture, these techniques were generally sensitive and not specific (32,70,95,106). Mohr *et al.* (70) showed that sensitivity was dependent on the enrichment broth and incubation period used; for instance, better recovery of *Salmonella* organisms was obtained from tetrathionate enrichment than from selenite F broth [although disappointing results with the former were also observed previously (32)]. False-positive results may be explained in two ways. First, they could be due to background material in the specimen, much of which could be removed using additional broth cultures before and/or after the selective enrichment. Thus, Sperber and Deibel (95) observed excellent results with an experimental "M broth" (but not brain–heart infusion broth) used after the enrichment. Incidentally, enrichment serology was observed to be more specific than the fluorescent-antibody method, and is simpler and less expensive (70). Second, the lack of specificity in these studies may be attributed to the polyvalent antisera used, which Thomason and Hebert (106) found to cross-react with *Arizona, Citrobacter,* and *E. coli.*

Indeed, when monospecific antisera prepared against the synthetic disaccharide–protein antigens O-2, O-4, O-8, and O-9 (Section II,D), were used in immunofluorescence and coagglutination (COAG) studies, *Salmonella* organisms present in pure cultures and fecal materials were detected with 100% accuracy (98–101). In these studies, COAG (using protein A-rich staphylococcal cells sensitized with antibody) was found to be a 1000-fold less sensitive than immunofluorescence and required at least 10^8 bacteria for visible reaction. When the O-9 antiserum was later used in indirect immunofluorescence to detect *S. enteritidis* organisms in an outbreak (98), it was found to be extremely specific (100% of 27 control subjects), and the organism was identified correctly in fecal smears from 75% of 28 culturally proved cases. The false-negative results were chiefly from patients who had less than 10^4 viable salmonellae per milliliter of feces. Better detection was seen in the 18- to 24-hr enrichment broth cultures (89%) and colonies (100%) grown from these broths. Direct inoculation of fecal samples onto agar yielded *S. enteritidis* colonies in 89% of the cases that were all identifiable by the antiserum; by this means, however, Sanborn *et al.* (87) obtained only 50% recovery of *Salmonella* colonies in an investigation of a nursery outbreak caused by *S. oranienburg* (group C_1). These workers, using C_1, E, and Vi polyvalent antisera in COAG, observed good specificity (100% of

50 control subjects) in their system, and found best detection of the salmonellae in dulcitol selenite enrichment broth incubated for 20 hr. However, attempts to detect the organisms directly in fecal suspensions were not successful, as spontaneous agglutination occurred. Using a similar technique in which staphylococcal cells were sensitized with *Salmonella* A, D, and Vi polyvalent antisera, Mikhail *et al.* (67) detected *S. typhi* and *S. paratyphi* A organisms in ox bile cultures of blood clots as effectively as by conventional culture (95% agreement).

A different way that antibody can be used to simplify diagnosis is the direct identification of *S. typhi* colonies on culture agar (in which specific antiserum has been incorporated) due to the formation of haloes (immunoprecipitates) around the colonies. Although good specificity and sensitivity were claimed in a study (75), a generous use of antiserum is required, and MAbs may not function well with this technique.

2. Immunodiagnosis

The developments in the immunological (serological) diagnosis of typhoid— the most important and, in some areas (78), the most prevalent of the enteric fevers—will be discussed in this section. Two immunological markers (antibody or antigen) and two groups of subjects (patient or carrier) are considered; the description is divided accordingly and outlined in Table II.

    a. Antibody Detection in Patients. The Widal test, first described in 1896, is the earliest and still the most widely used test in typhoid immunodiagnosis. Serum antibodies to the O, H, and Vi antigens of *S. typhi* are detected by tube agglutination with the appropriate cell suspensions. Theoretically, the test is not sensitive (agglutination used which favors IgM antibodies) or specific (whole cells used). Indeed, results obtained from this test are often difficult to interpret (89), although demonstration of a fourfold or higher increase in titer from paired sera is usually regarded as diagnostically significant. However, such a rise is not always seen in patients (8), nor are paired sera always obtainable, especially in places with overcrowded hospitals. With single Widal readings, Levine *et al.* (56) stressed that these are only meaningful if they are derived from cases in nonendemic areas or from children under 10 years of age in endemic areas. In Peru, an endemic area, they found poor specificity with the test, particularly in the H titers, which decreased progressively with age till 15 to 19 years (34% specificity); better specificity (>90%, of both O and H titers in all ages) was recorded in Baltimore, a nonendemic region. Similar findings were seen in other endemic (110) and nonendemic (13) areas. There are no consistent observations on the frequencies of the Widal responses in typhoid patients; unlike others, including Levine *et al.* (56), Brodie (13) found better H responses than those to O antigens.

TABLE II

Recent Advances in the Immunodiagnosis of Typhoid Fever[a]

Test	Antigen used	Specificity[b] (%)	Sensitivity[c] (%)	Remarks	Reference
A. Detection of antibody in serum					
Widal	O-Antigens	99(86)	65(62)	TAB vaccinated	13
(nonendemic		96(140)	62(314)	Not vaccinated	13
area)		99(101)	—[d]	0–9 years	56
		96(23)	—	10–19 years	56
Widal (endemic	O-Antigens	98(16)	100(2)	0–4 years	56
area)		94(246)	92(12)	5–9 years	56
		97(209)	95(19)	10–14 years	56
		71(102)	89(9)	15–19 years	56
		77(62)	75(52)	adult	110
Widal	H Antigens	10(869	92(52)	TAB vaccinated	13
(nonendemic		89(140)	83(308)	Not vaccinated	13
area)		100(101)	—	0–9 years	56
		96(23)	—	10–19 years	56
Widal (endemic	H Antigens	100(16)	100(2)	0–4 years	56
area)		89(246)	92(12)	5–9 years	56
		78(209)	90(19)	10–19 years	56
		34(102)	67(9)	15–19 years	56
		68(62)	87(52)	adult	110
Widal	O + H Antigens	—	70(52)	Nonendemic, adult	56
		84(62)	73(52)	Endemic area, adult	110
	Vi	45(86)	90(106)	TAB vaccinated	13
		35(140)	91(334)	Not vaccinated	13
HA	Vi	98(170)	47(77)	Endemic area	6
CIE	Cell sonicate	100(23)	4(26)	Acute-phase	36
		—	100(18)	Convalescent sera	36
	Cell sonicate	100(23)	4(24)	Acute-phase	37
		—	100(13)	Convalescent sera	37
	VBE	100(62)	96(52)	Before staining	110
		90	98	After staining	110
	Cell sonicate	79(62)	75(52)	Before staining	110
		68	96	After staining	110
	Barber	98(62)	69(52)	Before staining	110
		95	98	After staining	110
XIE	Cell sonicate	100(30)	100(23)	"precipitin score"	27
	VBE	100(20)	85(20)	"antigen 28"	17
RIA (endemic	LPS	70(20)	90(31)	IgM	16
area)		95(20)	94(31)	IgG	16
		90(20)	94(31)	IgA	16
ELISA (endemic	LPS	100(120)	93(29)	IgM	71a
area)		98(120)	97(29)	IgG	71a
		96(120)	83(29)	IgA	71a

(continued)

TABLE II (*Continued*)

Test	Antigen used	Specificity[b] (%)	Sensitivity[c] (%)	Remarks	Reference
	Cell envelope	96(23)	83(84)	IgM, acute phase	8
		100(23)	92(84)	IgG, acute phase	8
		100(23)	88(77)	IgM, convalescent	8
		96(23)	97(77)	IgG, convalescent	8
	Vi	98(170)	52(77)	—	6

Test	Antibody used (specimen)	Specificity (%)	Sensitivity (%)	Remarks	Reference
B. *Detection of antigen in serum (s) or urine (u)*					
COAG	Monovalent D,d,Vi (u)	83(46)	97(61)	—	85
	Monovalent Vi (u)	86(159)	34(141)	Afebrile	104
		54(21)	—	Febrile control	
	Polyvalent (s)	100(10)	100(10)	—	91
CIE	Polyvalent (s)	100(23)	92(26)	Acute-phase	36
		—	0(18)	Convalescent sera	36
	Polyvalent (s)	100(18)	25(123)	—	97
ELISA	Monovalent Vi (u)	100(50)	67(6)	—	7
	Monovalent Vi (u)	87(159)	62(141)	Afebrile	104
		53(21)	—	Febrile	104
		35(34)	—	Paratyphoid control	104

[a] Abbreviations are defined in the text.

[b] Number of noninfected (culture-negative) people with a negative test/total number of noninfected people examined. Sample sizes are in parentheses.

[c] Number of infected (culture-positive) people with a positive test/total number of infected people examined. Sample sizes are in parentheses.

[d] Not done or not relevant.

Numerous attempts have been made to improve the immunodiagnosis of typhoid by more sensitive techniques, using antigenic extracts instead of whole bacteria. The extracts consist of crude preparations, such as ultrasonic cell lysate and VBE, as well as purified antigens (e.g., LPS and Vi). Some of these studies are discussed below.

Various immunoabsorbents sensitized with *Salmonella* antigens were utilized in agglutination assays, including red blood cells (72), and bentonite (20) or latex particles (62). Although good sensitivities were observed, these early systems were not used for human typhoid detection. Recently, however, Barrett *et al.* (6) used hemagglutination (HA) to detect Vi antibodies in typhoid patients in El Salvador. Although a response was found in only 47% of 77 typhoid patients, the test seemed specific, since 1.7% only of 170 healthy individuals were found positive.

A few investigators have used counterimmunoelectrophoresis (CIE) to diagnose typhoid. Gupta and Rao (36,37) found results obtained by this technique similar to those from the Widal test: antibodies to *S. typhi* cell lysate were observed in only 4% of 24 to 26 acute-phase sera, but in 100% of 13 to 18 convalescent-phase sera obtained from proved typhoid patients; none of the 23 control sera used were positive with the test. In another endemic area, good sensitivity (96% of 52 patients) and specificity (100% of 62 control subjects) were also observed with the technique by Tsang and Chau (110), using VBE as antigen. They had found disappointing results with the Widal test done in parallel. However, less satisfactory results were obtained by these workers if other antigenic extracts were used, or if the slides were stained.

Using a sonicated preparation of *S. typhi*, Espersen *et al.* (27) employed XIE to determine the antibody response in a group of Danish patients with typhoid fever. They found no qualitative difference in response between these patients (*n* = 9) and normal persons (*n* = 30); however, if the responses were quantitated in terms of the total number and titer of precipitins present (''precipitin score''), then all the patients were significantly different from the normals. On the other hand, similar studies by Chau *et al.* (17), using *S. typhi* VBE, revealed a unique precipitin (antigen no. 28, Fig. 2) in the sera of 17 (85%) of 20 typhoid patients and in 4 typhoid carriers, which was absent in 8 nontyphoid septicemic patients, 12 normal persons, and rabbit anti-VBE serum. The discrepancy between the two studies is unexplained, and surprising.

Radioimmunoassays (RIAs) are little used in typhoid serology (16) and are largely superseded by enzyme-linked immunosorbent assays (ELISA). One of the first applications of these latter assays to typhoid diagnosis was a study by Carlsson *et al.* (15) on 41 typhoid patients and 36 healthy blood donors (including 12 paratyphoid A patients). They found a significant difference between the serum ELISA titers of the two groups, measured against *S. typhi* LPS. The assay itself was more reproducible and 100-fold more sensitive than the Widal test, although results from the two methods correlated. Later studies substantiated the high sensitivities and specificities seen with ELISA, whether chemically modified LPS and sera from a nonendemic area (98) or a cell envelope fraction and sera from endemic areas (8,90) were used in the assay. Similar observations were made by Nardiello *et al.* (71a) using LPS. These studies also showed the simplicity of the system and the advantage that IgM, IgG, and IgA antibodies could be individually determined. It was found that all three classes of specific antibodies could be produced in the serum of typhoid patients (13a,16,71a), which had different diagnostic potentials. More recently, Calderon *et al.* (13a) showed that IgG antibodies to *S. typhi* porins could be used for diagnosis in an endemic area. There were instances, however, where ELISA systems proved disappointing, but these were probably related to the antigens used. Thus, Barrett *et al.* (6) detected only 52% of 77 typhoid patients using purified Vi in an ELISA, which was no better than a parallel HA assay.

b. Antigen Detection in Typhoid Patients. Antigen detection is a recent development in diagnosis (Table II). Rockhill *et al.* (85), using D, Vi, or d antisera coupled to staphylococci, detected *S. typhi* antigens in the urine of 97% of 61 confirmed typhoid patients in Indonesia, compared with 17% of 46 healthy control subjects. In contrast, Taylor *et al.* (104) detected urinary Vi in only 62.4% (by ELISA) or 34% (COAG) of 141 proved typhoid patients in Chile, compared with 13.2% (ELISA) or 14% (COAG) of 159 afebrile control subjects. The specificities were not as good if febrile control subjects were used: 64.7% (ELISA) of 34 paratyphoid A or B patients and 47.1% (ELISA) or 46% (COAG) of 21 patients with other nontyphoidal febrile illnesses were (false) positive. Earlier, Barrett *et al.* (7) also observed low sensitivities with ELISA (67%) and COAG (17%) in similar investigations on (only) 6 patients; however, specificity of the ELISA appeared good (100%), although the 50 control subjects chosen were mostly healthy individuals or those with urinary tract infections.

Detection of *S. typhi* antigens in serum has been investigated by Indian workers using antisera raised against whole-cell lysate. Thus, Gupta and Rao (36) detected circulating antigens by CIE in 24 (92%) of 26 acute-phase sera of typhoid patients, but not in any of the 18 convalescent-phase sera obtained from these people, or from 23 normal control subjects. However, in a similar study, Sundararaj *et al.* (97) detected antigen from only 25% of 123 typhoid patients in the first 2–10 days of the disease, although good specificity (100% of 18 control subjects) was seen. Recently, Sivadasan *et al.* (91), using COAG, confirmed that circulating *S. typhi* antigens could be found in all 10 confirmed cases of typhoid during the first week of illness, but generally not later on, nor in any of the control patients ($n = 10$) with other febrile illnesses.

c. Detection of Typhoid Carriers. Since 1935, the immunological detection of chronic typhoid carriers has been based on the presence of Vi antibodies in these people. Agglutination using Vi-rich strains of *S. typhi* or *Citrobacter* and, later, HA using purified Vi (53) were used. However, there were difficulties in interpreting the HA titers (30); further, Bokkenhauser *et al.* (9) questioned the usefulness of the test, as they found 14% false-positives and 67% false-negatives in 1358 food handlers examined in Bantu. Among attempts by others to improve diagnosis, Chitkara and Urquhart (18) described a fluorescent-antibody technique that detected 11 (91.6%) of 12 typhoid carriers, and also had good specificity (98.3% of 119 normal subjects). Using highly purified Vi in an HA, Nolan *et al.* (74) detected 71% of 31 current typhoid carriers; none of the 22 normal persons tested were positive. More recently, an ELISA based on Vi antibody detection enabled Engleberg *et al.* (25) to identify a typhoid carrier as the cause of a typhoid outbreak. A similar assay used by Losonsky *et al.* (59a) detected 87% of 47 Chilean typhoid carriers, and the specificity achieved, based on 22 healthy American volunteers, was 100%.

D. Monospecific Antisera and Monoclonal Antibodies to *Salmonella*

Antisera specific for the individual *Salmonella* antigens are conventionally prepared by immunizing rabbits with whole cells of the desired serotypes and subsequently absorbing the antisera obtained with appropriate serotypes to remove cross-reacting antibodies [see (24)]. For instance, monospecific O-9 serum is obtained from rabbit antiserum to *S. gallinarum* (O-9, O-12) by absorption with *S. paratyphi A* (O-2, O-12) and *S. typhimurium* (O-4, O-12). Another way to remove these cross-reacting antibodies is by affinity chromatography (33). Monospecific sera can also be prepared by immunizing rabbits with synthetic disaccharide–protein conjugates (98–101). Monospecific O-9 serum thus obtained using tyvelose–mannose coupled to bovine serum albumin (BSA), was found to be more specific than that obtained conventionally (44).

The monospecific sera, though specific, are polyclonal. MAbs, on the other hand, are derived from single clones of cells, from the myelomas (81) or hybridomas (49). Only few MAbs with reactivities to *Salmonella* have been described to date; these are listed in Table III.

The *Salmonella*-specific myeloma proteins [reviewed by Potter (80,81)] are all IgA and generally have broad specificities that do not conform to the Kauffmann–White scheme. For example, MOPC 467 binds a common flagellar determinant present in many salmonellae (93), while MOPC 384 reacts with the LPS of various serotypes. The specificity of the latter was determined from inhibition studies to be α-methyl-D-galactoside, while analogs such as β-methyl-D-galactoside and α-methyl-D-mannoside were found to be unreactive. The fine specificity of MOPC 406, which binds *S. weslaco* LPS, was similarly determined to be 2-acetamido-2-deoxy-D-mannose (86), and that of MOPC 252 to be β-D-galactosyl-1,3-N-acetylgalactosamine, present as a terminal determinant in *S. worthington,* and as an internal determinant in *S. kingabwa.* In two pairs of proteins (MOPC 467 and MOPC 570; MOPC 384 and McPC 870), members of each share the same specificity despite independent origins.

Hybridoma antibodies have been produced against *S. typhi* and *S. typhimurium* (Table III). The former group of antibodies will be described in the next section. Of the latter which were used for immunological studies other than diagnosis, Komisar and Cebra (50) obtained nine MAbs, three of which showed cross-reactions with *Proteus morganii.* Based on binding to various *Salmonella*

TABLE III

Monoclonal Antibodies against *Salmonella*

Antibody	Isotype	Specificity	Reference
From myelomas			
MOPC 406	IgA	*S. weslaco* (O-42a)[a] LPS	80,81,86
		S. kampala (O-1,42) LPS	
		E. coli (O-31) LPS (2-acetamido-2-deoxy-D-mannose)	
MOPC 467	IgA	Many *Salmonella* serotypes	80,81,84,93
MOPC 570		e.g. *S. milwaukee* (O-43)	
		Pasteurella pneumotropica	
		Herellea vaginicola (flagellar protein)	
MOPC 384	IgA	*Salmonella* group E3 (O-34) LPS	80,81
McPC 870		*Salmonella* group M (O-28) LPS	
		S. tranoroa (O-55) LPS	
		Proteus mirabilis sp2 LPS	
		E. coli (O-70/O-80) LPS (α-methyl-D-galactoside, for MOPC 384)	
MOPC 252	IgA	*S. worthington* (O-1,13,23) LPS	80,81
		S. kingabwa (O-43) LPS (β-D-galactosyl-1,3-*N*-acetylgalactosamine)	
From hybridomas			
?	IgM	*S. typhimurium* (O-1,4,5,12)	12
7A11	IgG$_1$	*S. typhimurium* LPS	65
12F6	IgG$_{2b}$	*S. typhimurium* LPS	50
15G11	IgM	*S. typhimurium* LPS	
16G11	IgG$_1$	*S. typhimurium* LPS	
16H11	IgG$_{2b}$	*S. typhimurium* LPS	
5D5	IgG$_1$	O-1	65
3D9	IgG$_{2b}$	O-1	
12D4	IgG$_3$	α-galactosyl-1,2-mannose	50
12F4	IgM	O-1	
16F11	IgG$_{2b}$	O-4	
20E10	IgG$_3$	O-4	
17F3	IgG$_3$	O-5	
1c	IgM	O-9	59
3d	IgM	O-9	
8c	IgM	O-9	
7c	IgG	O-9	
2G6/1H11	IgG3	Lipid A	24a
865	IgM	Enterobacterial common antigen	79a
898	IgG2$_a$	Enterobacterial common antigen	

[a] Kauffmann–White antigens.

LPS and oligosaccharides, the specificities of 12F4, 16G11, as well as 20E0, 17F3, and 12D4, were presumed to be O-1, O-4, O-5, and α-galactosyl- 1,2,-mannose, respectively. Metcalf *et al.* (65) obtained three MAbs that reacted strongly with *S. typhimurium* but not with *E. coli* LPS. None were found specific for O-4 or O-12, but two (5D5, 3D9) reacted with *S. dublin* (O-1, O-9, O-12), and hence were presumed to be O-1 specific. More recently, an IgG MAb was described that bound well to purified lipid A obtained from *S. minnesota,* and a lipid A precursor from *S. typhimurium,* but not to whole cells or LPS of the latter (24a). Peters *et al.* (79a) obtained two MAbs that recognized the enterobacterial common antigen present in *Salmonella* and other members of *Enterobacteriaceae;* however, one of these (no. 865) cross-reacted with the capsular polysaccharide of *E. coli* K5, and consequently, its specificity is believed to involve the residue, α-*N*-acetylglucosamine.

III. RESULTS AND DISCUSSION

To illustrate the different diagnostic uses of MAbs to *Salmonella,* two studies will be discussed here. One concerns the detection of *Salmonella* antigens in food using a myeloma protein, and the other, the detection of specific antibodies in typhoid patients using a hybridoma antibody. In both, however, the MAb was conjugated with enzyme and used in solid-phase ELISA.

A. Detection of *Salmonella* in Food

The results presented are taken from a study by Robison *et al.* (84). The reagent MAb was produced from a myeloma, MOPC 467 (see Section II), in mouse ascitic fluid, and was purified by fractionation with 50% saturated ammonium sulfate. This partially purified material was then labeled with alkaline phosphatase.

Salmonella organisms were detected from their growth in M broth after 18 hr. A flagellar extract was prepared from the bacteria obtained by incubating the washed cells (resuspended in phosphate-buffered saline, PBS) in a boiling-water bath for 1 hr. The dissociated flagellar antigens were collected in the supernatant after centrifugation and used without further purification.

In the test, the flagellar extracts were coated on MICROELISA plates, and the presence of the specific antigen was detected directly with the enzyme-labeled MAb. An *E. coli* extract was used as reference. Of 100 *Salmonella* serotypes tested in pure cultures, 94 gave an absorbance of at least 0.10 units higher than that of the *E. coli* strain, and hence was considered positive. The serotypes not detected by the test were *S. typhi, S. paratyphi A, S. paratyphi B, S. kirkee, S. tennessee,* and *S. newington.* Part of the results are shown in Table IV (statistics

TABLE IV

**ELISA Absorbance Readings
of Pure Cultures**[a]

Organism	Absorbance (405 nm)
S. enteritidis	2.165
S. heidelberg	0.612
S. newport	2.010
S. saint paul	1.864
S. infantis	0.598
S. agona	2.311
S. derby	1.688
S. montevideo	2.311
S. typhimurium	0.533
S. typhi	0.029
S. tennessee	0.029
E. coli	0.021
Negative control	0.023

[a]Reproduced with permission from Robison *et al.* (84).

not available). Thus, the test detected a wide range of salmonellae, irrespective of their Kauffmann–White antigens. These serotypes accounted for 89% of the total cases (31,123) of human salmonellosis in the United States in 1979.

The antibody seemed specific for *Salmonella* since it did not react with *Escherichia* (three strains), *Citrobacter* (four), *Edwardsiella* (one), *Klebsiella* (five), *Enterobacter* (five), *Serratia* (five), *Providencia* (three), or *Proteus* (one). However, it bound to *Arizona hinshawii,* but this organism is presently classified under *Salmonella* (29).

Quantitation experiments determined the lower limit of sensitivity to be about 10^6 organisms per milliliter of broth. In experiments involving mixed cultures, it was found that *Salmonella* organisms could be detected when outnumbered by *E. coli* in the initial culture by 10-fold, but not 100-fold or greater; this paralleled observations made by culture. *Salmonella* organisms, when introduced intentionally into powdered infant formula at more than 100 organisms per liter to simulate food contamination, could be detected in the test as efficiently as by culture; success was especially good if the organisms were first grown in a preenrichment broth, followed by tetrathionate broth, and then in the M broth.

The study thus demonstrates the high specificity achievable by a MAb-based ELISA. Unfortunately, important pathogens such as *S. typhi, S. paratyphi A,* and *S. paratyphi B* are not recognized by this antibody. Could a better antibody be found from hybridomas? While this is possible, it may be easier to find another antibody (or antibodies) to complement MOPC 467 (see Section IV). Apparently, such an antibody has been presently obtained from hybridomas that also recognizes a determinant in flagellar extracts (B. Robison, personal communication; see 23a).

A cumbersome feature of the test, unfortunately, is the need to prepare flagellar extracts from the organisms, since attempts to use whole bacterial cells as immunoabsorbent were not successful. This can in fact introduce variability to the system, since Kenny and Dunsmoor (48) showed that components of an antigenic mixture could compete for absorption sites, so that an antigen present in less than 1% of the total could be a disadvantage. One possible way to avoid this problem would be to use an antibody capture system, such as that used for adenovirus detection (3). Alternatively, more direct methods of detection, such as COAG, which has been successfully used in this regard (87,100,101), could be explored.

B. Immunodiagnosis of Typhoid Fever

Hybridoma antibodies were made to *S. typhi* following the somatic cell hybridization procedure of Kohler and Milstein (49), using NS1 myeloma cells and 50% polyethylene glycol (MW 1500, British Drug Houses, Dorset) as a fusing partner and reagent, respectively. The spleen cells used in the hybridization came from BALB/c mice that were immunized with a Barber antigen of *S. typhi*. This antigen was obtained from buffer extracts of the organisms by precipitation with 10% trichloroacetic acid, and contained both LPS and protein. The immunization protocol used that resulted in good circulating antibodies in the animal was as follows: 0.1 mg of the antigen was first given intraperitoneally in incomplete Freund's adjuvant, followed 3 weeks later by an intravenous booster of the antigen (100 ng) in saline, and, subsequently, by another similar booster 2 weeks later. The animal was sacrificed for use 4 days after the last injection.

The fusion mixture was cultured in 96-well microtiter plates (Falcon Plastics) in RPMI 1640 medium (GIBCO Laboratories) containing 15% fetal calf serum and, as feeders, normal BALB/c thymus cells. After 2 weeks, 32 clones appeared, of which 8 (25%) clones produced antibodies reactive to *S. typhi*, as detected by HA. Monoclonality of selected clones was ensured by repeated cloning of the cells, using limiting dilution. Four of the clones that produced high-titered antibodies at the screening stage were expanded for antibody production in culture. Propagation of the hybridoma cells was found to be better in six-well Costar plates than in flasks, as growth here seemed less affected by cell densities.

Of the four MAbs examined by immunodiffusion, three were IgM and the fourth IgG. One of the IgM antibodies (no. 3d) was characterized first and found to be specific for O-9 This was determined from direct-binding studies using crude cell wall preparations extracted from various salmonellae and other bacteria. Thus, it only reacted with *S. typhi, S. sendai,* and *S. enteritidis,* but not with other *Salmonella* serotypes (*S. paratyphi A, S. paratyphi B, S. paratyphi C, S. stanley,* and *S. chester*) or *E. coli, P. aeruginosa, Klebsiella pneumoniae,* and *Staphylococcus aureus* (Fig. 5), or *T. spiralis.* This specificity was confirmed in absorption experiments using the above *Salmonella* types, showing that only the same three serotypes were able to absorb the antibody. Since these organisms belong to group D_1 of the Kauffmann–White scheme and share O-9 and O-12, the antibody must be specific for one of these determinants. However, since it did not bind to salmonellae that possess O-12 only (e.g., *S. paratyphi A* and *S. paratyphi B*), it consequently must be reactive against O-9. Similar results were obtained in studies in which the antibody was found to agglutinate cell suspensions of *S. typhi* and *S. pullorum,* but not those of *S. paratyphi A* (S. G. Hadfield, personal communication). It was further shown in these studies that group D_2 salmonellae, such as *S. haarlem, S. marylebone,* and *S. strassbourg,* were not agglutinated by the antibody unless high concentrations of cells were used, and even then the reactions were weak. Since O-9 in these organisms is partial (see Section II,B), the antibody consequently recognizes not only the tyvelose–mannose structure, but also the linkages of mannose in the main chain.

The specificities of the other three MAbs were similarly deduced to be, surprisingly, also O-9 (Fig. 6). Note that no O-12 antibody was found here or in the MAbs made against *S. typhimurium* (Table III). It is possible that O-12 is not very immunogenic in BALB/c mice, as indeed, based on absorption experiments, very little O-12 antibodies were found in the sera of our *S. typhi*-immunized mice.

The possibility of using MAb 3d to diagnose typhoid fever by detection of specific antibodies was considered. Although it could be employed to isolate the specific antigen from crude mixtures by affinity chromatography for use in immunoassays, we have, however, used it directly in competition (inhibition) assays that utilized only a partially purified antigen (LPS) that is easily obtainable. In such assays, which are infrequently used for this purpose (38,69) compared with their application to antigen detection, the test antibody (competitor) is detected by its effect on the reaction between the labeled, reagent antibody and its antigen. We initially used ^{125}I to label the antibody; high specific (~3000 cpm/ng) and functional activities were obtained using the lactoperoxidase technique of Thorell and Johannsson (108), but not with the chloramine-T method, as denaturation occurred. For the iodination, affinity-purified material was used. This was obtained using an LPS–Sepharose 4B absorbent, and as eluent, 50% ethylene glycol in 0.1 M NaOH–glycine buffer (pH 10.5); the common eluting media such as glycine–HCl buffer (pH 2.5) and $3M$ KSCN, were found unsuit-

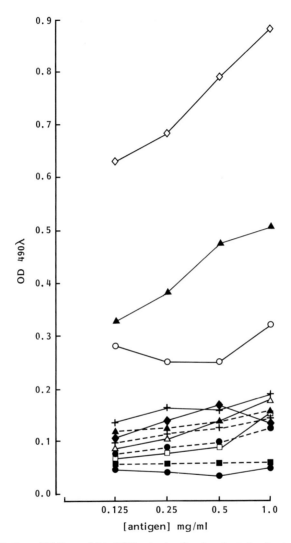

Fig. 5. Binding of MAb no. 3d to VBE extracts of various bacteria, developed with peroxidase-labeled anti-mouse IgG. (Undiluted MAb in spent culture medium used in all wells.) ◇——◇, *S. typhi;* ▲——▲, *S. sendai;* ○——○, *S. enteritidis;* +——+, *S. paratyphi A;* △——△, *S. paratyphi B;* ●- - -●, *S. paratyphi C;* □——□, *S. stanley;* +- - -+, *S. chester;* ◆——◆, *Escherichia coli;* ■- - -■, *Klebsiella pneumoniae;* ●——●, *Pseudomonas aeruginosa;* ▲- - -▲, *Staphylococcus aureus.* Reprinted with permission from Lim and Ho (59).

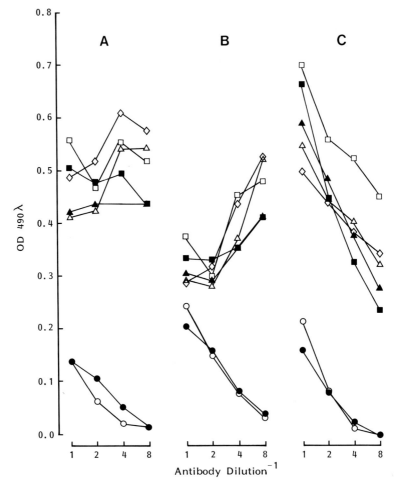

Fig. 6. Specificities of MAb no. 7c (A), 8c (B), and lc (C), determined by residual binding to *S. typhi* LPS (2.5 μg/ml) after absorption with *S. typhi* (○), *S. paratyphi A* (■), *S. paratyphi B* (△), *S. enteritidis* (●), *S. stanley* (◇), or *S. london* (▲) cells, or unabsorbed (□). Developed with peroxidase-labeled anti-mouse IgG.

able (58). In later studies however, an enzyme label (horseradish peroxidase) was used for convenience, which required only a partially purified fraction of the antibody obtained by precipitation of spent culture medium with 50% cold saturated ammonium sulfate. For conjugation, the two-step glutaraldehyde method (5) was followed.

In developing the competition assay, the binding characteristics of the enzyme-labeled antibody was first established, using *S. typhi* LPS insolubilized on 96-well MICROELISA plates (Immunon 2, Dynatech Lab). This involved a checkerboard analysis of a range of antigen and antibody concentrations. To achieve sensitivity in the assay, nonsaturating concentrations of both reagent antibody (conjugate) and antigen (~500 ng per ml) were chosen. For competition, dilutions of the test serum and conjugate were incubated together for 3 hr at 37°C. A variation of this that we experimented with was inhibition, in which the test serum was first allowed to react with the antigen for 3 hr at 37°C and then discarded, after which the conjugate was added and incubated for a further 3 hr at 37°C. Theoretically, this method has the advantage that it obviates any effect the test serum may have on the reagent antibody and, further, it favors the test antibody. Indeed, when the two systems were compared in parallel using two known typhoid sera, three normal (Widal-negative) sera, and the homologous unlabeled MAb, the inhibition assay showed better resolution (Fig. 7). In this assay, which was adopted henceforth, it is apparent that although the normal sera showed no significant binding inhibition, even at low dilutions, both the typhoid sera did. If inhibition is based on the free binding of the conjugate in buffer, then dilutions of these positive sera, as high as 1 : 64 or 1 : 128, gave greater than 80% inhibition. At this level, the amount of inhibitory antibody present, as determined from the unlabeled MAb, was about 300 ng/ml [this was overestimated previously (59)].

When applied to a larger pool of known typhoid patients ($n = 32$) and non-typhoid control subjects ($n = 100$), the inhibition test showed good discrimination between the groups. Figure 8 illustrates these results, based on the inhibitory activities of the sera used at a single dilution of 1 : 8. Thus, the typhoid sera showed greater inhibition ($88.0 \pm 4.4\%$ inhibition) than any of the control samples obtained from 27 febrile patients whose sera were found to be Widal-negative ($26.3 \pm 10.8\%$), 27 healthy blood donors ($44.6 \pm 13.9\%$), and 46 patients examined for syphilis but found negative in the VDRL test ($31.2 \pm 13.3\%$). If greater than 80% inhibition is considered significant, then no false-positives are observed in the test. However, some normal sera, particularly those from the blood donors, showed marked, albeit insignificant, inhibition. This could be due to previous exposure to *S. typhi* through natural infection (e.g., subclinically), or from vaccination. Indeed, two of three recent TAB (typhoid, paratyphoid A, and paratyphoid B) vaccinees included in the study were positive in the test. Consequently, the test cannot differentiate between patients with active infection from vaccinees, unless the sera are titrated and a rising titer is seen in the patients.

One false-negative serum of 33 examined was encountered. This was a sample obtained early in the disease, but a repeat sample obtained 2 weeks later from the patient showed significant inhibition. Two other early samples examined were,

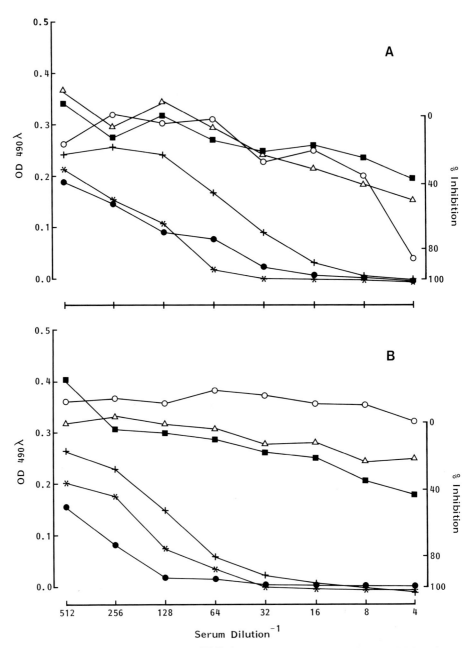

Fig. 7. Reactivities of normal sera (■,○,△), typhoid sera (+,*), and the unlabeled homologous MAb (●, antibody concentration ~60 μg/ml) in direct competition (A) or inhibition (B). ELISA expressed as absorbance (OD_{490}) or percentage inhibition of binding in PBS controls.

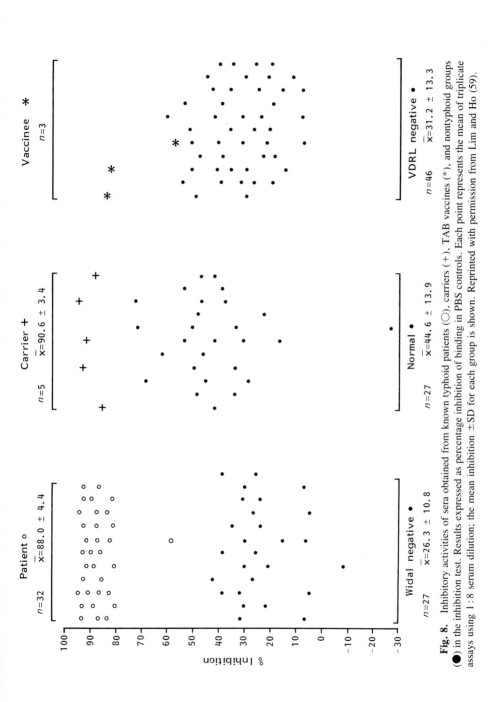

Fig. 8. Inhibitory activities of sera obtained from known typhoid patients (○), carriers (+), TAB vaccines (*), and nontyphoid groups (●) in the inhibition test. Results expressed as percentage inhibition of binding in PBS controls. Each point represents the mean of triplicate assays using 1:8 serum dilution; the mean inhibition ±SD for each group is shown. Reprinted with permission from Lim and Ho (59).

however, strongly positive in the test. The detection of low-titered antibodies in early serum samples will no doubt be a concern here, as has also been found by others (36,37).

A surprising finding was the strong reactivities (90.6 ± 3.4% inhibition) observed in all five sera obtained from known typhoid carriers (Fig. 8), including one which was negative by HA and CIE (*S. typhi* LPS and VBE used, respectively). Thus, the inhibition test is potentially useful for screening typhoid carriers for the presence of antibodies other than those to Vi; the pathogenic significance of this is unclear.

The inhibition seen with sera obtained from all typhoid patients, carriers, TAB vaccinees, and blood donors examined were specific, since it could be removed by absorbing the sera with *S. typhi* but not *E. coli* cells.

Specificity of the inhibition test was also investigated by examining sera obtained from septicemic patients infected with *E. coli* and other salmonellae. As expected, no significant inhibition was observed in infections caused by *E. coli* (two cases), *S. choleraesuis, S. senftenburg,* or *S. johannesburg* due to the absence of O-9 antibodies in these cases; on the other hand, a patient infected with *S. sendai* (O-1, O-9, O-12) showed marked, albeit insignificant, inhibition (76.3%). However, in two cases of paratyphoid A infection, strong inhibition (99.6–100%) was seen, which was unexpected, since *S. paratyphi A* organisms do not possess O-9 but have instead O-1, O-2, and O-12. Although the diagnosis in both cases was bacteriologically confirmed, it was necessary to rule out the possible presence in these patients of O-9 antibodies as well that can arise from *S. typhi* infection or vaccination. This was done in one of the cases. The serum was absorbed with *S. typhi, S. paratyphi A,* or, as control, *E. coli* bacteria; the absorbed sera thus obtained were examined for residual reactivity against cell wall extracts of *S. typhi* or *S. paratyphi A*. The results shown in Fig. 9 indeed confirm that the patient developed responses to *S. paratyphi A* and lacked O-9 antibodies. Further studies indicated that the cross-reactivity could be removed if the serum was preabsorbed with salmonellae containing antigen O-12 (e.g., *S. typhi, S. paratyphi A, S. paratyphi B., S. sendai, S. stanley,* and *S. chester*) but not those lacking it (e.g., *E. coli, S. paratyphi C, S. newport,* and S. london). This indicates that $O-12_2$ antibodies, in addition to O-9 antibodies, could inhibit the test. Based on structural considerations (Fig. 3), these antibodies presumably inhibit by steric hindrance by virtue of the juxtaposition of O-9 and O-12 and, also, the bulkiness of the (IgM) conjugate. It is interesting to note in this regard that Svenungsson *et al.* (98) had also observed, circumstantially, cross-reactions between an antiserum to O-2 (*S. paratyphi A*) and *S. enteritidis* (O-1, O-9, O-12). It was postulated that since the immunodominant sugar of O-2, paratose, is a product of the subterminal step in the biosynthesis of tyvelose (in O-9), O-2 specificities could consequently exist in O-9 organisms. This, however, is not the explanation in our case.

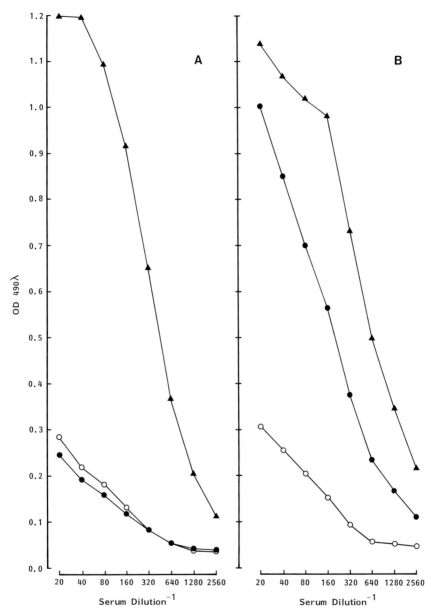

Fig. 9. Serological confirmation of the status of a paratyphoid A patient. Serum was absorbed with *S. typhi* (●), *S. paratyphi A* (○), or *E. coli* (▲) cells, and then examined for binding activity against *S. paratyphi A* (A) or *S. typhi* (B) cell extracts. Developed with peroxidase-labeled anti-human Ig.

Advantage was taken of the dual specificities in the test. Typhoid patients and carriers were examined for contents of the individual O-9 and O-12 antibodies in their sera to see if they differ in their responses. Each serum was absorbed with *S. typhi, S. paratyphi A,* and, as control, *E. coli* cells. The residual activity in the treated serum was then measured in the inhibition test. It appeared from a few selected cases studied (four to five each), that while patients generally made predominant amounts of O-12 antibodies that were removable by both *S. typhi* and *S. paratyphi A* cells, the response of the carriers, on the other hand, was largely directed against O-9. Previously, Brodie (13) observed that only 30–40% of typhoid patients developed O-12 antibodies as measured by the agglutination of *S. paratyphi B* organisms; however, this could be underestimated since even by *S. typhi* O-bacteria agglutination, less than 65% of these patients were considered positive. Although more cases need to be studied to see if indeed there is a sequential development of antibody responses to these antigens, it is clear that immunoassays that monitor only single responses will miss a number of cases. This may be a reason for the failure of an ELISA designed to detect O-9 antibodies to diagnose *S. enteritidis* infection in an outbreak (98). Indeed, Hewitt *et al.* (38) showed that tuberculous patients developed different patterns of antibody responses to mycobacterial antigens as defined by five non-cross-reacting MAbs in a competitive RIA; detection by the individual antibodies was poor, and even combinations of two or three MAbs together could detect no more than 71% of the 41 patients. Using a similar technique, Mitchell *et al.* (69) also observed that one of their MAbs (I.134) could detect only 90% of infected patients with schistosomiasis, while another antibody (P.41) was found to be mutually exclusive with it in diagnostic potential.

Since the test detects both O-9 and O-12 antibodies, it is not specific for typhoid but potentially detects all infections caused by the 216 or so salmonellae in groups A, B, and D. However, not many of these organisms invade and stimulate systemic antibody production, nor are they frequently encountered in nature. Of those that do, *S. typhi* is one of the more common. In theory, to diagnose typhoid specifically, it would be necessary to separate the O-9 and O-12 responses. Even then, there are 67 serotypes that possess O-9, and another 29 have a partial O-9 (24). Of other useful markers in *S. typhi,* H-d exists in 97 serotypes and Vi in 3, but neither per se has been shown to be diagnostically satisfactory (7,13,56,110). However, in combination with O-9 (including partial), H-d is present in 7 serotypes only (e.g., *S. ndolo, S. strassbourg*), while the combination of O-9, H-d, and Vi is unique to *S. typhi.* Thus, an ideal test for diagnosing typhoid fever may be one composed of individual tests that detect responses to O-9, O-12, H-d, and Vi. Indeed, such a panel would ensure a high predictive value in diagnosis (34).

The inhibition test was designed for routine use. Simplicity was thus intended; for example, a single dilution of the test serum in triplicates was used instead of

TABLE V

Evaluation of the Inhibition ELISA Test

Attribute	Remarks[a]
Specificity	All (100%) of 100 normal control subjects negative; detects O-9 and O-12 antibodies (i.e., presumably only those systemic infections caused by salmonellae with the corresponding antigens).
Sensitivity	One (3%) early serum sample from 33 typhoid sera was false-negative.
Resolution	Except for borderline cases, negative (OD_{490} 0.2–0.4) and positive ($OD_{490} < 0.01$) cases distinguishable by naked eye. Success due to separate incubations of test serum and conjugate, specificity of conjugate, and property of LPS (as adsorbent)?
Reproducibility	Intraplate, SE < 10% (of triplicates); interplate, requires careful standardization of reagents and inclusions of appropriate standards and controls.
Reagent antibody	IgM, stable at 37°C for 11 days (S. G. Hadfield, personal communication); easily conjugated with horseradish peroxidase; conjugate stable at 4°C for at least a month, binds well to antigen.
Reagent antigen	LPS, easily prepared or obtainable commercially; insolubilized easily on MICROELISA plates, keeps well in this state (after methanol fixation) for at least 4 months.
Versatility	Simple, can be automated; may be used routinely, especially for mass screening.
Cost	Potentially cheap, since mass production of reagents and 30 tests per MICROELISA plate possible.
Speed	7 hr to complete.

[a]OD_{490}, Optical density at 490 nm. Other abbreviations are defined in the text.

titration. Unfortunately, a reservation about its routine application is the need to standardize reagents and optimize conditions that are crucial to the test. However, this problem may be alleviated by preparing both conjugate and antigen-coated plates in bulk, and the inclusion of suitable controls and standards in the test. Indeed, it seems ideal for mass screening, as the majority of results can be gauged by the naked eye. Other features of the test are summarized in Table V.

IV. CONCLUSIONS

1. MAbs can be conjugated with enzymes and used to establish efficient diagnostic tests for *Salmonella*. Further, immunoglobulins other than IgG (often considered the choice isotype in immunoassays) can be utilized whether they are IgA (e.g., MOPC 467) or IgM (e.g., 3d). There is no doubt that many useful MAbs to *Salmonella* will be found in future, which will be successfully employed in a variety of diagnostic procedures.

2. High specificities were observed in the tests developed. Thus, MOPC 467 binds to a common flagellar determinant present in 94 of 100 *Salmonella* serotypes studied irrespective of their Kauffmann–White antigens, but not to non-*Salmonella* enterobacteria.

3d is specific for antigen O-9 present in group D salmonellae only. However, the inhibition test based on this antibody is less specific, as it detects not only O-9 but also O-12 antibodies, by virtue of steric hindrance of the latter. Thus, the test potentially detects all systemic infections caused by salmonellae that possess O-9 or O-12, that is, those in groups A, B, and D. In practice, all 32 cases of typhoid fever and 2 cases of paratyphoid A were diagnosed. Septicemia caused by *E. coli* and other *Salmonella* serotypes (e.g., *S. choleraesuis*) were negative in the test. As these results were obtained from an endemic area, there is reason to believe that similar specificity will be observed in nonendemic regions.

3. The sensitivities of the tests were less ideal. MOPC 467 could not detect 6 of 100 salmonellae examined, notably, *S. typhi, S. paratyphi A,* and *S. paratyphi B.* However, this deficiency can be compensated for by using a complementary antibody—and one has apparently been found. With the positive strains, the technique could detect as few as 10^6 organisms per milliliter of medium.

In the inhibition test using 3d to diagnose typhoid fever, one early serum sample of 33 examined was found to be false-negative; however, the extent of this problem will not be realized until more cases are examined, particularly from nonendemic areas where the subjects have no previous exposure to *S. typhi.* Undoubtedly, underestimation would have been greater if not for the fact that the test detects antibodies to both O-9 and O-12, the major antigens of *S. typhi.* From absorption studies, it seems some typhoid patients make predominantly O-12 and little O-9 antibodies. Thus, systems monitoring responses to single markers may not be sensitive, and a compromise between specificity and sensitivity may be required for an ideal test. Alternatively, a panel of tests could be used to detect individual responses to O-9 and O-12 including, if possible, H-d and Vi. There could be a sequential development of responses to these markers.

4. The inhibition test seems excellent for detecting chronic typhoid carriers, presumably by virtue of O-9 antibodies present in these people. However, more work is required to clarify the immune status of carriers, since they usually possess Vi antibodies.

V. PROSPECTS FOR THE FUTURE

This is only the beginning. It is envisaged that more MAbs will be used for the rapid detection of *Salmonella* organisms in foods, feeds, and clinical specimens. A definite use of MAbs to *Salmonella* is in serotyping; one can expect the whole range of conventional antisera presently utilized for the Kauffmann–White scheme to be replaced by MAbs. Whether MAbs too, can be used in lieu of phage typing, by virtue of newfound specificities, is an interesting thought. What are the MAbs we can expect? How are they best utilized for diagnosis?

A. The Antibody

The repertoire size of MAbs to *Salmonella* must be immeasurably large. With LPS alone, not only will MAbs be found to the Kauffmann–White antigens, new specificities can be expected as well. Even to each "conventional" antigen, a myriad of MAbs can be expected that differ in isotype, idiotype, and affinity, such as observed for α-1,6-linked dextran (45); on the other hand, idiotypically similar MAbs to the same antigen can also be found (69). These antibodies could also differ in the size (disaccharide, tetrasaccharide, etc.) and shape (groove, pocket, etc.) of the combining site (45), or in the recognition of different parts of the antigen (e.g., $O-9_1$, $O-9_2$). However, the number of such specificities that can be distinguished in practice depends on the availability of bacterial mutants and the sensitivity of assays (110a) used to study them. As demonstrated in our study, even MAbs made to closely linked antigens, such as O-9 and O-12, could not be distinguished in the inhibition test. Furthermore, the range of specificities that can be generated in an animal may be restricted by its genetic makeup; for example, horse or goat antisera to *Salmonella* O antigens were found to be more cross-reactive than the corresponding rabbit antisera (60).

Of the many MAbs that can be made to *Salmonella,* what are the useful ones in diagnosis? For most purposes, the isotype should not matter too much, although an IgG would still be preferred for precipitation reactions or immunofluorescence, and is easier to purify. If necessary, it should be possible in the future, with the advent of gene cloning techniques, to reconstruct useful hybridomas to secrete the desired isotype (77). The antibody should be stable, and, most importantly, have high affinity for the antigen. In terms of specificity, the choice of antibody will depend on the purpose for which it is intended. In addition to MAbs to the various Kauffmann–White antigens for identification (serotyping) purposes, it would be desirable to have an antibody that is specific for *S. typhi* only to diagnose typhoid fever, another that could recognize all the salmonellae but not other bacteria for routine food analysis, and yet another to detect endotoxin in patients suffering from gram-negative sepsis [i.e., with the potential of the limulus lysate test (111), but with better specificity]. Can such MAbs be found? Assuming the specificity of a MAb mirrors that of the antigen (defined by conventional antisera) to which it is made (which is not necessarily true), then, based on present knowledge (Section II,B), the more specific MAbs are likely to be directed against the O antigens, whereas MAbs of broad specificities are probably those relating to the LPS core, proteins such as Braun's lipoprotein and flagella, and the common antigens described in Section II,B,6. Admittedly, immunological studies on the proteins have been relatively limited. In contrast, polysaccharide antigens have been widely studied, not only in *Salmonella* but also in other bacteria and tissues. MAbs made against these antigens in *Shigella flexneri* (14), for example, were shown to be more specific than conventional antisera in bacterial identification. Further, MAbs produced against cell surface glycosphingolipids were found to exhibit extremely fine discrimination against structurally related di- and trisaccharide compounds that differed from the respective homologs in a single linkage or sugar residue only (117); this is reminiscent of studies that demonstrated the fine specificities of both rabbit antisera and the myeloma proteins to the *Salmonella* O antigens.

It is necessary that a MAb to be used for the immunodiagnosis of typhoid fever be not only specific for the causative bacterium, but also relevant diagnostically. That is, it must be specific for an antigen which all or most patients respond to, if the purpose is to detect specific antibodies in these patients. On the other hand, if antigen detection is intended, then it may be preferable to use an antibody which patients do not produce. The diagnostically relevant antigens may be identified in tests developed with sera obtained from the infected subjects, for example using XIE (17,27) or Western blot (26). Alternatively, relevant MAbs may be produced directly from human cells obtained from, say, typhoid patients, through cell immortalization (105). As discussed previously (Section III), the important diagnostic markers of *S. typhi* are O-9, O-12, Vi, and H-d, which are all exposed on the cell surface; consequently, MAbs to these antigens would be useful. Since both Vi and H-d are multiantigenic, it is possible that immunoassays developed with suitable MAbs to these antigens individually will be more specific than those seen previously. It would be ideal to monitor the responses in typhoid patients to all four markers, and better yet, in terms of predictive value and specificity, to monitor these separately (by inhibition or direct-binding) rather than as a combined (direct-binding) test. If this proves too cumbersome, the O-9 and O-12 antibody detection could perhaps be combined, as in our inhibition test.

A single MAb may also prove inadequate for the detection of common antigens in the case of endotoxemia or in food analysis. It may be more worthwhile, instead, to use mixtures of MAbs in a combined (direct-binding) system for this purpose. The judicious use of such mixtures may in fact be beneficial (107). A useful antibody for combination is one with O-12 specificity, since this antigen is present in many of the common and important salmonellae.

B. The Technique

MAbs are best applied to the M broth (food) or enrichment broth (stool) cultures for detecting salmonellae. Blood cultures, too, should be examined directly, because of previous successes seen with polyvalent antisera (23,67,113). If necessary, colonies obtained from the primary broths can also be examined. In the diagnosis of enteric fever, antigen detection should be given greater emphasis, and, for this, urine seems a convenient and useful source (19,40).

Among the techniques available, the system of enzyme labels will remain useful. The enzyme-conjugated antibody can be used to detect organisms directly in smears (64a), or employed in serological assays. However, the possibility of improving these techniques should be considered. For example, antigen or antibody insolubilization on MICROELISA plates is not always satisfactory, compared to its behavior in solution (47), or when coupled to polyacrylamide or sepharose beads (4). Further, the use of avidin–biotin as an indirect and more versatile means of coupling enzyme to antibody (114) and the use of fluorogenic substrates for enzymes (4) may be rewarding.

Another technique that is simple and rapid which can be used as a bedside kit is latex agglutination. It was found to be highly specific and 100-fold more sensitive than COAG or CIE in a comparative study on the detection of *Haemophilus influenzae* antigens in cerebrospinal fluid (64). Unlike the problem of spontaneous agglutination seen with COAG (87), latex agglutination was successfully used to detect rotavirus directly in fecal samples (88); it also detected *Staphylococcus aureus* in blood cultures with high (94.4%) efficiency (23). Thus, it seems a suitable method for detecting salmonellae in foods and clinical materials and is indeed an efficient and economical way of using MAbs that are otherwise poorly agglutinating. We have, in fact, examined an experimental latex suspension of our O-9 MAb (3d) developed by Wellcome Diagnostics (Beckenham, England). Preliminary studies indicated that the antibody kept in this state was stable for over a year, and was 100% accurate in identifying group D *Salmonella* colonies grown on MacConkey agar (C. Pang and P. L. Lim, unpublished observations). Moreover, it detected *S. typhi* bacteria in simulated blood culture at a sensitivity of 10^8 organisms per milliliter. It could also detect as little as 1 μg of *S. typhi* LPS per milliliter of (spiked) human serum. We are presently examining the possibility of using it to detect antigen and antibody in typhoid patients. Interestingly, O-12 antibodies also appeared to inhibit in the antibody detection system.

VI. SUMMARY

About a dozen hybridoma antibodies to *Salmonella* have been described with known specificities directed against the O antigens, including O-1, O-4, O-5, and O-9. Of these, the O-9 monoclonal antibody (MAb) has been used to develop an enzyme-linked immunosorbent assay (ELISA) to diagnose typhoid fever, based on the inhibition of binding between the peroxidase-labeled MAb and *S. typhi* lipopolysaccharide, in sera obtained from typhoid patients and carriers.

This was found to be specific and sensitive, although it detected not only O-9 antibodies, but O-12 antibodies as well, the latter due to steric hindrance. Six myeloma proteins are known that bind to *Salmonella*. One of these (MOPC 467) was utilized in a direct ELISA to detect salmonellae in food; the results obtained were encouraging. There is potential for the use of MAbs in the direct identification of *Salmonella* organisms in pure cultures (serotyping) as well as in clinical materials and foods (rapid methods), and in establishing better immunoassays for diagnosing the enteric fevers. Some of the future possibilities based largely on a knowledge of the *Salmonella* antigens and the conventional methods used to detect these organisms and their infections are discussed in this review.

ACKNOWLEDGMENTS

I am grateful to Dr. B. J. Robison of Bionetics, Charleston, South Carolina, and to Miss S. G. Hadfield of Wellcome Diagnostics, Beckenham, England, for use of information cited in the text. The gift of latex particles from Wellcome Diagnostics is also gratefully acknowledged. Most of the writing was done while on leave at the University of Texas Health Science Center at Dallas; I thank Dr. P. W. Tucker for his hospitality and his secretary, Miss Marilyn Gardner, for help with the manuscript.

REFERENCES

1. Abram, D., Koffler, H., and Vatter, A. E. (1965). Basal structure and attachment of flagellin in cells of *Proteus vulgaris*. *J. Bacteriol.* **90**, 1337–1354.
2. Ames, G. F., Spudich, E. N., and Nikaido, H. (1974). Protein composition of the outer membrane of *Salmonella typhimurium*: Effect of lipopolysaccharide mutations. *J. Bacteriol.* **117**, 406–416.
3. Anderson, L. J., Godfrey, E., McIntosh, K., and Hierholzer, J. C. (1983). Comparison of a monoclonal antibody with a polyclonal serum in an enzyme-linked immunosorbent assay for detecting adenovirus. *J. Clin. Microbiol.* **18**, 463–468.
4. Avrameas, S. (1981). Heterogeneous enzyme immunoassays. *In* "Immunoassays for the 80's" (A. Voller, A. Bartlett, and D. Bidwell, eds.), pp. 85–90. Univ. Park Press, Baltimore, Maryland.
5. Avrameas, S., and Ternynck, T. (1971). Peroxidase labelled antibody and Fab conjugates with enhanced intracellular penetration. *Immunochemistry* **8**, 117–1179.
6. Barrett, T. J., Blake, P. A., Brown, S. L., Hoffman, K., Liort, J. M., and Feeley, J. D. (1983). Enzyme-linked immunosorbent assay for detection of human antibodies to *Salmonella typhi* Vi antigen. *J. Clin. Microbiol.* **17**, 625–627.
7. Barrett, T. J., Snyder, J. D., Blake, P. A., and Feeley, J. D. (1982). Enzyme-linked immunosorbent assay for detection of *Salmonella typhi* Vi antigen in urine from typhoid patients. *J. Clin. Microbiol.* **15**, 235–237.
8. Beasley, W. J., Joseph, S. W., and Weiss, E. (1981). Improved serodiagnosis of *Salmonella* enteric fever by an enzyme-linked immunosorbent assay. *J. Clin. Microbiol.* **13**, 106–114.
9. Bokkenhauser, V., Smithy, P., and Richardson, N. (1964). A challenge to the validity of the Vi test for detection of chronic typhoid carriers. *Am. J. Public Health* **54**, 1501–1503.

10. Brade, H., and Galanos, C. (1983). Common lipopolysaccharides from different families of gram-negative bacteria. *Infect. Immun.* **42**, 250–256.
11. Braun, V. (1977). Lipoprotein from the outer membrane of *Escherichia coli* as antigen, immunogen, and mitogen. *In* "Microbiology 1977" (D. Schlessinger, ed.), pp. 257–261. Am. Soc. Microbiol., Washington, D.C.
12. Briles, D. E., Claflin, L. J., Schroer, K., Forman, C., Basta, P., Lehmeyer, J., and Benjamin, W. H., Jr. (1981). The use of hybridoma antibodies to examine antibody-mediated antimicrobial activities. *In* "Monoclonal Antibodies and T-cell Hybridomas" (G. J. Hammerling, U. Hammerling, and J. F. Kearney, eds.), pp. 285–290. Elsevier/North-Holland, Amsterdam.
13. Brodie, J. (1977). Antibodies and the Aberdeen typhoid outbreak of 1964. I. The Widal reaction. *J. Hyg.* **79**, 161–180.
13a. Calderon, I., Lobos, S. R., Rojas, H. A., Palomino, C., Rodriguez, L. H., and Mora, G. C. (1986). Antibodies to porin antigens of *Salmonella typhi* induced during typhoid infections in humans. *Infect. Immun.* **52**, 209–212.
14. Carlin, N. I. A., and Lindberg, A. A. (1983). Monoclonal antibodies specific for O-antigenic polysaccharides of *Shigella flexneri*: Clones binding to II, II:3,4, and 7,8 epitopes. *J. Clin. Microbiol.* **18**, 1183–1189.
15. Carlsson, H. E., Lindberg, A. A., Hammerstrom, S., and Ljunggren, A. (1975). Quantitation of *Salmonella* O-antibodies in human sera by enzyme-linked immunosorbent assay (ELISA). *Int. Arch. Allergy Appl. Immunol.* **48**, 485–494.
16. Tsang, R. S. W., Chau, P. Y., Lam, S. K., LaBrooy, J. T., and Rowley, D. (1981). Antibody response to the lipopolysaccharide and protein antigens of *Salmonella typhi* during typhoid infection. I. Measurement of serum antibodies by radioimmunoassay. *Clin. Exp. Immunol.* **46**, 508–514.
17. Chau, P. Y., Wan, K. D., and Tsang, R. S. W. (1984). Crossed immunoelectrophoretic analysis of anti-*Salmonella typhi* antibodies in sera of typhoid patients and carriers: Demonstration of the presence of typhoid-specific antibodies to a non-O, non-H, non-Vi antigen. *Infect. Immun.* **43**, 1110–1113.
18. Chitkara, Y. K., and Urquhart, A. E. (1978). Fluorescent Vi antibody test in the screening of typhoid carriers. *Am. J. Clin. Pathol.* **72**, 87–89.
19. Coonrod, J. D. (1983). Urine as an antigen reservoir for diagnosis of infectious diseases. *Am. J. Med.* **75**, 85–92.
20. Diena, B. B., Wallace, R., and Greenberg, L. (1963). A flocculation test for *Salmonella* antibodies using sensitized bentonite particles. *Can. J. Microbiol.* **9**, 281–226.
21. DiPauli, R. (1977). Natural history of the immune response to *Salmonella* polysaccharides in inbred strains of mice. *In* "Microbiology 1977" (D. Schlessinger, ed.), pp. 280–285. Am. Soc. Microbiol., Washington, D.C.
22. DiRienzo, J. M., Nakamura, K., and Inouye, M. (1978). The outer membrane proteins of gram-negative bacteria: Biosynthesis, assembly, and functions. *Annu. Rev. Biochem.* **47**, 481–532.
23. Doern, G. V., and Robbie, L. I. (1982). Direct identification of *Staphylococcus aureus* in blood culture fluid with a commercial latex agglutination test. *J. Clin. Microbiol.* **16**, 1048–1051.
23a. Eckner, K., Flowers, R. S., Robison, B. J., Mattingly, J. A., Gabis, D. A., and Silliker, J. H. (1986). Comparison of *Salmonella* Bio-EnzaBead™ immunoassay method and conventional culture procedure for detection of *Salmonella* in foods. *ASM 86th Ann. Meeting* Abstr.
24. Edwards, P. R., and Ewing, W. H. (1972). "Identification of Enterobacteriaceae," 3rd Ed. Burgess, Minneapolis, Minnesota.
24a. Elkins, K., and Metcalf, E. S. (1985). Binding activity of a murine anti-lipid A monoclonal antibody. *Infect. Immun.* **48**, 597–600.

25. Engleberg, N. D., Barrett, T. J., Fisher, H., Porter, B., Hurtado, E., and Hughes, J. M. (1983). Identification of a carrier by using Vi enzyme-linked immunosorbent assay serology in an outbreak of typhoid fever on an Indian reservation. *J. Clin. Microbiol.* **6**, 1320–1322.
26. De Jongh-Leuvenink, J., Vreede, R. W., Marcelis, J. H., de Vos, M., and Verhoef, J. (1985). Detection of antibodies against lipopolysaccharides of *Escherichia coli* and *Salmonella* R and S strains by immunoblotting. *Infect. Immun.* **50**, 716–720.
27. Espersen, F., Hertz, J. B., Holby, N., and Mogensen, H. H. (1980). Quantitative immunoelectrophoretic analysis of *Salmonella typhi* antigens and of corresponding antibodies in human sera. *Acta Pathol. Microbiol. Scand., Sect. B* **88B**, 237–242.
28. Espersen, F., Holby, N., and Hertz, J. B. (1980). Cross-reactions between *Salmonella typhi* and 24 other bacterial species. *Acta Pathol. Microbiol. Scand., Sect. B* **88B**, 243–248.
29. Farmer, J. J., III, McWhorter, A. C., Brenner, D. J., and Morris, G. K. (1984). The *Salmonella*-Arizona group of Enterobacteriaceae: Nomenclature, classification, and reporting. *Clin. Microbiol. Newsl.* **6**, 63–69.
30. Forrest, C. R., Matthews, R. N., Robertson, M. J., and Hanley, W. P.(1967). Vi reaction in Hong Kong. *Br. Med. J.* **ii**, 472–475.
31. Galanos, C., Freudenberg, M. A., Luderitz, O., Rietschel, E. T., and Westphal, O. (1979). Chemical, physicochemical and biological properties of bacterial lipopolysaccharides. *In* "Progress in Clinical and Biological Research: Biomedical Applications of the Horseshoe Crab (Limulidiae)" (E. Cohen, ed.), Vol. 29, pp. 322–332. Alan R. Liss, New York.
32. Gibbs, P. A., Patterson, J. T., and Murray, J. G. (1972). The fluorescent antibody technique for the detection of *Salmonella* in routine use. *J. Appl. Bacteriol.* **35**, 405–415.
33. Girard, R., and Goichot, J. (1981). Preparation of monospecific anti-*Salmonella* lipopolysaccharide antibodies by affinity chromatography. *Ann. Immunol. (Paris)* **132C**, 211–217.
34. Glynn, A. A., and Ison, C. (1981). Enzyme Immunoassays in Bacteriology. *In* "Immunoassays for the 80's" (A. Voller, A. Bartlett, and D. Bidwell, eds.), pp. 431–440. Univ. Park Press, Baltimore, Maryland.
35. Guinee, P. A. M., and van Leewen, W. J. (1978). Phage typing of *Salmonella*. *In* "Methods in Microbiology" (T. Bergan and J. R. Norris, eds.), Vol. 2, pp. 157–191. Academic Press, New York.
36. Gupta, A. K., and Rao, K. M. (1979). Simultaneous detection of *Salmonella typhi* antigen and antibody in serum by counterimmunoelectrophoresis for an early and rapid diagnosis of typhoid fever. *J. Immunol. Methods* **30**, 349–53.
37. Gupta, A. K., and Rao, K. M. (1981). Radial counterimmunoelectrophoresis for rapid serodiagnosis of typhoid fever. *J. Immunol. Methods* **40**, 373–376.
38. Hewitt, J., Coates, A. R. M., Mitchison, D. A., and Ivanyi, J. (1982). The use of murine monoclonal antibodies without purification of antigen in the serodiagnosis of tuberculosis. *J. Immunol. Methods* **55**, 205–211.
39. Ichiki, A., and Parish, C. R. (1971). Cleavage of bacterial flagellin with proteolytic enzymes. I. Physicochemical and antigenic properties of the tryptic and peptic peptides. *Immunochemistry* **9**, 153–167.
40. Ingram, D. L., Suggs, D. M., and Pearson, A. W. (1982). Detection of group B streptococcal antigen in early-onset and late-onset group B streptococcal disease with the Wellcogen strep B latex agglutination test. *J. Clin. Microbiol.* **16**, 656–658.
41. Izard, D., Husson, M. O., Vincent, P., Leclerc, H., Monget, D., and Boeufgras, J. M. (1984). Evaluation of the four-hour rapid 20E system for identification of members of the family Enterobacteriaceae. *J. Clin. Microbiol.* **20**, 51–54.
42. Jann, K., and Westphal, O. (1975). Microbial Polysaccharides. *In* "The Antigens" (M. Sela, ed.), Vol. 3, pp. 1–125. Academic Press, New York.

43. Johns, M. A., Whiteside, R. E., Baker, E. E., and McCabe, W. R. (1973). Common entero-bacterial antigen. I. Isolation and purification from *Salmonella typhosa* 0:901. *J. Immunol.* **110,** 781–790.
44. Jorbeck, H., Carlsson, H. E., Svenson, S. B., Lingberg, A. A., Alfredsson, G., Garegg, P. J., Svensson, S., and Wallin, N. H. (1979). Immunochemistry of *Salmonella* O-antigens. Specificity and cross-reactivity of factor 09 serum and of antibodies against tyvelose (1,3:α) mannose coupled to bovine serum albumin. *Int. Arch. Allergy Appl. Immunol.* **58,** 11–19.
45. Kabat, E. A. (1983). The antibody combining site. *In* "Progress in Immunology V" (Y. Yamamura and T. Tada, eds.), pp. 67–85. Academic Press, New York.
46. Kamio, Y., and Nikaido, H. (1977). Outer membrane of *Salmonella typhimurium*. Identification of proteins exposed on cell surface. *Biochim. Biophys. Acta* **464,** 589–601.
47. Kennel, S. J. (1982). Binding of monoclonal antibody to protein antigen in fluid phase or bound to solid supports. *J. Immunol. Methods* **55,** 1–12.
48. Kenny, G. E., and Dunsmoor, C. L. (1983). Principles, problems, and strategies in the use of antigenic mixtures for the enzyme-linked immunosorbent assay. *J. Clin. Microbiol.* **17,** 655–665.
49. Kohler, G., and Milstein, C. (1975). Continuous cultures of fused cells secreting antibodies of predefined specificity. *Nature (London)* **256,** 495–497.
50. Komisar, J. L., and Cebra, J. J. (1983). Monoclonal antibodies to *Salmonella typhimurium* and *Escherichia coli* lipopolysaccharides. *Adv. Exp. Med. Biol.* **162,** 303–311.
51. Kuusi, K., Nurminen, M., Saxen, H., Valtonen, M., and Makela, P. H. (1979). Immunization with major outer membrane proteins in experimental salmonellosis of mice. *Infect. Immun.* **25,** 857–862.
52. Kuusi, N., Nurminen, M., Saxen, H., and Makela, P. H. (1981). Immunization with major outer membrane protein (porin) preparations in experimental murine salmonellosis: Effect of lipopolysaccharide. *Infect. Immun.* **34,** 328–332.
53. Landy, M., and Lamb, E. (1953). Estimation of Vi antibody employing erythrocytes treated with purified antigen. *Proc. Soc. Exp. Biol. Med.* **82,** 593–598.
54. LeMinor, L, Vernon, M., and Popoff, M. (1982). Proposition pour une nomenclature des *Salmonella. Ann. Microbiol. (Paris)* **133B,** 245–254.
55. Levine, M. M., Black, R. E., Lanata, C., and the Chilean Typhoid Committee (1982). Precise estimation of the numbers of chronic carriers of *Salmonella typhi* in Santiago, Chile, an endemic area. *J. Infect. Dis.* **146,** 724–725.
56. Levine, M. M., Gredos, O., Gilmon, R. H., Woodward, W. E., Solis-Plaza, R., and Waldman, W. (1978). Diagnostic value of the Widal test in areas endemic for typhoid fever. *Am. J. Trop. Med. Hyg.* **27,** 795–800.
57. Mak, M. H. H. (1985). "The Medical Directory of Hong Kong," 3rd Ed. Fed. Med. Soc. Hong Kong, Hong Kong.
58. Lim, P. L. (1986). The isolation of specific IgM monoclonal antibodies by affinity chromatography using alkaline buffers. *Molec. Immunol.* (in press).
59. Lim, P. L., and Ho, M. Y. (1983). Diagnosis of enteric fever by inhibition assay using peroxidase-labelled monoclonal antibody and *Salmonella typhi* lipopolysaccharide. *Aust. J. Exp. Biol. Med. Sci.* **61,** 687–704.
59a. Losonsky, G. A., Kaintuck, S., Kotloff, K. L., Ferreccio, C., Robbins, J. B., and Levine, M. M. (1986). Evaluation of an enzyme linked immunosorbent assay (ELISA) for detection of chronic typhoid carriers. *ASM 86th Ann. Meeting* Abstr. C-279.
60. Luderitz, O., Staub, A. M., and Westphal, O. (1966). Immunochemistry of O and R antigens of *Salmonella* and related Enterobacteriaceae. *Bacteriol. Rev.* **30,** 192–255.
61. Luderitz, O., Westphal, O., Staub, A. M., and Nikaido, H. (1971). Isolation and chemical and

immunologic characterization of bacterial lipopolysaccharides. *In* "Microbial Toxins" (G. Weinbaum, S. Kadie, and S. J. Ajl, eds.), Vol. 4, pp. 145–233. Academic Press, New York.

62. Magwood, S. E., and Annau, E. (1961). The absorption of somatic antigens of *Salmonella* by polystyrene latex particles. *Can. J. Comp. Med. Vet. Sci.* **25,** 69–73.

63. Makela, P. H., and Mayer, H. (1976). Enterobacterial common antigen. *Bacteriol. Rev.* **40,** 591–632.

64. Marcon, M. J., Hamoudi, A. C., and Camon, H. J. (1984). Comparative laboratory evaluation of three antigen detection methods for diagnosis of *Haemophilus influenzae* type b disease. *J. Clin. Microbiol.* **19,** 333–337.

64a. McRill, C. M., Kramer, T. T., and Griffith, R. W. (1984). Application of the peroxidase-antiperoxidase immunoassay to the identification of salmonellae from pure culture and animal tissue. *J. Clin. Microbiol.* **20,** 281–284.

65. Metcalf, E. S., O'Brien, A. B., Laveck, M. A., and Biddison, W. E. (1983). Characterization of monoclonal antibodies which recognize specific cell surface determinants on *Salmonella typhimurium*. *Adv. Exp. Med. Biol.* **162,** 313–317.

66. Michael, J. G., and Maliah, I. (1981). Immune response to parental and rough mutant strains of *Salmonella minnesota*. *Infect. Immun.* **33,** 784–787.

67. Mikhail, I. A., Sanborn, W. R., and Sippel, J. G., (1983). Rapid, economical diagnosis of enteric fever by a blood clot culture coagglutination procedure. *J. Clin. Microbiol.* **17,** 564–565.

68. Miller, J. M. (1983). New genera and species of Enterobactericeae. *Clin. Microbiol. Newsl.* **6,** 149–153.

69. Mitchell, G. F., Garcia, E. G., and Cruise, K. M. (1983). Competitive radioimmunoassays using hybridoma and antiidiotype antibodies in identification of antibody responses to and antigens of *Schistosoma japonicum*. *Aust. J. Exp. Biol. Med. Sci.* **61,** 27–36.

70. Mohr, H. K., Trenk, H. L., and Yeterion, M. (1974). Comparison of fluorescent-antibody methods and enrichment serology for the detection of *Salmonella*. *Appl. Microbiol.* **27,** 324–328.

71. Morrison, D. C., and Ryan, J. L. (1979). Bacterial endotoxins and host immune responses. *Adv. Immunol.* **28,** 293–423.

71a. Nardiello, S., Pizzella, T., Russo, M., and Galanti, B. (1984). Serodiagnosis of typhoid fever by enzyme-linked immunosorbent assay determination of anti-*Salmonella typhi* lipopolysaccharide antibodies. *J. Clin. Microbiol.* **20,** 718–721.

72. Neter, E., Gorzynski, E. A., Gine, R. M., Westphal, O., and Luderitz, O. (1956). The enterobacterial hemagglutination test and its diagnostic potentialities. *Can. J. Microbiol.* **2,** 232–244.

73. Ngheim, O., Bagdian, G., and Staub, A. M. (1967). Etudes immunochimiques sur les *Salmonella*. 13. Determination de la structure du poloside specifique d'une *Salmonella* du groupe D_2 (*S. strasbourg*). *Eur. J. Biochem.* **2,** 392–398.

74. Nolan, C. M., Feeley, J. C., White, P. C., Jr., Hambie, E. A., Brown, S. L., and Wong, K. H. (1980). Evaluation of a new assay for Vi antibody in chronic carriers of *Salmonella typhi*. *J. Clin. Microbiol.* **12,** 52–56.

75. Nolan, C. M., LaBorde, E. A., Howell, R. T., and Robbins, J. B. (1980). Identification of *Salmonella typhi* in faecal specimens by an antiserum–agar method. *J. Med. Microbiol.* **13,** 373–377.

76. Nossal, G. J. V., Ada, G. L., and Austen, C. M. (1964). Antigens in immunity. II. Immunogenic properties of flagella, polymerised flagellin and flagellin in the primary response. *Aust. J. Exp. Biol. Med. Sci.* **42,** 283–294.

77. Ochi, A., Hawley, R. G., Hawley, T., Schuloran, M. J., Traunecker, A., Kohler, G., and Hozumi, N. (1983). Functional immunoglobulin M production after transfection of cloned

immunoglobulin heavy and light chain genes into lymphoid cells. *Proc. Natl. Acad. Sci. U.S.A.* **80**, 6351–6355.

78. Olitzki, A. (1972). "Enteric Fevers causing Organisms and Host's Reactions." Karger, Basel.
79. Orskov, I., Orskov, F., Jonn, B., and Jann, K. (1977). Serology, chemistry, and genetics of O and K antigens of *Escherichia coli*. *Bacteriol. Rev.* **41**, 667–710.
79a. Peters, H., Jurs, M., Jann, B., Jann, K., Timmis, K. N., and Bitter-Suermann, D. (1985). Monoclonal antibodies to enterobacterial common antigen and to *Escherichia coli* lipopolysaccharide outer core: Demonstration of an antigenic determinant shared by enterobacterial common antigen and *E. coli* K5 capsular polysaccharide. *Infect. Immun.* **50**, 459–466.
80. Potter, M. (1970). Mouse IgA myeloma proteins that bind polysaccharide antigens of enterobacterial origin. *Fed. Proc., Fed. Am. Soc. Exp. Biol.* **29**, 85–91.
81. Potter, M. (1977). Antigen-binding myeloma proteins of mice. *Adv. Immunol.* **25**, 141–211.
82. Riley, L. W., DiFerdinando, G. T., Jr., DeMelfi, T. M., and Cohen, M. L. (1983). Evaluation of isolated cases of salmonellosis by plasmid profile analysis: Introduction and transmission of a bacterial clone by precooked roast beef. *J. Infect. Dis.* **148**, 12–17.
83. Ristori, C. (1981). Epidemiologia de la fiebre tifoidea en Chile. *Bol. Vigil. Epidemiol. Minist. Salud Chile* **8**, 8–11.
84. Robison, B. J., Pretzman, C. I., and Mattingly, J. A. (1983). Enzyme immunoassay in which a myeloma protein is used for detection of salmonellae. *Appl. Environ. Microbiol.* **45**, 1816–1821.
85. Rockhill, R. C., Rumans, L. W., Lesmana, M., and Dennis, D. T. (1980). Detection of *Salmonella typhi* D, Vi, and d antigens, by slide coagglutination, in urine from patients with typhoid fever. *J. Clin. Microbiol.* **11**, 213–216.
86. Rovis, L., Kabat, E. A., and Potter, M. (1972). Immunochemical studies on a mouse myeloma protein having specific binding affinity for 2-acetamido-2-deoxy-D-mannose. *Carbohydr. Res.* **23**, 223–227.
87. Sanborn, W. R., Lesmana, M., and Edwards, E. A. (1980). Enrichment culture coagglutination test for rapid, low-cost diagnosis of salmonellosis. *J. Clin. Microbiol.* **12**, 151–155.
88. Sanekata, T., Yoshida, Y., and Okada, H. (1981). Detection of rotavirus in faeces by latex agglutination. *J. Immunol. Methods* **41**, 377–385.
89. Shroeder, S. A. (1968). Interpretation of serologic tests for typhoid fever. *J. Am. Med. Assoc.* **270**, 889–840.
90. Sippel, J. E., Mamoy, H. K., Weiss, E., Joseph, S. W., and Beasley, W. J. (1978). Outer membrane protein antigens in an enzyme-linked immunosorbent assay for *Salmonella* enteric fever and meningococcal meningitis. *J. Clin. MIcrobiol.* **7**, 372–378.
91. Sivadasan, K., Kurien, B., and John, T. J. (1984). Rapid diagnosis of typhoid fever by antigen detection. *Lancet* **1**, 134–135.
92. Smit, J., Kamio, Y., and Nikaido, H. (1975). Outer membrane of *Salmonella typhimurium*: Chemical analysis and freeze–fracture studies with lipopolysaccharide mutants. *J. Bacteriol.* **124**, 942–958.
93. Smith, A. M., Miller, J. S., and Whitehead, D. S. (1979). M467: A murine IgA myeloma protein that binds a bacterial protein. I. Recognition of common antigenic determinants on *Salmonella* flagellins. *J. Immunol.* **123**, 1715–1720.
94. Sompolinsky, D., Hertz, J. B., Hoiby, N., Jensen, K., Maneo, B., and Samra, Z. (1980). An antigen common to a wide range of bacteria. *Acta Pathol. Microbiol. Scand. Sect. B* **85B**, 143–149.
95. Sperber, W. H., and Deibel, R. H. (1969). Accelerated procedure for *Salmonella* detection in dried foods and feeds involving only broth cultures and serological reactions. *Appl. Microbiol.* **17**, 533–539.
96. Staub, A. M., and Bagdian, G. (1966). Etudes immunochimiques sur les *Salmonella*. XII.

Analyse immunologuique des facteurs 27_A, 27_B, et 27_D. *Ann. Inst. Pasteur, Paris* **110**, 849–860.

97. Sundararaj, T., Hango, B., and Subramanian, S. (1983). A study of the usefulness of counterimmunoelectrophoresis for the detection of *Salmonella typhi* antigen in the sera of suspected cases of enteric fever. *Trans. R. Soc. Trop. Med. Hyg.* **77**, 194–97.

98. Svenungsson, B., Jorbeck, H., and Lindberg, A. A. (1979). Diagnosis of *Salmonella* infections: Specificity of indirect immunofluorescence for rapid identification of *Salmonella enteritidis* and usefulness of enzyme-linked immunosorbent assay. *J. Infect. Dis.* **140**, 927–936.

99. Svenungsson, B., and Lindberg, A. A. (1978). Synthetic disaccharide–protein antigen for production of specific O2 antiserum for immunofluorescence diagnosis of *Salmonella*. *Acta Pathol. Microbiol. Scand., Sect. B* **36B**, 35–40.

100. Svenungsson, B., and Lindberg, A. A. (1978). Identification of *Salmonella* bacteria by co-agglutination, using antibodies against synthetic disaccharide–protein antigens O2,O4 and O9, absorbed to protein A-containing staphylococci. *Acta Pathol. Microbiol. Scand., Sect. B* **86B**, 283–290.

101. Svenungsson, B., and Lindberg, A. A. (1979). Diagnosis of *Salmonella* bacteria: Antibodies against synthetic *Salmonella* O-antigen 8 for immunofluorescence and co-agglutination using sensitized protein A-containing staphylococci. *Acta Pathol. Microbiol. Scand., Sect. B* **87B**, 29–36.

102. Szewczyk, B., and Taylor, A. (1980). Immunochemical properties of Vi antigen from *Salmonella typhi* Ty2: Presence of 2 antigenic determinants. *Infect. Immun.* **29**, 534–544.

103. Szewczyk, B., and Taylor, A. (1983). Purification and immunochemical properties of *Escherichia coli* B polysaccharide cross-reacting with *Salmonella typhi* Vi antigen: Preliminary evidence for cross-reaction of the polysaccharide with *Escherichia coli* K1 antigen. *Infect. Immun.* **41**, 224–231.

104. Taylor, D. N., Harris, J. R., Barrett, T. J., Hargrett, N. T., Prentzel, J., Valdiviese, C., Palomino, C., Levine, M. M., and Blake, P. A. (1983). Detection of urinary Vi antigen as a diagnostic test for typhoid fever. *J. Clin. Microbiol.* **18**, 872–876.

105. Teng, N. N. H., Calvo-Riera, F., Lam, K. S., and Kaplan, H. S. (1983). Construction of heteromyelomas for human monoclonal antibody production. *In* "Monoclonal Antibodies and Cancer" (B. D. Boss, R. Langman, I. Trowbridge, and R. Dulbecco, eds.), pp. 135–142. Academic Press, Orlando, Florida.

106. Thomason, B. M., and Hebert, O. A. (1974). Evaluation of commercial conjugates for fluorescent antibody detection of salmonellae. *Appl. Microbiol.* **27**, 862–869.

107. Thompson, R. J., and Jackson, A. P. (1984). Cyclic complexes and high avidity antibodies. *Trends Biochem. Sci.* **9**, 1–3.

108. Thorell, J. I., and Johannson, B. G. (1971). Enzymatic iodination of polypeptide with ^{125}I to high specific activity. *Biochim. Biophys. Acta* **251**, 363–369.

109. Tokunaga, H., Tokunaga, M., and Nakae, T. (1979). Characterization of porins from the outer membrane of *Salmonella typhimurium*. *Eur. J. Biochem.* **95**, 433–439.

110. Tsang, R. S. W., and Chau, P. Y. (1981). Serological diagnosis of typhoid fever by counterimmunoelectrophoresis. *Br. Med. J.* No. 282, 1505–1507.

110a. Underwood, P. A. (1985). Practical considerations of the ability of monoclonal antibodies to detect antigenic differences between closely related variants. *J. Immunol. Methods* **85**, 309–323.

111. Watson, S. W., Levin, J., and Novitsky, T. J. (1982). "Progress in Clinical and Biological Research. Vol. 93: Endotoxin and Their Detection with the Limulus Amoebocyte Lysate Test." Alan R. Liss, New York.

112. Weiner, L. M., and Neely, J. (1963). The nature of the antigenic relationship between *Trichinella spiralis* and *Salmonella typhi*. *J. Immunol.* **92**, 908–911.

113. Wetkowski, M. A., Peterson, E. M., and de la Maza, L. M. (1982). Direct testing of blood cultures for detection of streptococcal antigens. *J. Clin. Microbiol.* **16,** 86–91.
114. Wilchek, M., and Bayer, E. A. (1984). The avidin–biotin complex in immunology. *Immunol. Today* **5,** 39–43.
115. Wong, K. H., Feeley, J. C., Northrup, R. S., and Forlines, M. E. (1974). Vi antigen from *Salmonella typhosa* and immunity against typhoid fever. I. Isolation and immunologic properties in animals. *Infect. Immun.* **9,** 348–353.
116. Woodward, T. E., and Woodward, W. E. (1982). A new oral vaccine against typhoid fever. *J. Infect. Dis.* **145,** 289–291.
117. Young, W. W., Portoukalian, J., and Hakomori, S. (1981). Two monoclonal anticarbohydrate antibodies directed to glycosphingolipids with a lacto-*N*-glycosyl Type II chain. *J. Biol. Chem.* **256,** 10967–10972.

3

Monoclonal Antibodies and Immunodetection Methods for *Vibrio cholerae* and *Escherichia coli* Enterotoxins

ANN-MARI SVENNERHOLM, MARIANNE WIKSTRÖM,
LEIF LINDHOLM, AND JAN HOLMGREN

Department of Medical Microbiology
University of Göteborg
Göteborg, Sweden

I. INTRODUCTION

Diarrheal diseases constitute a major health problem in many parts of the world, particularly in developing countries. Children are especially severely afflicted by these diseases, and there are estimates that one-third to one-half of all deaths in children under 5 years old in Asia, Africa, and Latin America are due to diarrhea (24).

77

MONOCLONAL ANTIBODIES
AGAINST BACTERIA
Volume III

Most diarrheal episodes in humans are due to enteric infections by bacteria or viruses. In the youngest age groups (birth to 2 years) enterotoxin-producing bacteria, and in particular enterotoxin-producing *Escherichia coli* (ETEC), are the second most common etiological agent, and after the age of 3 such bacteria are by far the most important enteric pathogens in most parts of the world (32). Recent epidemiological studies suggest that ETEC is responsible for up to 25% of acute diarrheas in children in the developing world and for about 50 to 70% of diarrheas affecting travelers in these countries (24). ETEC infection is also a common cause of diarrhea in animal husbandry, with a high proportion of newborn piglets and calves experiencing fatal diarrhea during the first weeks of life (26). The enterotoxin-producing bacteria, which include *Vibrio cholerae*, ETEC, and several other gram-negative organisms such as *Aeromonas, Klebsiella, Serratia, and Yersinia* (43), may give rise to diarrheal disease with symptoms varying from a few episodes of watery stools to, in the most severe cases, fatal dehydration. The enterotoxins formed by human as well as animal pathogens may either be heat-labile (LT) or heat-stable (ST), and in many instances both types of toxins may be produced by a single strain (32).

There is at present a great need for sensitive and specific methods to allow rapid identification of disease caused by enterotoxin-producing bacteria, particularly in less well-equipped laboratories or in the field. Since most enterotoxin-producing bacteria cannot be differentiated from normal inhabitants of the intestinal flora by conventional bacterial isolation procedures, these methods have to be based on identification of enterotoxins produced by fecal cultures or demonstration of preformed toxin in stool. To permit differentiation of the immunologically cross-reactive enterotoxins (3,5,19), such methods have to depend on the initial isolation and identification of the causative agent before enterotoxin testing or on the specific demonstration of the toxin produced by using immunoreagents directed against unshared enterotoxin antigen determinants. The hybridoma technology which permits production of unlimited quantities of monoclonal antibodies (MAbs) with high specificity for bacterial enterotoxins offers unique possibilities for the development of such specific and sensitive immunodetection methods.

In this review we describe the production and characterization of MAbs against different heat-labile enterotoxins and the development of immunodiagnostic methods based on utilization of MAbs directed against shared as well as unique enterotoxin epitopes.

II. BACKGROUND

Cholera is the prototype for the enterotoxic enteropathies, that is diarrheal diseases caused by bacteria producing exoenterotoxins. These enterotoxins may induce fluid and electrolyte secretion in the small intestine, which in the most severe cases results in copious diarrhea and lethal dehydration. The causative agent of cholera, *Vibrio cholerae,* produces a potent enterotoxin, cholera toxin (CT), which has structural, functional, and immunological similarities to the heat-labile enterotoxin (LT) produced by ETEC (16). Both CT and LT consist of two types of subunits, and each toxin contains one A and five B subunits (3,16). By means of amino acid sequence studies it has been shown that both subunits of each toxin have varying degrees of homology in their primary structure (5,45). The B subunits are responsible for binding the toxin molecules to specific receptors on the surface of the intestinal mucosal cells; the ganglioside GM1 has been shown to be the receptor for CT (16), and, probably, this ganglioside together with structurally related glycoprotein(s), also function as receptors for LT (17). The A subunit of each toxin, on the other hand, has enzymatic activity and activates intracellular adenylate cyclase, resulting in increased levels of cyclic AMP (16). Immunologically, LT and CT have both shared and unique antigenic determinants which extend to both the A and B subunits (3,19,21). Slight differences have been observed in the amino acid composition between LTs synthesized by human and porcine ETEC isolates, although in general their primary structural homology is extensive; 98% of the amino acids of the B subunits of human LT (LT_h) and porcine LT (LT_p) are identical (42,45).

In addition to, or instead of producing LT, ETEC bacteria may produce ST. This toxin is a small hormonelike and ordinarily nonimmunogenic contiguous polypeptide chain with a molecular weight of less than 5000 (30). Two classes of *E. coli* STs have been described: STa, which is active in infant mice and is elaborated from ETEC strains of human and porcine origin, and STb, which is active in pig loops and is produced by porcine *E. coli* only (1). DNA hybridization tests provide evidence for slight molecular heterogeneity among STas, and two different STas (STaI and STaII) are produced by human *E. coli* isolates and only differ in a few amino acids (27,33). At variance with *E. coli* LT, ST exerts its effect by stimulating guanylate cyclase, and it also binds to receptors unrelated to those for LT (30). Furthermore, ST is not immunogenic unless coupled to a carrier molecule or cross-linked (11).

A number of diagnostic methods for the demonstration of LTs have been described. Initially methods that either required animals [ileal loops (6), rabbit skin (4)] or tissue culture cells [adrenal cells (8), Chinese hamster ovary cells (12)] were employed. These methods were later complemented by, or even overtaken by, immunoassays [enzyme-linked immunosorbent assay, ELISA (46), GM1-ELISA (35), ELEC test (20), or DNA hybridization (27) tests].

Due to problems in purifying *E. coli* LT in great quantities, immunodiagnostic methods for the demonstration of this toxin have been based either on antisera raised against crude LT (35,45) or against purified CT (31). In general, these anti-LT antisera have proved to be reliable for detection of LT when used in conjunction with GM1-ganglioside, which specifically binds the LT before the immunodetection step (GM1-ELISA) (31,35,38). The anti-CT antisera, on the other hand, have tended to detect LT (in contrast to CT), with insufficient sensitivity to demonstrate LT production in many *E. coli* isolates. Neither type of antiserum has permitted differentiation between LTs produced by different bacterial species or between cholera toxin and *E. coli* LT.

Demonstration of STs has until very recently been entirely dependent on an animal model, the infant mouse assay (10). However, simple immunodetection methods based on MAbs against ST are now available. (36,40).

The ideal method for the demonstration of enterotoxins in the field should be sensitive, specific, simple, and rapid. Furthermore, it should be based on stable, readily available, and inexpensive reagents, and it should be possible to read the results without any complicated equipment. Although many of the immunoassays hitherto described have fulfilled these criteria, they have not been entirely based on commercially available reagents and they have not permitted differentiation of enterotoxins produced by different bacterial species. By utilizing MAbs, which have unique uniformity and specificity, in the immunodetection step, diagnostic methods which seem to fulfill the criteria of being ideal tools for enterotoxin demonstration have also been developed in less well-equipped laboratories.

III. RESULTS AND DISCUSSION

A. Production of Monoclonal Antibodies (MAbs)

Inbred 8 to 14-week-old BALB/c mice of either sex were immunized with purified CT (Schwartz-Mann, Orangeburg, Pennsylvania), LT_h purified according to the procedure described by Tayot *et al.* (39) for the purification of CT, or purified LT_p (14) by different immunization schedules (Table I). Three to four days after the last immunization the animals were killed and spleen cell suspensions were prepared. Hybridomas were then produced according to De St. Groth and Scheidegger (7), fusing exponentially growing Sp2/0 myeloma cells with spleen cells from the immunized mice with the aid of polyethylene glycol. Stable hybrid cell lines were selected with hypoxanthine–aminopterine–thymidine medium, and 10–14 days after fusion culture fluids were tested for the presence of antitoxin antibodies by means of ELISA (18) or GM1-ELISA methods (35). Specific antitoxin-producing hybrids were cloned and expanded, and culture fluid from established antitoxin-secreting clones was harvested and frozen in aliquots at −30°C until further testing.

TABLE I

Immunization Schemes Employed for Production of MAbs against *Vibrio cholerae* and *Escherichia coli* Enterotoxins

Immunogen	Number of immunizations	Immunization scheme		
		Interval (weeks)	Route	Dose (μg)
CT[a]	6	2–3	iv	1 + 2.5 + 5 + 5 + 10 + 10
CT	6	1–3	ip + iv	2 + 2 + 2 + 2 + 2 + 2
LT$_h$[b]	4	2, 2, and 5	ip + iv	2 + 2 + 1 + 2.5
LT$_h$	2	4	ip + iv	2 + 2
LT$_p$[c]	4	7, 2, and 2	ip + iv	2 + 1 + 1 + 1

[a] Purified cholera toxin, Schwarz-Mann, Orangeburg, Pa.

[b] Purified human LT prepared from *E. coli* strain 286 C2 of human origin by a sequence of affinity chromatography of crude LT on GM1-cellulose and gel filtration on a Sephacryl column (39).

[c] Purified porcine LT kindly obtained from Dr. T. R. Hirst, and purified by him from an *E. coli* strain carrying a plasmid coding for porcine LT (14).

Since initial experiments showed that immunization by the intravenous (iv) route resulted in lower percentages of antitoxin-producing cell hybrids (~5% of the hybrids tested were antitoxin-producing) than a sequence from intraperitoneal (ip) and iv antigen administrations (25–35% of tested hybrids were antitoxin-producing), a sequence of ip and iv immunizations was chosen in all subsequent experiments. Only hybridomas which after expansion and cloning continued to produce good amounts of antitoxin antibodies were further characterized with regard to their MAb product. Seventy hybridomas from four cell fusion experiments, using lymphocytes from mice receiving CT by one of two immunization schedules (Table I), 24 hybridomas from two cell fusions using cells from mice receiving LT$_h$ in two or four injections, and 20 hybridomas from one cell fusion with lymphocytes from mice given three immunizations with LT$_p$ were thus selected for further studies.

B. Isotype

By means of single radial immunodiffusion (SRID;23), using isotype-specific antisera for mouse immunoglobulin (IgM, IgA, IgG$_1$, IgG$_{2a}$, IgG$_{2b}$; Meloy Laboratories Inc., Springfield, Virginia and IgG$_3$; Sigma, St. Louis, Missouri), it was found that most of the antitoxin-producing clones obtained after immunization with either CT, LT$_h$, or LT$_p$ produced antibodies of IgG$_1$ class (Table II) (22,37). Immunization with CT also frequently gave rise to MAbs of IgG$_2$ type,

TABLE II

Isotypes of Monoclonal Antienterotoxin Antibodies

MAb specificity	Total number	Number with isotype specificity				
		IgG_1	IgG_2	IgG_3	IgA	IgM
CT	70	39	29	2	0	0
LT_h	24	19	1	0	0	4
LP_p	20	15	0	0	1	4

but only one such MAb was found after immunization with the two LT preparations. Whereas the anti-CT MAbs were restricted to the IgG class, some IgA-
and IgM-producing clones were also induced by immunization with LT_h or LT_p
(Table II). The isotype of the MAbs was also determined with a specific-antibody
ELISA (22), using isotype-specific antisera for mouse Ig in the immunodetection
step. These antisera were used in dilutions chosen to suppress their weak cross-
reactivity with other isotypes. Results from these ELISA tests were confirmed by
those obtained with SRID testing of the hybridoma culture medium in isotype-
specific antiserum-containing agar (22). The isotype distribution of the MAbs
obtained differed markedly from that of the original immunized mouse spleen
cells used for fusion with myeloma cells. In the CT-immunized mice, 26% of the
spleen cells produced IgM and 27% produced IgA antitoxin, as studied by a
plaque-forming cell assay (22). This selection of IgG-secreting clones may be
due to the fact that only spleen cells of hyperimmunized mice were used for the
hybridization experiments. In contrast, Remmers et al. (28) found that cell
hybrids obtained after immunization with a single dose of CT produced MAbs
that were only of the IgM class. Furthermore, our own data show that immunization with LT, which was given in two to four doses, resulted in a higher proportion of MAbs of IgM class than the six-dose immunization regimen with CT.

C. Subunit Specificity

The GM1-ELISA method (15,19,35), in which either holotoxin, containing
both A and B subunit, or isolated B subunits were attached to plastic-adsorbed
GM1-ganglioside was used to study the subunit specificity of the antienterotoxin
MAbs. Of the 70 anti-CT-producing hybrids tested, as many as 61 produced
MAbs that reacted equally well with GM1-bound holotoxin and with B subunit,
suggesting that they were specific for the B-subunit complex of the CT molecule.
The remaining 9 clones produced antibodies that bound to CT but not to isolated
B subunit, suggesting that they might be directed against the A-subunit portion of
the molecule. This was confirmed by ELISA titrations against purified cholera A
subunit (List Laboratories, Campbell, California), in which the 9 MAbs that did

not bind to GM1-attached B subunit reacted strongly with solid-phase bound A subunit even after absorption with high concentrations of purified B subunit (22). These subunit specificities were in all cases supported by ELISA inhibition tests: the 9 MAbs reacting with A subunit in the ELISA were all completely inhibited from reacting with the solid-phase CT by preincubation with high concentrations (30 μg/ml) of CT but not with corresponding concentrations of purified cholera B subunit, whereas the B subunit-reactive MAbs were inhibited by both these proteins. The formation of a considerably large number of MAbs with specificity for the B rather than the A subunit of CT supports the notion of a greater immunogenicity of the B as compared to the A portion of the toxin molecule (34). The 7:1 ratio of anti-B- to anti-A-producing MAbs in the present study corresponds to the considerably higher titers of anti-B than anti-A subunit antibodies seen both in sera from CT-immunized rabbits (34) and in human sera after experimental cholera infection (36).

By comparing the binding of the anti-LT_h MAbs to LT_h and corresponding B subunits attached to plastic-absorbed GM1-ganglioside, the subunit specificity of these MAbs was also studied. It was found that all of the 24 LT_h MAbs tested reacted equally well with the isolated B subunits as with the holotoxin, implying that all of the LT_h MAbs were directed against the B-subunit molecule (Table III) (37). In subsequent studies, an intensified search for hybridomas producing antibodies specific for the A subunit of LT_h was undertaken. Tissue culture fluids from all hybrids obtained in four different cell fusion experiments were screened for reactivity with LT_h holotoxin and isolated B subunit. In more than 2000 culture fluids tested from 34 stable cell hybrids, antibodies that reacted with GM1-bound holotoxin but not with corresponding B subunit were not found. One possible explanation for this failure to induce MAbs against the A subunit may be that this portion of the LT_h molecule had been subjected to partial degradation or loss during storage at −70°C. Shortly after purification the LT_h preparation used contained both A and B subunits as studied with GM1-ELISA

TABLE III

Subunit Specificity of MAbs against CT, LT_h, and LT_p

Immunogen	Experiment	Number of immunizations	Subunit B	Subunit A
CT	1	6	61	9
LT_h	1	4	17	0
	2	2	7	0
	3[a]	4	34	0
LT_p	1	4	9	11

[a] Four cell fusions.

and had almost the same biological activity in rabbit loops (6) and in rabbit skin tests (4) as corresponding amounts of purified CT. However, these analyses of LT_h were not repeated immediately before the mouse immunizations performed 1–2 years later.

With regard to the LT_p MAbs, 11 of 20 reacted with GM1-coupled holotoxin but not with the corresponding isolated B subunits, suggesting that they were specific for the A-subunit portion of LT_p or, perhaps directed against conformational A-attachment induced "novel" epitopes in the B subunit. By testing the 11 non-B-reactive LT_p MAbs for subunit specificity by means of the Western blot technique (41), the A-subunit specificity could be verified in each case (Table III).

D. Immunological Cross-Reactivity

Cross-reactions of the monoclonal antienterotoxin antibodies with heterologous LT enterotoxins were studied by the GM1-ELISA method in which the reactivity of the anti-CT MAbs with corresponding concentrations of GM1-attached CT and LT_h and of the anti-LT MAbs with GM1-bound CT, LT_h, and LT_p was compared. In these experiments, 0.5 μg/ml of either toxin was attached to polystyrene-adsorbed GM1-ganglioside and each MAb tested was diluted 1 : 2 in parallel against the different toxins. Based on the absorbance readings, the anti-CT MAbs were categorized as being fully cross-reactive with LT, partly cross-reactive (reacting stronger with CT than LT_h), or CT-specific, and the anti-LT MAbs in an analogous manner were categorized as reacting with each of the three toxins, cross-reacting with one of the heterologous toxins, or reacting exclusively with the homologous toxin. In addition, most of the anti-LT MAbs were titrated in parallel against the three toxins and the end point titer was determined, that is, the interpolated dilution of the MAbs giving an absorbance value at 450 nm of 0.2 above the background level when reacting the enzyme with its substrate for 20 min.

These experiments showed that as many as 63% of the anti-CT MAbs were of the cholera type only, 17% reacted more strongly with CT than with LT_h, and only 20% were fully cross-reactive, that is, gave similar reactions with GM1-absorbed CT and LT (22). This pattern differed somewhat for the MAbs produced against the LT_h; in this case as many as 13 of 25 (55%) reacted with all three enterotoxins, whereas only 7 of 25 (28%) reacted with the homologous toxin only (Table IV; 37). Similarly, 5 of 20 (25%) of the MAbs against LT_p reacted with LT_p only. However, very few of the MAbs raised against LT_p cross reacted with CT (10%), the remaining 13 MAbs reacting with LT_p and LT_h (Table IV).

Parallel titration of the anti-LT_h MAbs against the three toxins showed that most (15 of 25) of these MAbs reacted equally well with the two LT toxins; that

TABLE IV

Reactivity of Monoclonal Anti-LT Antibodies with Shared and Specific LT Epitopes

	MAbs against	
Reactivity	LT_h ($n = 25$)	LT_p ($n = 20$)
LT_h, LT_p, CT	13	2
LT_h, LT_p	4	13
LT_h, CT	1	0
LT_p, CT	0	0
LT_h	7	0
LT_p	0	5

is, they had similar GM1-ELISA titer against LT_h and LT_p when tested in alternate wells on the same day (Fig. 1; 37). Although as many as 13 of the 25 anti-LT_h MAbs cross-reacted with CT in initial experiments, only 8 of them had about the same antibody titer against CT as against LT_h. Similarly, as many as half (9 of 18) of the anti-LT_p MAbs had the same titer against the two LT toxins, whereas only one of them reacted equally well with CT and LT_p (Fig. 2). By means of immunodiffusion analyses the presence of unique as well as shared determinants on LT and CT relating to both types of subunits has been demon-

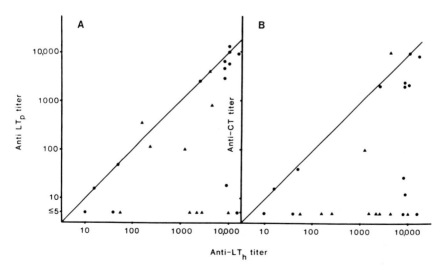

Fig. 1. Comparison of GM1-ELISA antitoxin titers against LT_h and LT_p (A) and against LT_h and CT (B) of monoclonal anti-LT_h antibodies; four immunizations with LT_h (●); two immunizations with LT_h (▲).

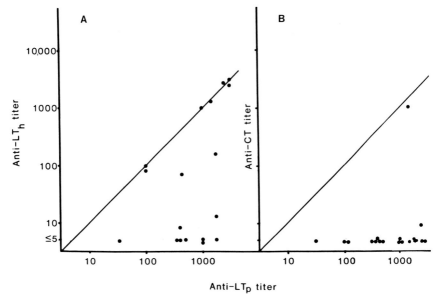

Fig. 2. Comparison of GM1-ELISA antitoxin titers against LT_p and LT_h (A) and against LT_p and CT (B) of monoclonal anti-LT_p antibodies.

strated (2,44). Separation of cross-reactive from non-cross-reactive antitoxin has also been reported (21). By means of the hybridoma technology, the degree and nature of the immunological cross-reactivity between CT and *E. coli* LTs could be further elucidated. Our results, showing that most of the anti-CT B MAbs did not cross-react with *E. coli* LT, indicate a substantial conformational difference between the two toxins despite a very close amino acid sequence homology between their B subunits, with 83 of 103 residues being identical (5). However, the finding of relatively fewer MAbs against unique determinants by immunization with LT_h or LT_p than with CT is in agreement with previous studies showing that the species-specific determinants on cholera B subunit are relatively stronger immunogens than those of LT B (3,13,19).

E. Neutralizing Capacity

The capacity of the different MAbs to neutralize active toxin was evaluated by the rabbit skin test (4). Undiluted or fivefold serial dilutions of antitoxin-containing culture medium in phosphate-buffered saline (PBS) supplemented with 0.1% bovine serum albumin (BSA), were mixed with an equal volume of CT (20 ng/ml), LT_h (60 ng/ml), or LT_p (50 ng/ml), and after incubation at room temperature for 60 min the mixtures (0.1 ml) were injected intracutaneously and studied for toxic activity. The neutralizing titer of the different MAbs was determined as the interpolated dilution giving a blueing zone of 4 mm in diameter; the toxin concentrations used for the neutralization studies gave a blueing zone of 8 to 10 mm when injected in non-antibody-containing medium.

All but 1 of 25 studied anti-CT MAbs that were specific for the B-subunit portion had detectable and usually strong CT-neutralizing activity (Fig. 3). The anti-CT MAbs with specificity for the A-subunit portion, on the other hand, all lacked significant toxin-neutralizing capacity even after fivefold concentration of the tissue culture fluids (22). The neutralizing capacities of the different B subunit-reactive MAbs varied considerably in relation to their immunoglobulin contents, and there was no statistically significant correlation with the corresponding ELISA titer against purified CT (Fig. 3).

Most (17 of 20) of the anti-LT_h MAbs, all of which had specificity for the B-subunit portion of the molecule, were also effective in neutralizing the homologous toxin. At variance with the anti-CT MAbs, there was a highly significant correlation ($p < .01$) between the toxin-neutralizing titer and the corresponding GM1-ELISA titer (Fig. 4; 37). Similarly, the anti-LT_p MAbs were effective in

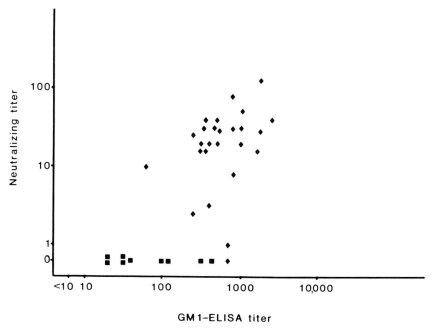

GM1–ELISA titer

Fig. 3.   Specific CT-neutralizing activity (neutralizing titer per SRID unit of immunoglobulin) of monoclonal anti-cholera A subunit (■) and anti-cholera B subunit (♦) antibodies in relation to the specific antigen-binding capacity (ELISA titer per SRID unit of Ig).

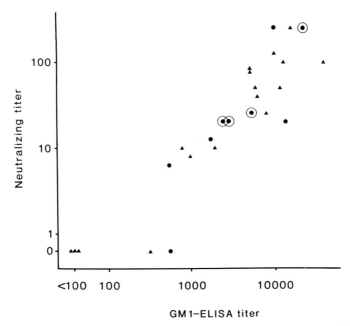

Fig. 4.   *E. coli* LT-neutralizing activity of monoclonal anti-LT$_h$ (●) and anti-LT$_p$ (▲) antibodies in relation to the GM1-ELISA titer against the homologous toxin.

neutralizing the homologous toxin in proportion to their GM1-ELISA titer, and these MAbs were effective irrespective of whether they were directed against the A- or the B-subunit portion of the toxin molecule.

Antibodies of IgG$_1$ and IgG$_2$ isotypes did not differ with regard to neutralizing capacity in any of the three toxin-neutralizing systems tested. MAbs of IgM and IgA isotypes were produced in too low concentrations to be detectable in the neutralizing systems studied.

F. Identification of Enterotoxin-Producing Bacteria

The usefulness of anti-enterotoxin MAbs in the immunodetection step for demonstration of heat-labile enterotoxins (CT, LT$_h$, and LT$_p$) by diagnostic GM1-ELISA methods (35,38) was evaluated. Eighty-two *E. coli* strains isolated from humans with diarrhea (33 representing LT only or LT plus ST, 21 ST only, and 28 non-enterotoxin-producing strains), kindly provided by Dr. Y Takeda, Japan, and 18 *E. coli* strains isolated from piglets with diarrhea (11 LT/ST and 7 ST only), kindly provided by Dr. J. J. Morris, Weybridge, United Kingdom, were studied for enterotoxin production. In addition, 28 *V. cholerae* 01 strains representing Inaba as well as Ogawa serotypes, and the classical and El Tor biotypes, provided by Dr. H. Smith, Philadelphia, or by Dr. I. Huq, ICDDR,B, Dhaka, Bangladesh, were studied. All strains were cultured in CAYE medium (9) with shaking at 37°C overnight, and after continued incubation with polymyxin B for 45 min (38), the supernates of the cultures were analyzed for enterotoxin content by the GM1-ELISA using MAbs with different specificities.

In initial experiments the culture supernates were analyzed according to the rapid GM1-ELISA procedure previously described (38), except that a MAb with specificity for CT, LT_h, as well as LT_p diluted 1:25 was used in the immunodetection step and anti-mouse immunoglobulin coupled to horseradish peroxidase (Dakopatts, Copenhagen, Denmark) diluted 1:300 was used as the enzyme conjugate. In all instances, human as well as porcine *E. coli* strains previously shown to produce LT alone or in combination with ST were positive in the GM1-ELISA (Table V). Thus, all the LT producing strains gave a color reaction which was considerably stronger than that read visually in the negative-control wells, and gave an absorbance value that was significantly higher (i.e., A 450 nm ≥ 0.1) (38), than that registered in the negative controls. In no instance were cultures of the ST-only or nonenterotoxigenic human or porcine *E. coli* strains read as positive either by eye or spectrophotometrically (Table V). With regard to the *V. cholerae* strains, 26 of 28 were read as positive using the broadly cross-reactive enterotoxin MAb (Table V). When testing the two cultures that were negative in the GM1-ELISA by alternate methods, such as the ileal loop test (6), the intradermal toxicity test (4), and adrenal cells (8), they were all negative, suggesting loss of toxin-producing capacity or at least poor or absent toxin production in the actual cultures.

TABLE V

Enterotoxin Detection in *Vibrio cholerae* and *Escherichia coli* Cultures by GM1-ELISA Using MAbs against Shared and Unique Epitopes on CT, Human LT, and Porcine LT, Respectively, in the Immunodetection Step

Culture	n	Number of enterotoxin-positive cultures with MAb of indicated reactivity			
		CT, LT_h, LT_p	CT	LT_h	LT_p
V. cholerae	28	26	26	0	0
E. coli, human isolates					
LT + ST or LT only	33	33	0	33	0
ST only	21	0	0	0	0
non-LT/non-ST	28	0	0	0	0
E. coli, porcine isolates					
LT + ST	11	11	NT[a]	0	11
ST only	7	0	NT	0	0

[a] NT, Not tested.

The different cultures were also analyzed using species-specific MAbs in the immunodetection step. When using a MAb with strong reactivity with LT_h but no binding capacity either to LT_p or CT, all human *E. coli* isolates that had previously been found to produce LT or LT + ST were positive, whereas none of the porcine *E. coli* strains, the *V. cholerae* cultures, or any of the ST-only or non-enterotoxin-producing human *E. coli* isolates were positive (Table V).

Similarly, all the *V. cholerae* cultures that were positive when using the MAb reacting with shared enterotoxin epitopes were positive when using a MAb against unique CT epitopes, and all the LT-producing porcine *E. coli* isolates were positive when using a MAb with specificity for LT_p (Table V). In no instance did the toxin-specific MAbs show a positive reaction in the GM1-ELISA with cultures of strains producing heterologous toxins (Table V).

G. Direct-Culture MAb-GM1-ELISA

Based on the report by Ristaino *et al.* (29) describing the possibility of culturing strains for enterotoxin production directly in GM1-coated wells, we evaluated whether this simplified approach would improve the previously described MAb-GM1-ELISA. In initial experiments, we found that the procedure of culturing the strains directly in the GM1-coated plates not only simplified the diagnostic procedure but also resulted in increased sensitivity of the GM1-ELISA. After slight modifications of the culture procedure recommended by Ristaino *et al* (29), a MAb-GM1-ELISA procedure has been developed which permits species-specific demonstration of enterotoxin production within 24 hr after arrival of the clinical specimen. The detailed procedure is presented in Table VI.

On comparing the results of a number of LT-positive and LT-negative human and porcine *E. coli* isolates analyzed by the conventional and direct-culture MAb-GM1-ELISA, it was found that the latter procedure resulted in considerably stronger toxin reactions without any loss in specificity (Fig. 5). Preliminary studies have suggested that this procedure can also be used for demonstrating enterotoxin production using stool specimens rather than fecal isolates as inoculum in the GM1-coated wells.

Due to its relative simplicity, rapidity, dependence on stable and commercially available reagents only (except for the MAbs), and the possibility of reading results by eye, the MAb-GM1-ELISA methodology is not only suitable for use in conventional microbiological diagnostic laboratories but may also be used in less well-equipped laboratories and in the field.

Since prompt diagnosis, particularly of the more severe forms of enterotoxin-induced diarrheas, is desirable and may be vital, different approaches to speed up the demonstration of enterotoxin production even further should be evaluated. One obvious possibility is to analyze preformed enterotoxin in stool directly from

TABLE VI

**Rapid GM1-ELISA Procedure for Detection of Enterotoxin from
Cultures of Bacterial Isolates or Stool Specimens in
GM1-Coated Plates**

1. ELISA microtiter plates (Dynatech, Plochingen, West Germany or Nunc, Roskilde, Denmark) are coated with GM1-ganglioside (Supelco, Bellefonte, Pennsylvania), 2 μg/ml, at 37°C for 4 hr or at room temperature, $\cong 22$°C, overnight, 0.1 ml per well (plates could be stored at 4°C for at least 14 days).
2. Plates are washed twice with phosphate-buffered saline (PBS).
3. Plates are incubated with PBS containing 1% bovine serum albumin (BSA; Sigma, St. Louis, Missouri) at 37°C, 30 min, 0.2 ml per well.
4. Plates are washed twice with PBS.
5. Half a loopful of bacteria from an agar plate or 0.1 ml of fecal specimen is diluted in 1 ml of Casamino acid–yeast extract medium (9) containing 2.5 mg glucose + 45 μg lincomycin per milliliter. Then, 200 μl of each suspension is transferred to a GM1-coated and BSA-blocked well, and the plate is incubated, preferably on a shaker or a roller drum (200 rpm), at 37°C overnight.
6. Plates are washed three times with PBS containing 0.05% Tween 20.
7. Mouse anti-LT MAb diluted in PBS–Tween containing 0.1% BSA (antibody concentration is based on checkerboard titrations of antibody and toxin) is added and plates incubated at room temperature for 1 hr, 0.1 ml per well.
8. Plates are washed three times with PBS–Tween.
9. Plates are incubated with anti-mouse Ig conjugated with horseradish peroxidase (Dakopatts, Copenhagen, Denmark) diluted in PBS–Tween containing 0.1% BSA (conjugates are diluted according to results of checkerboard titrations, usually 1:250) at room temperature for 2 hr, 0.1 ml per well.
10. Plates are washed three times with PBS–Tween.
11. The chromogen *p*-phenylenediamine (PPD, Sigma) or *o*-phenylenediamine (OPD, Sigma) is diluted in citrate buffer, pH 4.5, to a final concentration of 1 mg/ml and H_2O_2 is added to 0.01% final concentration immediately before adding the substrate. Incubate at room temperature for 20 min, 0.1 ml per well.
12. The plates are read visually: brown or light-brown color reaction (PPD), or orange or yellow (OPD), suggests a positive reaction; compare with negative medium control and positive LT-producing strain or spectrophotometrically at 450 nm (an absorbance value of ≥ 0.1 above background indicates a positive reaction).

patients with watery diarrhea. By this approach, lengthy incubations for out-growth and toxin production of bacteria can be avoided.

By the access to species-specific antibodies in the immunodetection step, the MAb-GM1-ELISA may not only permit demonstration of heat-labile enterotoxin in stool but also of the origin of the toxin produced. In a preliminary study, a number of stool specimens collected from cholera patients and patients with mild to moderate ETEC-induced diarrhea at the cholera hospital of the ICDDR,B in Dhaka (kindly supplied by Dr. M. Jertborn, Göteborg, or by Dr. I. Huq, ICD-DR,B Dhaka) were analyzed for enterotoxin content by the MAb-GM1-ELISA

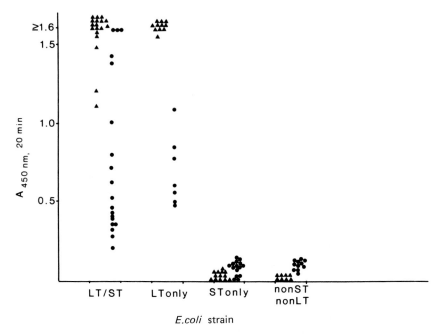

Fig. 5. GM1-ELISA activity of human and porcine fecal *E. coli* isolates, representing LT+ST (LT/ST), LT only, ST only, and non-ST, non-LT strains, after initial preparation of culture filtrates and measurement of enterotoxin in the supernates (●) and as determined after culture of the strain directly in GM1-coated ELISA plates (▲).

procedure. Immediately after collection the specimens were put on ice and brought to Sweden in a container kept at 0° to 4°C. All specimens were analyzed for enterotoxin content within 5 days of isolation. Despite this long delay of 3 to 5 days before analyses, as many as 13 of 17 stools from cholera patients were positive in the GM1-ELISA without prior culture of the stools when a CT-specific MAb was used in the immunodetection step. Similarly, LT could be demonstrated directly in 15 of 18 stools from patients with ETEC-induced diarrhea when a MAb with specificity for LT_h unique epitopes was used. This sensitivity of the MAb-GM1-ELISA is comparable to that found by Merson *et al.* (25) analyzing LT and CT in the stool of patients with moderate to severe cholera, or ETEC-induced diarrhea by the adrenal cell assay (8), or the ELISA method using anti-CT antibodies as catching antibody (45).

IV. CONCLUSIONS AND PROSPECTS FOR THE FUTURE

The results presented with MAbs against CT, *E. coli* LT_h, and *E. coli* LT_p have yielded new and more detailed insight into the nature and degree of immunological cross-reactivity between these enterotoxins. A general conclusion is that even though these toxins all cross-react to a significant extent, the degree of immunological cross-reactivity between them is less than would be predicted from their strikingly similar amino acid sequences, indicating that even a few nonhomologous residues can yield distinct strong conformational antigenic determinants. Indeed, the majority of the MAbs against CT which were directed against the B subunit did not cross-react with the LT B subunit despite 80% primary structural homology in the subunits (5,45). Conversely, only a few of the MAbs against LT_p cross-reacted with CT, although the majority of them reacted well with LT of human as well as the porcine type. Most strikingly, 25% of the MAbs against both LT_p and LT_h were entirely specific for the homologous type of LT, even though their B subunits differ from each other in only 4 of 103 amino acids (42).

The examinations performed on the neutralizing capacity of the various MAbs revealed some interesting differences between CT and the *E. coli* LTs. In the case of anti-CT MAbs, only those reacting with the B subunit had any significant neutralizing activity, whereas MAbs against the A subunits of *E. coli* LT could neutralize the LT enterotoxicity. Furthermore, among the anti-B MAbs those raised against *E. coli* LT neutralized the homologous enterotoxin in direct proportion to their titer in *in vitro* binding assays (GM1-ELISA), while MAbs against the B subunit of CT behaved with greater variability in regard to neutralizing capacity in relation to their GM1-ELISA titer. Nonetheless, virtually all MAbs reacting with B subunits of either CT or *E. coli* LTs had detectable neutralizing activity on their homologous enterotoxin despite apparent reactivity with different intrasubunit epitopes. Studies are in progress to determine whether all of these neutralizing anti-B-subunit MAbs interfere with the ability of the enterotoxins to bind to GM1-ganglioside and also whether the different intrasubunit epitopes are located to allow simultaneous binding and cooperative neutralization of two or more MAbs.

The practical goal, to identify antitoxin MAbs that were either completely specific for CT, LT_h, or LT_p, or were fully cross-reactive for all of these toxins, was fulfilled, as was the additional goal to develop simple yet sensitive and specific immunodiagnostic methods for toxin detection based on these MAbs. With almost 100% sensitivity and specificity it was possible to detect all forms of enterotoxin using a fully cross-reactive MAb, as well as to detect only the homologous enterotoxin by using species-specific MAbs in GM1-ELISA procedures. These procedures functioned well irrespective of whether they were performed on culture media from clinical isolates or from these isolates, or even from an unfractionated stool cultured directly in the GM1-coated ELISA wells. The "optimal test conditions" are described in this article. Furthermore, in preliminary experiments these MAb-based GM1-ELISA methods yielded results that also promise to be useful for sensitive toxin detection as well as for differentiation between different heat-labile enterotoxins directly in stool specimens from patients with diarrheal disease.

V. SUMMARY

Monoclonal antibodies (MAbs) against cholera toxin (CT) and E. coli heat-labile enterotoxin (LT) of human (LT_h) and porcine (LT_p) origin have been prepared. Most of the MAbs produced were directed against the B-subunit portion of the toxin molecules and were of the IgG_1 or IgG_2 isotypes. Both MAbs against the B-subunit portion of the CT and LT had toxin-neutralizing capacity, whereas none of 9 MAbs against the cholera A subunit had any detectable neutralizing ability. Of 70 anti-CT MAbs, no less than 44 reacted specifically with CT, the remaining ones showing full or partial cross-reactivity with LTs. Seven of the 25 MAbs against LT_h reacted only with LT_h (not with LT_p or CT), and 5 of 20 MAbs against LT_p were LT_p-specific. One MAb that showed full cross-reactivity between CT, LT_h, and LT_p and one MAb that was specific for each of these toxins were exploited for development of "diagnostic" LT detection methods based on the GM1-ELISA principle. These methods fulfilled the criteria of excellent sensitivity and specificity for the detection of "any" heat-labile toxin using the cross-reactive MAb, or for the detection of species-specific toxin using the "unique epitope" MAbs. By these methods, heat-labile enterotoxins could be demonstrated in overnight cultures of fecal isolates; the sensitivity of the methods could be further increased by inoculation of bacterial isolates or stools directly in GM1-coated microtiter plates.

ACKNOWLEDGMENTS

Financial support was obtained from the Swedish Agency for Research Cooperation with Developing Countries (SAREC), and the Swedish Medical Research Council.

The skilled technical assistance of Ms. Gudrun Wiklund, Ulla Karlsson, and Gun Lindholm is gratefully acknowledged.

REFERENCES

1. Burgess, M. M., Bywater, R. J., Cowley, C. M., Mullan, M. A., and Newsone, P. N. (1978). Biological evaluation of a methanol soluble, heat-stable *Escherichia coli* enterotoxin in infant mice, pigs, rabbits and calves. *Infect. Immun.* **21,** 526–531.
2. Clements, J. D., and Finkelstein, R. A. (1978). Immunological cross–reactivity between heat-labile enterotoxin(s) of *Escherichia coli* and subunits of *Vibrio cholerae* enterotoxin. *Infect. Immun.* **21,** 1036–1039.

3. Clements, J. D., and Finkelstein, R. A. (1978). Demonstration of shared and unique immunological determinants in enterotoxins from *Vibrio cholerae* and *Escherichia coli*. *Infect. Immun.*
   22, 709–713.
4. Craig, J. P. (1965). A permeability factor (toxin) found in cholera stools and culture filtrates and
   its neutralization by convalescent cholera sera. *Nature (London)* **207**, 614–616.
5. Dallas, W. S., and Falkow, S. (1980). Aminoacid sequence homology between cholera toxin
   and *Escherichia coli* heat-labile toxin. *Nature (London)* **288**, 499–501.
6. De, S. M., and Chatterje, D. N. (1953). An experimental study of the mechanism of action of
   Vibrio cholerae on the intestinal mucous membrane. *J. Pathol. Bacteriol.* **46**, 559–562.
7. De St. Groth, S. F., and Scheidegger, D. (1980). Production of monoclonal antibodies: Strategy
   and tactics. *J. Immunol. Methods* **35**, 1–21.
8. Donta, S. T., Moon, H. W., and Whipp, S. C. (1974). Detection of heat-labile *Escherichia coli*
   enterotoxin with the use of adrenal cells in tissue cultures. *Science* **183**, 334–336.
9. Evans, D. J., Evans, D. G., Richardson, S. H., and Gorbach, S. L. (1976). Purification of the
   polymyxin-released heat-labile enterotoxin of *Escherichia coli*. *J. Infect. Dis.* **133**, S92–S97.
10. Gianella, R. A. (1976). Suckling mouse model for detection of heat-stable *Escherichia coli*
    enterotoxin: Characteristics of the model. *Infect. Immun.* **14**, 95–99.
11. Gianella, R. A., Drake, K. W., and Luttrell, M. (1981). Development of a radioimmunoassay
    for *Escherichia coli* heat-stable enterotoxin: Comparison with the suckling mouse bioassay.
    Infect. Immun. **33**, 186–192.
12. Guerrant, R. L., Brunton, L. L., Schnaitman, T. A., Rebrun, L., and Gilman, A. G. (1974).
    Cyclic adenosine monophosphate and alteration of Chinese hamster ovary cell morphology: A
    rapid sensitive *in vitro* assay for enterotoxins of *Vibrio cholerae* and *Escherichia coli*. *Infect.
    Immun.* **10**, 320–327.
13. Gyles, C. L. (1974). Relationship among heat-labile enterotoxins of *Escherichia coli* and *Vibrio
    cholerae*. *J. Infect. Dis.* **129**, 277–283.
14. Hirst, T. R., Hardy, S. J. S., Lindblad, M., Sanchez, J., and Holmgren, J. (1986). Enterotoxin
    export mechanisms of *V. cholerae* and *Escherichia coli*: Implications for LT purification. *In*
    Proc. Joint U.S. Japan Cholera Conf., 20th, 1984, Nara, Japan. Nijhoff. (in press).
15. Holmgren, J. (1973). Comparison of the tissue-receptors for *Vibrio cholerae* and *Escherichia
    coli* enterotoxins by means of gangliosides and natural cholera toxoid. *Infect. Immun.* **8**, 851–
    859.
16. Holmgren, J. (1981). Actions of cholera toxin and the prevention and treatment of cholera.
    Nature (London), **7**, 759–763.
17. Holmgren, J., Fredman, P., Lindblad, M., Svennerholm, A.-M., and Svennerholm, L. (1982).
    Rabbit intestinal glycoprotein receptor for *Escherichia coli* heat-labile enterotoxin lacking af-
    finity for cholera toxin. *Infect. Immun.* **38**, 424–433.
18. Holmgren, J., and Svennerholm, A.-M. (1973). Enzyme-linked immunosorbent assay for chol-
    era serology. *Infect. Immun.* **7**, 759–763.
19. Holmgren, J., and Svennerholm, A.-M. (1979). Immunologic cross-reactivity between *Esche-
    richia coli* heat-labile enterotoxin and cholera toxin A and B subunits. *Curr. Microbiol.* **2**, 55–
    58.
20. Honda, T., Taga, S., Takeda, Y., and Miwatani, T. (1981). Modified ELEC test for detection of
    heat-labile enterotoxin of enterotoxigenic *Escherichia coli*. *J. Clin. Microbiol.* **13**, 1–5.
21. Honda, T., Takeda, Y., and Miwatani, T. (1981). Isolation of special antibodies which react
    only with homologous enterotoxin from *Vibrio cholerae* and enterotoxigenic *Escherichia coli*.
    Infect. Immun. **34**, 333–336.
22. Lindholm, L., Holmgren, J., Wikström, M, Karlsson, U., Andersson, K., and Lycke, N.
    (1983). Monoclonal antibodies to cholera toxin with special reference to cross-reactions with
    Escherichia coli heat-labile enterotoxin. *Infect. Immun.* **40**, 570–576.
23. Mancini, G., Carbonara, A. O., and Heremans, J. F.(1965). Immunochemical quantitation of
    antigens by single radial immunodiffusion. *Immunochemistry* **2**, 235–254.

24. Merson, M. H., and Black, R. E. (1981). Enterotoxigenic *Escherichia coli* diarrhea. *In* "Acute Enteric Infections in Children: New Prospects for Treatment and Prevention" (T. Holme, J. Holmgren, M. H. Merson, and R. Möllby, eds.), pp. 81–92. Elsevier/North-Holland, New York.

25. Merson, M. H., Yolken, R. H., Sack, R. B., Froehlich, J. L., Greenberg, H. B., Huq, I., and Black, R. B. (1980). Detection of *Escherichia coli* enterotoxins in stools. *Infect. Immun.* **29**, 108–113.

26. Moon, H. W. (1981). Enterotoxigenic *Escherichia coli* infections in animals. *In* "Acute Enteric Infections in Children: New Prospects for Treatment and Prevention" (T. Holme, J. Holmgren, M. H. Merson, and R. Möllby, eds.), pp. 93–95. Elsevier/North-Holland, New York.

27. Moseley, S. L., Huq, I., Alim, A., So, M., Sammadpor-Motalebi, M., and Falkow, S. (1980). Detection of enterotoxigenic *Escherichia coli* by DNA colony hybridization. *J. Infect. Dis.* **142**, 892–898.

28. Remmers, E. F., Colwell, R. R., and Goldsby, R. A. (1982). Production and characterization of monoclonal antibodies to cholera toxin. *Infect. Immun.* **37**, 70–76.

29. Ristaino, P. A., Levine, M. M., and Young, C. R. (1983). Improved GM1-enzyme-linked immunosorbent assay for detection of *Escherichia coli* heat-labile enterotoxin. *J. Clin. Microbiol.* **18**, 808–815.

30. Robertson, D. C., and Alderete, J. F. (1980). Chemistry and biology of the heat-stable *Escherichia coli* enterotoxin. *In* "Cholera and Related Diarrhoeas" (Ö. Ouchterlony and J. Holmgren, eds.), pp. 115–126. Karger, Basel.

31. Sack, D. A., Huda, S., Neogi, P. K. B., Daniel, R. R., and Spira, W. M. (1980). Microtiter ganglioside enzyme-linked immunosorbent assay for *Vibrio* and *Escherichia coli* heat-labile enterotoxins and antitoxin. *J. Clin. Microbiol.* **11**, 35–40.

32. Sack, R. B. (1975). Human diarrheal disease caused by enterotoxigenic *Escherichia coli*. *Annu. Rev. Microbiol.* **29**, 333–353.

33. So, M., and McCarthy, B. J. (1980). Nucleotide sequence of bacterial transposone Tn1681 encoding heat-stable toxin (ST) and its indentification in enterotoxigenic *Escherichia coli* strains. *Proc. Natl. Acad, Sci. U.S.A.* **77**, 4011–4015.

34. Svennerholm, A.-M. (1980). The nature of protective immunity in cholera. *In* "Cholera and Realted Diarrheas" (Ö. Ouchterlony and J. Holmgren, eds.), pp. 171–184. Karger, Basel.

35. Svennerholm, A.-M., and Holmgren, J. (1978). Identification of *Escherichia coli* heat-labile enterotoxin by means of a ganglioside immunosorbent assay (GM1-ELISA) procedure. *Curr. Microbiol.* **1**, 19–23.

36. Svennerholm, A.-M., Wikström, M., Lindblad, M., and Holmgren, J. (1986). Monoclonal antibodies against *Escherichia coli* heat-stable toxin (STa) and their use in a diagnostic ST ganglioside GM1-enzyme-linked immunosorbent assay. *J. Clin. Microbiol.* (in press).

37. Svennerholm, A.-M., Wikström, M., and Holmgren, J. (1986). Monoclonal antibodies to *Escherichia coli* heat-labile enterotoxin: Neutralising activity and differentiation of human and porcine LT_s and cholera toxin. *Med. Biol.* **64**, 23–30.

38. Svennerholm, A.-M., and Wiklund, G. (1983). Rapid GM1 enzyme-linked immunosorbent assay with visual reading for identification of *Escherichia coli* heat-labile enterotoxin. *J. Clin. Microbiol.* **17**, 596–600.

39. Tayot, J.-L., Holmgren, J., Svennerholm, L., Lindblad, M., and Tardy, M. (1981). Receptor-specific large-scale purification of cholera toxin on silica beads derivatized with lyso-GM1 ganglioside. *Eur. J. Biochem.* **113**, 249–258.

40. Thompson, M. R., Brandwein, H., Labine-Racke, M., and Gianella, R. A. (1984). Simple and reliable enzyme-linked immunosorbent assay with monoclonal antibodies for detection of *Escherichia coli* heat-stable enterotoxin. *J. Clin. Microbiol.* **20**, 59–64.

41. Towbin, H., Staehelin, E., and Gordon, J. (1979). Electrophoretic transfer of proteins from polyacrylamide gels to nitrocellulose sheets: Procedure and some applications. *Proc. Natl. Acad. Sci. U.S.A.* **76**, 4350–4354.

42. Tsuji, T., Taga, S., Honda, T., Takeda, Y., and Miwatani, T. (1982). Molecular heterogeneity of heat-labile enterotoxins from human and porcine enterotoxigenic *Escherichia coli*. *Infect. Immun.* **38**, 444–448.

43. Wadström, T., Aust-Kettis, A., Habte. D., Meeuwisse, G., Holmgren, J., Möllby, R., and Söderlind, O. (1976). Enterotoxin-producing bacteria and parasites in stools of Ethiopian children with diarrhoeal disease. *Arch Dis. Child.* **51**, 865–870.

44. Wolk, M., Svennerholm, A.-M., and Holmgren, J. (1980). Isolation of *Escherichia coli* enterotoxin by affinity chromatography: Characterization of subunits. *Curr. Microbiol.* **3**, 339–344.

45. Yamamoto, T., Tamura, T., and Yokota, T. (1984). Primary structure of heat-labile enterotoxin produced by *Escherichia coli* pathogenic for humans. *J. Biol. Chem.* **259**, 5037–5044.

46. Yolken, R. H., Greenberg, H. B., Merson, M. H., Sack, R. B., and Kapickian, A. Z. (1977). Enzyme-linked immunosorbent assay for detection of *Escherichia coli* heat-labile enterotoxin. *J. Clin. Microbiol.* **6**, 439–444.

4

Monoclonal Antibodies against *Campylobacter* Strains

TIMO U. KOSUNEN AND MIKKO HURME

Department of Bacteriology and Immunology
University of Helsinki
Helsinki, Finland

I. INTRODUCTION

Interest in campylobacters first arose in the early 1900s in veterinary medicine, when these bacteria were found to cause infertility and abortion in cattle and sheep (42). But it was only after King's report in 1957 (14) of human patients with enteritis, whose blood culture showed similar curved and spiral bacteria (''related *Vibrio*'s'') that it became clear that the group of *Vibrio*-like organisms included thermophilic strains pathogenic to humans. It was in the 1970s that Butzler *et al.* (7) and Skirrow (38) first showed that thermophilic campylobacters were among the most common bacterial causes of human diar-

MONOCLONAL ANTIBODIES
AGAINST BACTERIA
Volume III

rheal diseases. Skirrow's selective medium for stool cultures was the key factor for intensive worldwide research into campylobacters. Because campylobacters were gram-negative enteric pathogens, it was natural that in the early studies the same methods and analogous ideas were applied as in the successful and sophisticated investigations on coliform enterobacteria. Very soon, however, it became evident that the classical identification and typing methods were ineffective when applied to these microaerophilic bacteria, which also proved to be inactive in most biochemical tests.

The simultaneous expansion of research into campylobacters and the availability of the knowledge, skill, and material for handling hybridomas have led a few laboratories to explore the possibility of producing monoclonal antibodies against components of *Campylobacter* spp. The first attempts aimed at clarifying the various antigenic structures which had been shown by polyclonal antisera to vary greatly, not only from subspecies to subspecies but also from strain to strain (16,19,21,33). A number of interstrain cross-reactions and the rather limited knowledge of the chemical structures of the antigens have hampered serotyping by polyclonal antisera and increased the temptation to avoid difficult absorptions by producing monoclonal reagents known to have unique specificity. The available literature has reports from only three laboratories (15,26,31). The purpose of this review is to give background information and to present and discuss the principal findings and experiences to date, as well as to consider the possible future applications of monoclonal antibodies against campylobacters.

II. BACKGROUND

A. Taxonomy and Pathological Features

All campylobacters commonly regarded as pathogenic are catalase-producing gram-negative curved rods with a flagellum at one or both ends. The present classification, originally presented by Véron and Chatelain (49) and accepted for the "Approved Lists of Bacterial Names" (37), will, according to Karmali and Skirrow (13), also be the one used in the ninth edition of *Bergey's Manual*. Since the present names are not those given in the eighth edition of the manual (41), and since both present and former names are found in recent literature, both sets of names are given in Table I. This table also gives the main differences between the results of the tests for identifying the strains. A further recently described subspecies with definite criteria, *C. laridis* (2), is also included. The latest candidate for the group of human pathogens is *C. pyloridis* (not included), which has been found in patients with gastritis in particular (39,50). For other strains and methods for their identification, see the review by Karmali and Skirrow (13).

Campylobacter coli and *C. jejuni* are frequently isolated from patients with

TABLE I

Nomenclature and Differential Characteristics of Catalase-Producing *Campylobacters*

		Growth at		Growth in 1% glycine	Nalidixic acid resistance	Hippurate hydrolysis
Present name	Former name	25°C	43°C			
C. coli	*C. fetus* subsp. *jejuni*	−	+	+	−	−
C. jejuni	*C. fetus* subsp. *jejuni*	−	+	+	−	+
C. laridis	NARTC group	−	+	+	+	−
C. fetus subsp. *venerealis*	*C. fetus* subsp. *fetus*	+	−	−	+	−
C. fetus subsp. *fetus*	*C. fetus* subsp. *intestinalis*	+	v[a]	+	+	−

[a] Variable.

gastroenteritis. Both are commonly regarded as normal flora in some farm animals: *C. coli* in swine and *C. jejuni* in cattle, sheep, and chickens (42). *Campylobacter jejuni* is known also as a cause of enteritis in cattle (47), abortion in sheep, and hepatitis in chickens (42). *Campylobacter laridis* owes its name to the sea gull (*Larus*), in which it is normally found (2). It has occasionally been isolated from human stools as well (2).

Campylobacter fetus subsp. *venerealis* causes infertility in cows, and its name describes the transmission of the infection through symptomless bulls (42). It has not been recorded as a human pathogen. *Campylobacter fetus* subsp. *fetus* in humans is mainly an opportunistic cause of septic infections (35). Originally it was identified as a cause of abortion in cattle, and the former name, *C. fetus* subsp. *intestinalis,* better described its occurrence in their intestinal flora (42).

B. *Campylobacter coli* and *Campylobacter jejuni*

1. General Characterization

Campylobacter coli is differentiated from *C. jejuni* by the hippurate hydrolysis test, in which *C. jejuni* is positive. *Campylobacter jejuni* can be divided into two biotypes by a H_2S test (40). No biotypes have been reported for either *C. coli* or *C. laridis*. Variation in susceptibility to some antibiotics, such as metronidazole, erythromycin, or tetracycline, has some value in differentiating strains within subspecies, particularly when it shows that strains which in other tests appear similar are not identical (17). Further tests have been applied to differentiate thermophilic campylobacters (10,22), but there are no reports from other laboratories confirming their usefulness. The surface structures of *C. jejuni* have been studied from outer membrane preparations isolated by sodium–lauryl sarcosinate extraction (5,24), which in *E. coli* selectively dissolves the cytoplasmic membrane (8). Sodium dodecyl sulfate–polyacrylamide gel electrophoresis (SDS–PAGE) strips stained with Coomassie Blue showed six to eight outer membrane proteins. One of these had a molecular weight of 41,000 to 45,000 and was suspected by Logan and Trust of being porin (24). According to Blaser *et al.*(5), there were nine variants in this molecular size, which were stable for each strain and could thus be used in epidemiological follow-up of strains.

Some outer-membrane proteins are surface-exposed, as shown by Logan and Trust (25) with lactoperoxidase labeling. The finding of antibodies against some of them in normal human sera (6) indicates either earlier contacts with campylobacters or the presence of cross-reacting antigens in other bacteria. The fact that these antibodies increase during *Campylobacter* infections makes them interesting for diagnostic serology, but which if any of them are specific and common enough for campylobacters remains to be determined. One of the strong bands with a molecular weight of 63,000 was shown by Logan and Trust (24) to be flagellin and it was antigenically cross-reactive in a few strains. An acid glycine extract of 10 *C. jejuni* strains was first used as antigen by Svedhem *et al.* (45) to show antibodies in patients with gastroenteritis. Later it was shown that similar extracts from one or two strains contained antigens against which most patients with gastroenteritis with positive stool cultures for campylobacters developed antibodies (18,20,46). Logan and Trust (24) found an abundance of a 31-kDa protein in this extract, which was antigenically cross-reactive in the six thermophilic strains studied. Unexpectedly they did not find any 98-kDa component, although this was the principal component found in the original studies by Winter *et al.*in *C. fetus* subsp. *fetus* (54). However, in outer-membrane preparations of *C. jejuni* VC 74 strain, Logan and Trust (25) saw a 94-kDa protein, which differed antigenically from other strains. By staining SDS–PAGE strips with a sensitive silver method (48), they characterized the lipopolysaccharide (LPS) profile of 24 thermophilic *Campylobacter* strains (27). All the strains appeared to have low molecular weight LPS, which had few if any demonstrable carbohydrate structures. Such structures are known to be responsible for the specific O antigens in smooth salmonellae and they appear as washboardlike lines in the silver staining (32). The low carbohydrate content was in agreement with the high lipid A: neutral sugar ratio found in the LPS of the two *C. jejuni* strains Logan and Trust (27) analyzed chemically. Despite its low carbohydrate content, this low molecular weight LPS showed antigenic heterogeneity (11,27).

Due to the limited number of useful biochemical and biotyping tests available for identifying *Campylobacter* strains, several laboratories have directed their studies to the use of antigenic markers. As with enterobacteria, there is wide antigenic heterogeneity in both heat-labile and heat-stable antigens (16,19,21,33).

As the final internationally approved typing system is still being developed, the preliminary serotypes reported by the various laboratories are currently described by the first three letters of the senior author's name, followed by the type strain number (e.g., Jon 7, Kos 372, Lau 5, Lio 2, Pen 6, Rog 12).

2. Serotyping on the Basis of Heat-Labile Antigens

These serotypes are determined using live bacteria in slide (16,21) or latex agglutination (16) tests. The immune sera produced separately for each individual strain are first absorbed with heated homologous bacteria and then, in the case of strong cross-reactions, with live heterologous strains. The largest collection of different type strains and antisera is that of Lior *et al.* (22) and consists of more than 50 different serotypes. Most of these serotypes are specific for either *C. coli* or *C. jejuni* strains, but in some both subspecies are found. All tested *C. laridis* strains belong to the one serotype. Heat-labile antigens are supposedly proteins, but the role of flagellar, capsular, and cell wall proteins remains to be determined.

3. Serotyping on the Basis of Heat-Stable Antigens

The most popular method has been passive hemagglutination (PHA) in rabbit immune sera of sheep red cells (33) or human blood group O red cells (19) coated with boiled saline extracts of bacteria. The widest collection of different serotypes is that of Penner *et al.* (34), who have found altogether more than 50 different serotypes of *C. coli* and *C. jejuni*. Some serotypes include strains from both subspecies. At the present time the typing is carried out with nonabsorbed sera and there are some cross-reactions between certain serotypes. As stated above, LPS is antigenically different in different heat-stable serotypes (11,27), but whether the whole antigen is LPS alone or whether it is combined with other heat-stable structures, like polysaccharides and certain proteins, will be seen in the future.

C. *Campylobacter fetus* subsp. *fetus* and *Campylobacter fetus* subsp. *venerealis*

The inactivity of these subspecies in most tests used for differentiating gram-negative rods, and the limited number of useful tests reported, do not offer many possibilities for showing interstrain variations (Table I). The fact that only two different heat-stable antigens, A and B, had been reported led Berg *et al.* (3) to combine the biotyping (glycine and H_2S tests) and serotyping methods, but even so they were only able to record four types (see Table IV). Serotyping of the heat-stable antigens was by tube agglutination of boiled bacteria in immune sera from rabbits injected with formalinized bacteria. The heat-stable antigens responsible for the serotypes have not been defined. Among the isolated polysaccharides Ristic and Murty (36) noted at least two antigenic variants. The LPS that Winter (53) isolated, however, cross-reacted with antisera against the other strains in the agar gel precipitation test. Logan and Trust (24) applied the sensitive silver-staining method (48) also to the SDS–PAGE strip of isolated outer membrane of *C. fetus* subsp. *fetus* CIP 5396 strain and found polysaccharides of only intermediate length, in addition to lipid A and core components. When similar strips were stained for proteins, a number of lines were found as expected (24,29).

The acid extract that McCoy *et al.* (28) obtained with glycine–HCl buffer (pH 2.2) was antiphagocytic and prevented O agglutination. The authors thought that the main component was a glycoprotein that formed a part of the microcapsule which "in vesicles derived from sheared cells appeared to exist in complex with lipopolysaccharide." Its molecular weight was about 98,000.

By absorbing rabbit immune sera against formalinized bacteria, Berg *et al.* (3) found seven different heat-labile antigens, each strain having one to five. The nature of these was not clarified and the classification has not found further application. Wiidik and Hlidar (52) presented evidence for the existence of capsular antigens in 1955 but no further studies have been reported.

III. RESULTS AND DISCUSSION

A. Monoclonal Antibodies against *Campylobacter jejuni*

1. Heat-Labile Antigens

The number and quality of the antigens to be studied by monoclonal antibodies is decisive when the donor animals are immunized. Purified antigenic components are likely to result in several clones whose specificity focuses mainly against the determinants of the purified immunogen, whereas the use of whole bacteria is more likely to result in clones which are specific to any antigen of the immunizing strain.

Newell (31) as well as Logan and Trust (26) studied monoclonal antibodies against flagellar antigens. Newell first immunized mice with an outer-membrane preparation, then boosted them with purified flagella (31). She screened the products of the hybridomas by enzyme immune assay (EIA) with flagella as antigen and obtained 14 active clones. The antiflagellar properties of the antibodies were confirmed by comparing their binding to flagellate and aflagellate bacteria in EIA, by their binding to 62-kDa flagellar protein in immunoblotting, and by radioimmunoprecipitation of ^{125}I-labeled flagella. Although the antibodies were of IgM class, they did not immobilize live bacteria (31), neither did they have any effect on the pathogenicity of the immunogen strain in an infant mouse model (D. G. Newell, personal communication). Using competitive radioimmunoassay, Newell distinguished at least four different epitopes in the flagellar antigen. Two of them were specific for the Lio 6 strain which she used as immunogen (31). These antibodies would thus be suitable for serotyping, but until a more practical test is found for typing, their use will be limited to research purposes. The lack of reactivity of the clones against the aflagellar variant of the same strain implies that flagellar antigens are important heat-labile antigens, but the possible participation of other components is not excluded.

One clone produced antibodies against an epitope that was common to the flagella of several serotypes of *C. jejuni*. Another epitope was found to be common not only to all the *C. coli* and *C. jejuni* strains studied, but also to *C. laridis*, *C. fetus* subsp. *fetus*, *C. fetus* subsp. *venerealis*, and *C. pyloridis* strains (D. G. Newell, personal communication). The antibody against this epitope thus fulfills the criteria of a common reagent for identifying pathogenic *Campylobacter* spp., in particular because it functions in both EIA and immuno-dot antigen detection systems.

The ultrastructural immuno-gold labeling technique proved to be informative about the localization of the antigenic epitopes. All the monoclonal reagents failed to label the surface of intact flagella but reacted with the tips of broken flagella only (D. G. Newell, personal communication). This might also explain the failure of these reagents to immobilize live bacteria and to prevent gastrointestinal colonization in passively immunized infant mice, although unexpected failures of monoclonal antibodies in biological tests are by no means unknown (30).

Logan and Trust (26) used purified flagellin to immunize donor mice and screen the products of the hybridomas. They obtained 12 stable hybridomas which produced IgG antibodies, 11 of which were specific for flagellin, whereas one reacted with a heat-stable determinant located superficially on all the *C. coli* and *C. jejuni* strains studied as well as on the *C. fetus* subsp. *fetus* strain. Ten of the antiflagellin antibodies recognized surface-exposed epitopes, but only one was specific for the flagellin used as immunogen. Eight of them reacted with several different strains, indicating the complexity of the flagellin antigen, and another detected an epitope that was found in all thermophilic *Campylobacter* strains as well as in the *C. fetus* subsp. *fetus* strain studied. The one antibody specific for the flagella of the immunogen strain fulfills the criterion for reacting with a serotype-specific surface epitope. In practical serotyping the use of this reagent would be limited by the demanding techniques needed. EIA, immunoblotting, radioimmunoprecipitation, and indirect fluorescent antibody testing are often considered less suitable for routine laboratories than, for example, slide agglutination techniques.

2. Heat-Stable Antigens

We immunized donor mice with formalin-treated *C. jejuni* strain Wat 143843 (51) and subsequently tested the hybridoma products in EIA with live immunogen as antigen (15). We obtained 30 antibodies. One of these gave two lines in cellulose acetate electrophoresis, indicating that it was not monoclonal. Table II gives results of the antibodies which reacted in some agglutination tests with antigens obtained from the immunogen strain. Although six antibodies gave a positive slide agglutination result with live bacteria, we were unable to confirm their antiflagellar nature by tube agglutination of formalinized bacteria and immobilization tests. Two of the six clones (3 and 9) were against heat-stable purified polysaccharide preparation (23), thus showing the importance of careful absorptions in the preparation of serotyping reagents for heat-labile antigens. The antigen was so loosely bound to the bacteria that it could be extracted with saline even in room temperature. It could also have been removed by boiling, since these two antibodies did not agglutinate boiled bacteria in the tube test. Seven of the monoclonal antibodies reacted in the passive hemagglutination test most commonly used in the serotyping of heat-stable antigens of thermophilic *Campylobacter* spp. (33). Four of these were specific for the polysaccharide antigen thus confirming the contribution of these epitopes in the heat-stable serotyping antigen. Two of the three antibodies which failed to react with the polysaccharide

TABLE II

Agglutination Reactions of Ascitic Fluids with Different Antigenic Preparations of the Immunogen *Campylobacter jejuni* strain Wat 143483[a]

			Test results[b]			
				PHA[e]		
Ascites number	Slide agglutination[c]	Tube agglutination[d]	Saline extract	Boiled extract	Autoclaved extract	Polysaccharide
1				1:1.280		
3	+++		1:5.120	1:1.280	1:5.120	1:2.560
4		1:800		1:1.280		
5				1:640	1:2.560	1:640
9	+++		1:5.120	1:640	1:5.120	1:640
16		1:3.200				
18	++					
20				1:80	1:160	1:320
24		1:1.600		1:1.280		
26	+					
27	+					
28	++					

[a] Adapted from Kosunen *et al.* (15).
[b] Negative reaction was obtained unless otherwise indicated.
[c] Live bacteria antigen: ascitic fluid diluted 1:5.
[d] Boiled bacteria antigen; first dilution studied, 1:100.
[e] Passive hemagglutination. First dilution studied, 1:40.

agglutinated boiled bacteria in the tube test indicating that, although the determinant was extractable with saline, some of it still remained bound in the bacterial surfaces.

A surprising finding was the failure of the four antibodies which reacted with the polysaccharide to bind to the purified LPS preparation in EIA. The only hybridoma product which reacted with the LPS was the one that was not monoclonal, but this antibody was negative in the passive hemagglutination tests. Jones *et al.* (11) have shown the importance of LPS in the serotyping reactions of campylobacters based on heat-stable antigens by the passive hemagglutination (PHA) method. This is analogous to the dominance of O antigens in the antigenicity of LPS in salmonellae. The lack of repeating polysaccharide units in silver-stained SDS–PAGE strips of *Campylobacter* spp. reported by Logan and Trust (24,27) was also evident in the LPS prepared from our immunogen (15). Logan and Trust (27) noted that the situation resembled that of, for example, neisseriae (43), which also have low molecular weight LPS, although their antigenic variability seems to be less pronounced than that of *Campylobacter* spp. They suggested that the polysaccharide content in *Campylobacter* LPS could be so low that it escapes detection by standard methods. Another possibility is that the polysaccharides extracted in the purification were not tightly bound to LPS, or perhaps not at all.

When the seven PHA-positive monoclonal antibodies were tested in PHA with extracts from other type strains which had reacted with our rabbit antisera against the immunogen, several different reaction patterns were recorded (Table III). This implies that the immunogen has several antigenic determinants which induce specific antibody clones, which in turn recognize antigenically similar determinants in other strains. The use of several cross-reacting strains with different reaction patterns to the monoclonal antibodies can thus give the minimal number of antigenically different epitopes which contribute to the mosaiclike whole antigen responsible for the PHA results with rabbit antisera. Several cross-reactions in the serotyping results with these antisera have indicated that, at least in these strains, the PHA antigen is composed of several antigenic determinants. Whereas cross-reactions, on the one hand, are undesirable for any serotyping system, on the other hand, they are essential for picking up all the cross-reacting strains, thus ensuring that the hybridizations have produced clones for all antigenically relevant epitopes. The data in Table III show the presence of at least five epitopes, if we leave out the weak reaction of clone 20 and consider clones 3 and 9 as reagents for the same antigenic determinant. The strains studied to date have shown identical reaction patterns with the products of these clones, which have also given similar results in other tests with the immunogen (15). The titer of clone 1 in the PHA test with the immunogen has, in repeated tests, varied from negative (in 1 : 40 dilution) to 1 : 640. Until now we have not been able to show whether this variability is due to irregularities in production, availability, and

TABLE III

Reciprocals of Passive Hemagglutination Titers of Polyvalent Rabbit Antisera and Monoclonal Murine Antibodies against *Campylobacter jejuni* Strain Wat 143483

Antibody	Antigen										
	Wat 143483	Kos 1988	Pen 3	Pen 4	Lau 25	Lau 48	Lio 1	Jon 2	Jon 5	Jon 11	Aberdeen
Rabbit anti-											
Wat 143483	5120	1280	—[b]	5120	5120	5120	5120	10240	5120	2560	5120
Kos 1988	10240	20480	2560	2560	5120	10240	10240	5120	5120	20480	5120
Monoclonal murine anti-Wat 143483											
Clone 1	640(—)[c]	—	—	—	—	2560	—	2560	2560	5120	2560
4	1280	—	—	—	1280	2560	—	2560	1280	640	2560
3	1280	40	40	1280	1280	2560	640	1280	1280	—	1280
9	640	—	—	320	320	640	640	640	640	—	640
5	640	1280	—	—	320	1280	—	320	—	—	—
20	80	—	—	—	—	160	80	—	—	—	—
24	1280	—	—	—	640	>40 / <160	<320	<320	<320	<320	1280
			Pen 13[a] Pen 16 Lau 3 Lau 16 Lio 7	Lio 17			Raf				

[a] Other strains showing similar results.

[b] Starting dilution tested 1:40 unless otherwise indicated (Clone 24).

[c] See text.

stability of the antigen, to technical differences in coating the red cells, or to inherent characteristics of the antibody.

3. *Other Antigens of* Campylobacter jejuni

Reports from the three laboratories with monoclonal reagents have included data on antibodies which have reacted in tests not directly involved in serotyping. Some antibodies are strain-specific but several react with antigens of other strains as well. These latter have formed the basis for attempts to find and define common antigens which could be used for determining antibodies in patients. An acid glycine extract from *C. jejuni* strains was applied by Svedhem *et al.* (45) as antigen in the serological diagnosis of patients with *Campylobacter* enteritis. They used the same extraction method as McCoy *et al.* (28) had used on *C. fetus* subsp. *fetus*. We tested our monoclonal antibodies against a similar extract from the immunogen strain and found several strongly reacting clones in EIA. One of them cross-reacted strongly with other live *Campylobacter* strains in EIA, thus showing the presence of one or more common antigens. The usefulness of the acid extract in clinical serology has since been amply confirmed (4,12,18,20,46), but the antigen(s) responsible has still not been defined.

The fact that there are several monoclonal antibodies reactive in the screening tests applied to date shows that further studies with more refined methods are needed in the exploration of *Campylobacter* antigens.

B. Monoclonal Antibodies against Heat-Stable Antigens of *Campylobacter fetus* subsp. *venerealis*

In a fusion with *C. fetus* subsp. *venerealis* Fir 14840 strain we obtained eight clones which reacted in the PHA test with sheep red cells coated with a supernatant from bacteria autoclaved in saline (Table IV). When the same antibodies were used in PHA tests with four other *C. fetus* subsp. *venerealis* and *C. fetus* subsp. *fetus* strains, five different reaction patterns were obtained. In rabbit antisera the same strains, which all had the heat-stable antigen A of Berg *et al.* (3), gave PHA titers which did not differentiate the strains (Table IV). Four antibodies (2,26,28, and 30) also agglutinated sheep red cells coated with purified polysaccharide (23) from the immunogen. Their reactions with the other strains were similar, thus showing that the strains either have a common epitope and all four clones have the same specificity, or that there are several similar epitopes. These four antibodies also gave by far the highest EIA values with LPS extracted from the immunogen, implying that the polysaccharide contributes to the antigenicity of the LPS in this strain. The other four clones which did not react with the polysaccharide did not react with the LPS either, indicating the presence of further antigens in the autoclaved saline extract. Whether they are components that are lost in the purification of the polysaccharide and LPS or

TABLE IV

Reciprocals of Passive Hemagglutination Titers of Polyvalent Rabbit Antisera and Monoclonal Murine Antibodies against *Campylobacter fetus* subsp. *venerealis* Strain Fir 14840

	Antigen				
Antibody[a]	*C. fetus* subsp. *venerealis*	*C. fetus* subsp. *venerealis*	*C. fetus* subsp. *venerealis*	*C. fetus* subsp. *fetus*	*C. fetus* subsp. *fetus*
	Fir 14840 A sub-1[b]	Fir 13823 A-1[b]	Fir 17995 A-1[b]	Fir 13014 A-2[b]	Fir 14865 B[b]
Rabbit anti-					
Fir 14840	10,240	2,560	1,280	10,240	—
Fir 13014	10,240	2,560	1,280	10,240	—
Fir 13823	10,240	10,240	5,120	10,240	—
Fir 14865	—	—	—	—	1,280
Murine					
anti-Fir 14840					
Clone 2	5,120[c]	—	2,560	5,120	—
3	5,120	—	1,280	—	—
4	10,240	—	10,240	5,120	—
10	640[d]	—	—	—	—
14	2,560	2,560	—	5,120	—
26	2,560[c]	640	1,280	2,560	—
28	2,560[c]	—	640	2,560	—
30	1,280[c]	—	320	2,560	—

[a] Starting dilution tested 1:320.
[b] Heat-stable antigen and biotype (3).
[c] Also positive in PHA with polysaccharide antigen.
[d] Weak and nontypical agglutinations in all dilutions.

some other heat-stable structures is still unresolved. Silver staining of SDS–PAGE strips of this strain failed to show the washboard structure typical of the *O*-polysaccharides of smooth salmonellae (32).

IV. CONCLUSIONS

The number of laboratories working on monoclonal antibodies against *Campylobacter* spp. is small, and the number of hybridomas produced is likewise small. All results must be regarded as preliminary. The antibodies which have been reactive in tests have for the most part given clear-cut and valuable results. It is far too early to evaluate the negative results. All negative results need to be confirmed by other techniques, including those that measure the binding of antibodies directly and not only secondary manifestations like agglutination which are influenced strongly by both the class of immunoglobulin and such characteristics of the antigen as variability of antigenic determinants and density of identical epitopes.

The clearest results have been in the understanding of the basis of serotyping. Heat-labile antigens are determined mainly by slide agglutination of live bacteria with rabbit antisera absorbed with heat-resistant antigens (16,21). The first monoclonal antibodies produced against flagellar antigens were not useful for practical application by slide agglutination (26,31). This has been shown to be due both to their specificity to antigens all of which are not surface-exposed in intact flagella and to impractical detection methods which can be applied in research laboratories only. The monoclonal reagents, however, have shown clearly that the antigenicity of flagellin is determined by several epitopes, some of which are strain-specific and others which are so common that they may be useful for identification purposes.

Serotyping on the basis of heat-stable antigens gives many cross-reactions when rabbit antisera are used in PHA (19,33). This indicates the contribution of several antigenic determinants, at least in the strains reacting with several typing sera. In the first hybridization reported, the immunogen was selected on the basis that most sera from *Campylobacter* enteritis patients agglutinated bacteria of this strain (15,51). Several type strains from different laboratories reacted in PHA test with a rabbit antiserum against this immunogen strain. These cross-reacting strains could be divided into several groups by their reactions with the mono-clonal antibodies. In this way, antibodies resemble the antisera against antigenic factors used in the serotyping of *Salmonella* strains and strengthen the idea that several different epitopes together form the whole heat-stable antigen we deter-mine with rabbit antisera.

By 1983 the continuously growing number of different heat-stable serotypes of the *C coli* and *C. jejuni* group already exceeded 50 (34). This number is likely to grow considerably through the use of monoclonal antibodies. Although the char-acterization of strains by their antigenic factors is of scientific importance, it is questionable whether such information is needed in the majority of clinical laboratories involved, for instance, in transmission, virulence, identification, and diagnostic problems, as there are no clear data showing that any of the present serotypes would be more virulent than the others and thus responsible for severe clinical diseases or complications. In fact, it is questionable whether serotyping can at the moment give any valuable information at all in individual, sporadically appearing cases of *C. coli* and *C. jejuni* enteritis which tend to be the majority.

It is obvious that the situation is quite different for *C. fetus* subsp. *fetus* and *C. fetus* subsp. *venerealis,* since rabbit antisera divide these by heat-stable antigens into two types only. Our first PHA tests with monoclonal reagents indicate that the heat-stable antigen A may consist of several epitopes, but since the negative typing results have not yet been confirmed by other tests, the question is still open. The results have, however, shown definitely that, in the C. *fetus* subsp. *venerealis* strain we used, a polysaccharide determinant, which is also found in LPS, is part of the heat-stable antigen.

At this stage of development, monoclonal antibodies against *Campylobacter* spp. are beginning to become important tools for the analysis of antigens, but their use is still limited to specific research purposes.

V. PROSPECTS FOR THE FUTURE

The production of monoclonal antibodies against *Campylobacter* spp. is increasing and several laboratories are known to have started studies on them. It is easy to make a list of problems which monoclonal antibodies could help to solve, but it is very difficult to select those projects which would definitely benefit.

It is widely agreed that what is most urgently needed in *Campylobacter* research is progress in serotyping. To be commonly acceptable, the serotyping schemes should be based on known and defined structures, like the flagellar ones of the heat-labile antigens and the LPS and polysaccharides of the heat-stable ones.

The most extensive preliminary serotyping scheme for heat-labile antigens is based on slide agglutination of live bacteria (21,22). It is assumed that the antigens are proteins and that they could best be serotyped with IgM antibodies. Whereas most hybridomas produce IgG antibodies, the development of serotyping reagents of the IgM class would require large series of monoclonal antibodies or technical innovations that would favor IgM production. One solution to this problem could be the production of monoclonal antibodies of any class combined with typing methods in which both IgG and IgM antibodies function as in latex agglutination, or in which IgG antibodies alone operate as in coagglutination. If flagellin proves to be the antigen in the serotyping of heat-labile antigens, purified flagellin would be an excellent immunogen and screening antigen.

The preliminary serotyping system differentiates more than 50 heat-labile types, sufficient for most epidemiological studies (22). Thus the role of monoclonal reagents in the future will be to create the specific sera for mapping the epitopes in the different strains, thereby defining both the strain and the group-specific as well as the common heat-labile antigens.

Monoclonal antibodies function in the PHA test used in serotyping the heat-stable antigens of *Campylobacter* spp. (15). When rabbit antisera are used in serotyping, it is usual that several strains react with more than one typing serum (19,33). Due to the fact that these cross-reactions may vary from strain to strain, monoclonal reagents would be useful in dividing the present groups of more or less similarly behaving strains into smaller, antigenically more distinct types. Since LPS and polysaccharides contribute strongly if not entirely to the serotypes currently recorded with rabbit antisera (11,27), the production of hybridomas with these antigens would lead to reagents that would enable characterization of the type of antigen which the determinants represent. The rabbit antisera currently used differentiate more than 50 heat-stable serotypes (34). Since this number is sufficient for solving most epidemiological problems, the use of monoclonal reagents in the near future will be limited to laboratories working on the development of serotyping systems.

Well-characterized antigens will also have other uses besides serotyping. The fact that monoclonal antibodies can be used as immunosorbents makes it possible to purify antigens. It is tempting to speculate how such purified antigens could be used not only in basic science but also in practical applications such as the development of diagnostic antigens for clinical serology, production of vaccines, studies on the pathogenesis of infections, and development of immunity.

Monoclonal antibodies against well-defined group antigens could also be used in identifying strains isolated from various sources as campylobacters as well as in detecting the antigen directly in clinical samples. Such reagents have been sought after, for use in rapid diagnosis (1,9,44). In the case of *Campylobacter* infection a rapid test would detect the antigen directly in stool or other samples within minutes with, for example, latex or coagglutination reagents, or within hours with the more sensitive enzyme and radioimmunoassay methods. In the latter tests monoclonal antibodies could be used at either the capturing or the detecting phase. These types of rapid tests could also be of interest commercially, since a pattern of sensitive tests against, for example, common enteric pathogens could replace stool cultures, microscopy, and electron microscopy.

The antigen most commonly used in the determination of antibodies in patient sera is a crude acid extract from whole bacteria (28). The specificity of the test for IgG antibodies is not as high as that for IgM, indicating that the antigenic mixture obtained by the extraction procedure includes components against which many humans have detectable IgG antibodies. With the aid of monoclonal reagents it should be possible to discover which of these components are most specific to campylobacters, and they could then be purified and used as antigen in diagnostic serology.

In many laboratories the final decision on the use of monoclonal or polyclonal antibodies will be made on the basis of local resources, technical possibilities, cost–benefit estimates, and, not least, individual research interest. Commercial laboratories may be interested in guiding development toward profitable, practical solutions of diagnostic problems. In some cases the production of monoclonal antibodies may be favored because of outside criticism against the use of experimental animals in research and antiserum production. Most of these considerations are not specific to *Campylobacter* investigations and many of the problems and prospects associated with other microbes are not strange to laboratories working with campylobacters. What is specific to campylobacters and to other microbes discovered recently is the rather empty field of knowledge, and researchers should be ready to take full advantage of the modern and uniquely specific help offered by monoclonal antibodies.

VI. SUMMARY

Monoclonal antibodies have been produced against *C. jejuni* and *C. fetus* subsp. *venerealis*. Live bacteria can be used as antigen in the primary screening of culture fluid and ascites samples by enzyme immune assay. Although the results are still preliminary, they show that serotyping systems based on both heat-labile and heat-stable antigens can be established using monoclonal reagents against well-defined antigens.

Antibodies against *C. jejuni* have been produced by immunizing with flagellar preparations and with formalinized whole bacteria. The antiflagellar antibodies have shown the presence in flagella of several antigenic determinants—some strain-specific, some common to a few strains of the same subspecies, and some common to most *Campylobacter* spp. The techniques required, however, are complicated and demanding. Some monoclonal antibodies have functioned in passive hemagglutination tests used in the serotyping of heat-stable antigens with rabbit antisera and support the theory that these antigens are composed of several different epitopes per strain. At least some of them are polysaccharides, but this could not be shown in purified lipopolysaccharide (LPS). Similar results have been obtained in studies of heat-stable antigens of *C. fetus* subsp. *venerealis* with monoclonal antibodies, except that the polysaccharide component was present also in purified LPS.

ACKNOWLEDGMENTS

This study was financially aided by the Sigrid Jusélius Foundation and the Finnish Medical Research Council, Helsinki. The skillful technical assistance of Barbro Bång, Eila Kelo, Maire Laakso, and Maarika Weissmann is gratefully acknowledged.

REFERENCES

1. Beards, G. M., Campbell, A. D., Cottrell, N. R., Peiris, J. S. M., Rees, N., Sanders, R. C., Shirley, J. A., Wood, H. C., and Flewett, T. H. (1984). Enzyme-linked immunosorbent assays based on polyclonal and monoclonal antibodies for rotavirus detection. *J. Clin. Microbiol.* **19,** 248–254.
2. Benjamin, J., Leaper, S., Owen, R. J., and Skirrow, M. B. (1983). Description of *Campylobac-*

ter laridis, a new species comprising the nalidixic acid resistant thermophilic *Campylobacter* (NARTC) group. *Curr. Microbiol.* **8,** 231–238.

3. Berg, R. L., Jutila, J. W., and Firehammer, B. D. (1971). A revised classification of *Vibrio fetus. Am. J. Vet. Res.* **32,** 11–22.

4. Blaser, M. J., and Duncan, D. J. (1984). Human serum antibody response to *Campylobacter jejuni* infection as measured in an enzyme-linked immunosorbent assay. *Infect. Immun.* **44,** 292–298.

5. Blaser, M. J., Hopkins, J. A., Berka, R. M., Vasil, M. L., and Wang, W.-L. L. (1983). Identification and characterization of *Campylobacter jejuni* outer membrane proteins. *Infect. Immun.* **42,** 276–284.

6. Blaser, M. J., Hopkins, J. H., and Vasil, M. L. (1984). *Campylobacter jejuni* outer membrane proteins are antigenic for humans. *Infect. Immun.* **43,** 986–993.

7. Butzler, J. P., Dekeyser, P., Detrain, M., and Dehaen, M. (1973). Related *Vibrio* in stools. *J. Pediatr.* **82,** 493–495.

8. Filip, C., Fletcher, G., Wulff, J. L., and Earhart, C. F. (1973). Solubilization of the cytoplasmic membrane of *Escherichia coli* by the ionic detergent sodium-lauryl sarcosinate. *J. Bacteriol.* **115,** 717–722.

9. Frame, B., Mahony, J. B., Balachandran, N., Rawls, W. E., and Chernesky, M. A. (1984). Identification and typing of herpes simplex virus by enzyme immunoassay with monoclonal antibodies. *J. Clin. Microbiol.* **20,** 162–166.

10. Hebert, A. G., Hollis, D. G., Weaver, R. E., Lambert, M. A., Blaser, M. J., and Moss, C. W. (1982). 30 years of campylobacters: Biochemical characteristics and a biotyping proposal for *Campylobacter jejuni. J. Clin. Microbiol.* **15,** 1065–1073.

11. Jones, D. M., Fox, A. J., and Eldridge, J. (1984). Characterization of the antigens involved in serotyping strains of *Campylobacter jejuni* by passive hemagglutination. *Curr. Microbiol.* **10,** 105–110.

12. Kaldor, J., Pritchard, H., Serpell, A., and Metcalf, W. (1983). Serum antibodies in *Campylobacter* enteritis. *J. Clin. Microbiol.* **18,** 1–4.

13. Karmali, M. A., and Skirrow, M. B. (1984). Taxonomy of the genus *Campylobacter. In* "Campylobacter Infection in Man and Animals" (J. P. Butzler, ed.), pp. 1–20. CRC Press, Boca Raton, Florida.

14. King, E. O. (1957). Human infection with *Vibrio foetus* and a closely related vibrio. *J. Infect. Dis.* **101,** 119–128.

15. Kosunen, T. U., Bång, B. E., and Hurme, M. (1984). Analysis of *Campylobacter jejuni* antigens with monoclonal antibodies. *J. Clin. Microbiol.* **19,** 129–133.

16. Kosunen, T. U., Danielsson, D., and Kjellander, J. (1982). Serology of *Campylobacter fetus* ss. *jejuni.* 2. Serotyping of live bacteria by slide, latex and co-agglutination tests. *Acta Pathol. Microbiol. Scand., Sect. B* **90B,** 191–196.

17. Kosunen, T. U., Pöllänen, S., Hänninen, M. L., and Danielsson, D. (1982). Are the *Campylobacter jejuni* strains from different species similar? *In* "Campylobacter" (D. G. Newell, ed.), pp. 45–49. MTP Press, Lancaster, England.

18. Kosunen, T. U., Rautelin, H., Pitkänen, T., Pönkä, A., and Pettersson, T. (1983). Antibodies against an acid extract from a single *Campylobacter* strain in hospitalized *Campylobacter* patients. *Infection* **11,** 189–191.

19. Lauwers, S., Vlaes, L., and Butzler, J. P. (1981). *Campylobacter* serotyping and epidemiology. *Lancet* **i,** 158–159.

20. Lior, H., and Lacroix, R. (1983). Detection of *Campylobacter jejuni* and *Campylobacter coli* serum antibodies using paper enzyme-linked immunosorbent assay. *In* "Campylobacter II" (A. D. Pearson, M. B. Skirrow, B. Rowe, J. R. Davies, and D. M. Jones, eds.), pp. 72–73. Public Health Lab. Serv., London.

21. Lior, H., Woodward, D. L., Edgar, J. A., Laroche, L. J., and Gill, P. (1982). Serotyping of *Campylobacter jejuni* by slide agglutination based on heat-labile antigenic factors. *J. Clin. Microbiol.* **15,** 761–768.
22. Lior, H., Woodward, D. L., Laroche, L. J., Lacroix, R., and Edgar, J. A. (1983). Serotyping by slide agglutination and biotyping of *Campylobacter jejuni* and *Campylobacter coli*. *In* "Campylobacter II" (A. D. Pearson, M. B. Skirrow, B. Rowe, J. R. Davies, and D. M. Jones, eds.), p. 87. Public Health Lab. Serv., London.
23. Liu, T.-Y., Gotschlich, E. C., Jonssen, E. K., and Wysocki, J. R. (1971). Studies on the meningococcal polysaccharides. I. Composition and chemical properties of the group A polysaccharide. *J. Biol. Chem.* **246,** 2849–2858.
24. Logan, S. M., and Trust, T. J. (1982). Outer membrane characteristics of *Campylobacter jejuni*. *Infect. Immun.* **38,** 898–906.
25. Logan, S. M., and Trust, T. J. (1983). Molecular identification of surface protein antigens of *Campylobacter jejuni*. *Infect. Immun.* **42,** 675–682.
26. Logan, S. M., and Trust, T. J. (1983). Monoclonal antibody analysis of the surface antigens of *Campylobacter jejuni*. *In* "Campylobacter II" (A. D. Pearson, M. B. Skirrow, B. Rowe, J. R. Davies, and D. M. Jones, eds.), pp. 69–70. Public Health Lab. Serv., London.
27. Logan, S. M., and Trust, T. J. (1984). Structural and antigenic heterogeneity of lipopolysaccharides of *Campylobacter jejuni* and *Campylobacter coli*. *Infect. Immun.* **45,** 210–216.
28. McCoy, E. C., Doyle, D., Burda, K., Corbeil, L. B., and Winter, A. J. (1975). Superficial antigens of *Campylobacter (Vibrio) fetus:* Characterization of an antiphagocytic component. *Infect. Immun.* **11,** 517–525.
29. McCoy, E. C., Wiltberger, H. A., and Winter, A. J. (1976). Major outer membrane protein of *Campylobacter fetus:* Physical and immunological characterization. *Infect. Immun.* **13,** 1258–1265.
30. Milstein, C. (1982). Monoclonal antibodies from hybrid myelomas: Theoretical aspects and some general comments. *In* "Monoclonal Antibodies in Clinical Medicine" (A. J. McMichael, and J. W. Fabre, eds.), pp. 3–16. Academic Press, New York.
31. Newell, D. G. (1983). Monoclonal antibodies against *Campylobacter jejuni* flagella. *In* "Campylobacter II" (A. D. Pearson, M. B. Skirrow, B. Rowe, J. R. Davies, and D. M. Jones, eds.), pp. 70–71. Public Health Lab. Serv., London.
32. Palva, E. T., and Mäkelä, P. H. (1980). Lipopolysaccharide heterogeneity in *Salmonella typhimurium* analyzed by sodium dodecyl sulfate–polyacrylamide gel electrophoresis. *Eur. J. Biochem.* **107,** 137–143.
33. Penner, J. L., and Hennessy, J. N. (1980). Passive hemagglutination technique for serotyping *Campylobacter fetus* subsp. *jejuni* on the basis of soluble heat-stable antigens. *J. Clin. Microbiol.* **12,** 732–737.
34. Penner, J. L., Hennessy, J. N., Congi, R. V., and Pearson, A. D. (1983). Progress in the development of a serotyping scheme on the basis of thermostable antigens for *Campylobacter jejuni* and *Campylobacter coli*. *In* "Campylobacter II" (A. D. Pearson, M. B. Skirrow, B. Rowe, J. R. Davies, and D. M. Jones, eds.), p. 90. Public Health Lab. Serv., London.
35. Rettig, P. J. (1979). *Campylobacter* infections in human beings. *J. Pediatr.* **94,** 855–864.
36. Ristic, M., and Murty, D. K. (1961). Characterization of *Vibrio fetus* antigens, IV. Study of polysaccharide–antibody reactions by a rapid slide gel diffusion technique. *Am. J. Vet. Res.* **22,** 783–789.
37. Skerman, V. B. D., McGowan, V., and Sneath, P. H. A. (1980). Approved lists of bacterial names. *Int. J. Syst. Bacteriol.* **30,** 225–420.
38. Skirrow, M. B. (1977). *Campylobacter* enteritis: a "new" disease. *Br. Med. J.* **ii,** 9–11.
39. Skirrow, M. B. (1983). Report on the session taxonomy and biotyping. *In* "Campylobacter II" (A. D. Pearson, M. B. Skirrow, B. Rowe, J. R. Davies, and D. M. Jones, eds.), pp. 33–38. Public Health Lab. Serv., London.

40. Skirrow, M. B., and Benjamin, J. (1980). Differentiation of enteropathogenic *Campylobacter*. *J. Clin. Pathol.* **33**, 1122.

41. Smibert, R. M. (1974). *Campylobacter*. *In* "Bergey's Manual of Determinative Bacteriology" (R. E. Buchanan and N. E. Gibbons, eds.), 8th Ed., pp. 207–212. Williams & Wilkins, Baltimore, Maryland.

42. Smibert, R. M. (1978). The genus *Campylobacter*. *Annu. Rev. Microbiol.* **32**, 673–709.

43. Stead, A., Main, J. S., Ward, M. E., and Watt, P. J. (1975). Studies on lipopolysaccharides isolated from strains of *Neisseria gonorrhoeae*. *J. Gen. Microbiol.* **88**, 123–131.

44. Sugasawara, R. J., Prato, C. M., and Sippel, J. E. (1984). Enzyme-linked immunosorbent assay with a monoclonal antibody for detecting group A meningococcal antigens in cerebrospinal fluid. *J. Clin. Microbiol.* **19**, 230–234.

45. Svedhem, Å., Gunnarsson, H., and Kaijser, B. (1982). Serological diagnosis of *Campylobacter jejuni* infections using the enzyme-linked immunosorbent assay principle. *In* "Campylobacter" (D. G. Newell, ed.), pp. 118–121. MTP Press, Lancaster, England.

46. Svedhem, A., Gunnarsson, H., and Kaijser, B. (1983). Diffusion-in-gel enzyme linked immunosorbent assay for routine detection of IgG and IgM antibodies to *Campylobacter jejuni*. *J. Infect. Dis.* **148**, 82–92.

47. Taylor, D. J. (1982). Natural and experimental enteric infections with catalase-positive campylobacters in cattle and pigs. *In* "Campylobacter" (D. G. Newell, ed.), pp. 163–166. MTP Press, Lancaster, England.

48. Tsai, C. M., and Frasch, C. E. (1982). A sensitive silver stain for detecting lipopolysaccharide in polyacrylamide gels. *Anal. Biochem.* **119**, 115–119.

49. Véron, M., and Chatelain, R. (1973). Taxonomic study of the genus *Campylobacter* Sebald Véron and designation of the neotype strain for the type species, *Campylobacter fetus* (Smith and Taylor) Sebald and Véron. *Int. J. Syst. Bacteriol.* **23**, 122–134.

50. Warren, J. R., and Marshall, B. J. (1983). Unidentified curved bacilli on gastric epithelium in active chronic gastritis. *Lancet* **i**, 1273–1275.

51. Watson, K. C., Kerr, E. J. C., and McFadzean, S. M. (1979). Serology of human *Campylobacter* infections. *J. Infect.* **1**, 151–158.

52. Wiidik, R. W., and Hlidar, G. E. (1955). Untersuchungen über die antigene Struktur von *Vibrio fetus* vom Rind. Das Kapsel- oder K-Antigen von *Vibrio fetus*. *Zentralbl. Veterinaermed.* **2**, 238–250.

53. Winter, A. J. (1966). An antigenic analysis of *Vibrio fetus*. III. Chemical, biologic and antigenic properties of the endotoxin. *Am. J. Vet. Res.* **27**, 653–658.

54. Winter, A. J., McCoy, E. C., Fullmer, C. S., Burda, K., and Bier, P. J. (1978). Microcapsule of *Campylobacter fetus*: Chemical and physical characterization. *Infect. Immun.* **22**, 963–971.

5

Monoclonal Antibodies to the Lipopolysaccharide and Capsular Polysaccharide of *Bacteroides fragilis*

MATTI K. VILJANEN,* LINNÉA LINKO,*
PERTTI ARSTILA,† OLLI-PEKKA LEHTONEN,*
AND ANDREJ WEINTRAUB‡
*Department of Medical Microbiology
University of Turku
Turku, Finland
†Department of Virology
University of Turku
Turku, Finland
‡Department of Clinical Bacteriology
Huddinge University Hospital
Huddinge, Sweden

119

I. INTRODUCTION

Bacteroides fragilis has been studied extensively in recent years. One aim of these studies has been to identify the superficial and extracellular structures that account for the distinct pathogenicity of this organism. Another important aim has been to establish immunologic methods for rapid diagnosis of the usually severe infections caused by this fastidious organism. The immunologic analysis of the outer-membrane (OM) components and extracellular polysaccharides of *B. fragilis* has, until recently, been performed by means of polyclonal antibodies. Several factors, however, complicate the interpretation of results obtained by conventional antisera. These include the insurmountable difficulty of purification and the abundant phenotypic variation of the various cell wall and extracellular components, as well as the occurrence of natural antibodies to *B. fragilis* in animals used for antiserum production. Some of these problems can be overcome by using monoclonal antibodies (MAbs). Even relatively impure antigen preparations can be used for immunization, provided that reliable methods are available for demonstration of the specificity properties and target structures of the MAbs obtained. At least in theory, these antibodies can recognize a common antigenic epitope in an antigen with other varying determinants, and, on the other hand, they can reveal labile minor determinants that are never shown by polyclonal antibodies. A definite advantage of MAbs is that they can be produced in serum-free media *in vitro,* where the interference of natural antibodies can be avoided. We describe here the results of a study on MAbs to two pathogenetically interesting surface structures of *B. fragilis,* lipopolysaccharide (LPS) and capsular polysaccharide (CPS), both of them promising candidates for diagnostic antigen detection.

II. BACKGROUND

A. Immunologic Implications of the Structure of *Bacteroides fragilis* LPS and CPS

Bacteroides fragilis LPS has several unique structural features. It has been shown that the LPS lacks 3-deoxy-D-mannooctulosonic acid (dOclA, formerly termed KDO) and L-glycero-D-mannoheptose (18,26). Recently, however, strong evidence has been presented that *B. fragilis* LPS does contain a dOclA derivative that may differ from that found in Enterobacteriaceae (Brade H. and Weintraub A., unpublished observation). The lipid A of *B. fragilis* LPS does not contain 3-hydroxymyristic acid, a major fatty acid in aerobic gram-negative bacteria (49). This and other unique features in the lipid composition of *B. fragilis* LPS may be related to its low endotoxicity (26). However, from the immunologic point of view, the most prominent structural property of *B. fragilis* LPS is the absence of the long heteropolysaccharide chain (26,46). It thus resembles the rough-type LPSs of aerobic bacteria and can apparently not show serovariation to the extent that typical smooth-type LPSs can do. Since the O chains are absent, the more conservative parts of the LPS are immunologically exposed. Thus, production of antibodies cross-reactive with a large array of gram-negative bacteria can be expected to occur. The wide cross-reactivity of antibodies to the rough-type LPS of *Escherichia coli* strongly supports this allegation (36). A study using polyclonal antibodies has, however, shown that antibodies to *B. fragilis* only react with most *B. fragilis* strains and some other members of *B. fragilis* group (47). Therefore, the differences between the LPS of *B. fragilis* and that of aerobic bacteria are so profound that immunologically dominant antigenic determinants specific to *B. fragilis* do occur. The best candidates for these determinants are located in the oligosaccharide part of LPS comprising 8–10 sugar residues (48), which is probably comparable to the core of typical LPSs. In view of the low immunogenicity of lipids, it is hard to believe that differences in fatty acid composition could account for differences in immunologically important epitopes. In addition, fatty acids are closely linked to, and surrounded by, the hydrophobic parts of OM proteins (51). This makes them less easily available to the immune system.

The extreme complexity and variability of *B. fragilis* CPS makes it difficult to obtain valid information about the structure of the *B. fragilis* capsule. Particular care has to be taken during *in vitro* studies of laboratory-passaged *B. fragilis* strains (24). Both quantitative and qualitative changes occur in the capsule with consecutive cultures; the thickness of the capsule is decreased and the relative amount of glucose is increased at the expense of galactose and glucosamine. In parallel, the capsule is replaced by a glycan with a glycogenlike structure. That some of the original capsular antigens are retained is indicated by the fact that some binding of CPS antibodies to laboratory-passaged bacteria occurs (24). However, the antisera used in the immunologic studies of the *B. fragilis* capsule have been produced by immunization with killed and repeatedly washed organisms, or with highly purified CPS. It is possible that these methods only produce antibodies to the most resistant parts of the capsule. These antibodies cannot be used to detect the labile outermost structures occurring during natural infection. The best possible antibodies for the study of the capsule and other exopolysaccharides of *B. fragilis* are probably obtained from animals infected with bacterium. However, in the polyclonal antibody response, antibodies are produced both to superficial and deep capsular structures. Antibodies to resistant deep structures may far outnumber antibodies to superficial determinants. Investigation of the ultrastructure of bacterial capsule is further complicated by the collapse of this water-containing structure with the dehydration processes of electron microscopy. The shrinkage can, at lease partially, be prevented by cross-linking the CPS chains with antibodies (28). This conserves, however, only those parts of the CPS to which antibodies are available.

B. LPS and CPS as Virulence Factors of *Bacteroides fragilis*

Although *B. fragilis* accounts for only 0.5% of the colonic microflora, it is the anaerobic bacterial species most often isolated in cases of intraabdominal sepsis and the most common blood culture isolate in patients with anaerobic bacteremia (12). This strongly suggests that *B. fragilis* has unique virulence properties.

Bacteroides fragilis has an OM similar to that of aerobic gram-negative bacteria (28). An integral component of OM is LPS, which usually acts as endotoxin and is therefore an important virulence factor of aerobic bacteria. However, as mentioned above, *B. fragilis* LPS has very low biologic activity when tested in different *in vivo* models (26). Since its toxicity is low, patients with *B. fragilis* bacteremia rarely suffer from disseminated intravascular coagulation or purpural skin lesions, disorders clearly attributable to endotoxins (25).

Interestingly, although *B. fragilis* LPS is atoxic it still has a mitogenic activity on lymphocytes (21). The atoxic LPSs of *B. fragilis* and other members of the *B. fragilis* group may serve as stimulatory factors in the maturation of the immune system.

The capsule is probably the most important virulence factor of *B. fragilis*. Encapsulated *B. fragilis* strains produce abscesses in experimental infections, whereas unencapsulated strains can produce abscesses only when combined with aerobic bacteria (25). The growth of bacteria is not necessary for abscess formation, since abscesses can be produced in animals injected with heat-killed encapsulated *B. fragilis* strains or even with purified CPS (25). The antibody response to CPS occurring in various clinical and experimental infections, and the absence in CPS-immunized animals of early bacteremia and abscesses further emphasize the central pathogenetic role of the capsule (23,25).

The relationship between capsular and other exopolysaccharides of *B. fragilis* is poorly understood. The bacterial glycocalyx is known to mediate bacterial adhesion to surfaces (8), and confer resistance to bacteriophages (50), surfactants (13), specific antibodies (2), phagocytes (43), and certain antibiotics (14). The glycocalyx contains about 99% water (44), and it tends to be reduced to a sharply condensed residue after dehydration for ultrastructural studies. Lambe *et al.* (30), who used antibody cross-linking of exopolysaccharides, showed that *B.*

fragilis may have a large glycocalyx. The role of the glycocalyx in the pathogenesis of infections with *B. fragilis* can be shown by using antibodies to its outermost structures. More gentle techniques are needed for studying the glycocalyx in its natural conformation in the infection focus.

C. Serologic Variation of *Bacteroides fragilis* LPS and CPS

Earlier reports on the serologic heterogeneity of *B. fragilis* somatic antigens are highly discrepant. Hofstad (19), Cherniak *et al.* (4), and Elhag *et al.* (5,6) reported a pronounced multispecificity of *B. fragilis* somatic antigens. The results obtained by Rissing *et al.* (39) using an antibody-inhibition enzyme immunoassay (EIA) suggested that the LPS is a serogroup-specific antigen unsuitable for diagnostic purposes. Similar results were obtained by Abshire *et al.* (1), who used an antigen extracted from *B. fragilis* with trichloroacetic acid. On the other hand, Lambe and Moroz (31) observed that an antigen, designated as E antigen and having LPS-like properties, was present in 86% of isolates. Recently, Kasper *et al.* (27) and Weintraub *et al.* (46) showed that LPS rather than the capsular polysaccharide is common to most *B. fragilis* isolates, with 88% of strains positive in immunofluorescence assay with an antiserum to the LPS of prototype strain NCTC 9343.

Serogrouping of many bacteria is based on CPS antigens. However, the assessment of capsular heterogeneity is complicated by the large variation in the amount of capsular material. The early results of Kasper (22) indicated that CPS antigen could be used for differentiating *B. fragilis* from other subspecies of the *B. fragilis* group. Later results of antigen-specific immunofluorescence assays have shown that only 50% of clinical *B. fragilis* isolates yield a positive reaction with antiserum to CPS, in contrast to the 88% obtained with antiserum to *B. fragilis* LPS (46). When mouse-passaged *B. fragilis* reference strains (ATCC 23745 and NCTC 9343) were cultured in a rich medium supplemented with 1% glucose and 10% fetal calf serum, a high yield of CPS, apparently resembling that in a natural infection, was obtained (27). The CPSs of these strains definitely differed from each other chemically, and in an inhibition they only showed a very weak cross-reaction. The number of the immunologic varieties of *B. fragilis* CPS is not known. The above studies, however, indicate that CPS could have structural variation to a much larger extent than LPS.

D. *Bacteroides fragilis* LPS and CPS as Diagnostic Antigens

An ideal antigen for immunodiagnostic assays should be specific to a given bacterial species, it should not express antigenic variation, it should be excreted by the bacteria in sufficient amounts, and it should retain its immunologic reactivity in various body fluids. As discussed above, the specificity and serologic heterogeneity properties of LPS seem more suitable for immunologic diagnostic purposes than those of CPS (27,46). The most efficient assays can probably be established by combining the demonstrations of both of these antigens (46).

LPS is an essential structure for the integrity of gram-negative organisms and is abundant in the OM (34). As gram-negative bacteria grow *in vitro,* they shed LPS into the medium. LPS is usually associated with OM proteins and phospholipids (9,41), and it is likely that fragments of varying size are shed from OM. Rissing *et al.* (39) showed that *B. fragilis* LPS is excreted in an immunologically active form in the urine. For this to occur, it is necessary that the LPS be degraded to a monomeric form capable of being filtered into the urine. Excretion in the urine is enabled by the small molecular size of monomeric *B. fragilis* LPS, which makes it an exceptionally promising candidate for antigen detection. The LPS possibly reaggregates in the urine because of its amphipathic properties (26).

When antibodies to *B. fragilis* LPS are used in immunofluorescence assays, they efficiently stain most clinical isolates (47). However, it is not known whether a thick exopolysaccharide layer could prevent the binding of LPS antibodies to their targets and thus interfere with demonstration of *B. fragilis* in fresh clinical isolates. As mentioned above, the results obtained by studying strains grown *in vitro* may be misleading (24).

Recent studies on *B. fragilis* glycocalyx suggest that a large amount of exopolysaccharides is produced at the site of infection (30). These polysaccharides probably facilitate the attachment of the bacterium to surfaces and prevent the host's immune attacks. Thus, it is reasonable to think that an abundant amount of exopolysaccharides is released from the infection focus. It is not known whether *B. fragilis* capsular polysaccharides appear in body fluids in an immunologically active form, but the results of studies on other encapsulated bacteria are highly suggestive of this. Polysaccharide antigens are resistant to enzymes in tissues and body fluids and excreted through the kidneys (7). Pneumococcal antigens can even be released from phagocytes and return to the circulation and bind free antibodies (20). CPS antigens of streptococci and pneumococci have been detected in serum, urine, and sputum in the course of various infections (17,35,37).

III. RESULTS AND DISCUSSION

A. Production of Monoclonal Antibodies (MAbs)

B. fragilis was grown throughout this study on *Brucella* blood agar (BBA) plates supplemented with vitamin K_1 (10 μg/ml), and hemin (1 μg/ml) in anaerobic jars. In the production of MAbs to *B. fragilis* LPS, a Triton X-100-treated OM preparation originating from prototype strain ATCC 23745 was used for immunization of BALB/c mice (32). Since the immunogen was subjected to high-speed ultracentrifugation after Triton X-100 treatment, all membrane fragments were apparently eliminated. As Kuusi *et al.* (29) have shown, the treatment of *Salmonella typhimurium* OMs with this weak nonionic detergent does not break up protein–protein linkages, and LPS is a major component of the crude preparation obtained. Another possibility is that LPS binds to protein–Triton X-100 micelles (16), and that most hydrophilic structures are located on the surfaces of these micelles. Whatever the conformation obtained by this treatment, the LPS of *B. fragilis* appeared to be in a highly immunogenic form, since all the 19 clones that yielded a positive reaction in an EIA with *B. fragilis* sonicate produced antibodies to the LPS (32). This suggests that the complexes did not contain immunogenic OM proteins or that only the hydrophobic parts of the proteins were present. These parts seem to reassociate with lipid A and become embedded in the complexes (9).

Air-exposed *B. fragilis* organisms (ATCC 23745, 10^7 per injection) were used for immunization in the production of MAbs to CPS. The 12 clones yielding a positive reaction against crude *B. fragilis* antigen were identical in the primary specificity testing. Thus, the MAbs obtained by this method were exclusively directed against the capsular structures of *B. fragilis*. This suggests that either the prototype strain retains its essential capsular antigens during *in vitro* passages or that some live organisms were injected into the animals. The bacteria were briefly exposed to atmospheric oxygen during their manipulation in aerobic conditions, and fresh cultures were used for each immunization. Although the animals did not show any marked signs of peritoneal infection at the time of removal of their spleens, it is possible that the bacterium had started to regain its capsule but not to the extent that it could cause abscesses. However, it should be kept in mind that the assay used for the primary screening of the culture media may favor some antigenic structures but not others, and thus provide false information about the spectrum of antibodies originally produced.

B. Specificity of LPS MAbs

All 19 monoclonals reactive with *B. fragilis* LPS appeared to be almost equally reactive in the preliminary studies; four of those with the highest titers in the enzyme-linked immunosorbent assay (ELISA) were selected for further studies (32). The specificities of the MAbs selected were studied by an inhibition EIA against 14 anaerobic (134 strains) and 14 aerobic (49 strains) bacterial species (Table I) (32). Two MAbs gave a positive reaction with 68 (95.7%), and the other two with 66 (93.0%) of the 71 *B. fragilis* strains tested. Prototype strains ATCC 23745 and NCTC 9343 caused equal inhibitions (Table I). Three wild strains were negative with all MAbs. They were retested with API 20A, and patterns matching with *B. fragilis* were obtained. They also showed metabolite patterns typical of *B. fragilis* as analyzed by high-performance liquid chromatography and gas–liquid chromatography (15). The inhibitions by strains interpreted as positive showed some variation. This could be due to differences in the quantities of bacteria, although some rough equalization of bacterial amounts was attempted. However, the bacterial concentrations used in the inhibition EIA were so high that there should have been enough antigen for total inhibition. The variation in the inhibition figures may reflect slight differences in the target determinant. The fact that the reactivities to different *B. fragilis* strains of the four MAbs were not quite equal suggests some differences in their fine specificity. The main finding, however, was that *B. fragilis* LPS carries an immunodominant antigenic determinant common to almost all strains tested. This confirms earlier findings obtained by polyclonal antibodies (27,47).

The MAbs gave varying results with the nine *B. thetaiotaomicron* strains tested. One MAb (BF6) reacted with two strains, one (BF3) with four, one (BF5) with five, and one (BF7) with six strains (Table I). By contrast, the MAbs were identical in their reactions to the five *B. ovatus* strains, all of them giving a

TABLE I

Reaction of MAbs to *Bacteroides fragilis* LPS with Different Anaerobic and Aerobic Organisms Tested by Inhibition EIA

				MAb					
			BF3		BF5		BF6		BF7
Organism		n^a	Inhib.[b]	n	Inhib.	n	Inhib.	n	Inhib.
B. fragilis									
ATCC 23745			729		707		630		717
NCTC 9343			751		497		663		492
Clinical isolates	+	64	711 ± 131	66	648 ± 131	64	654 ± 155	66	580 ± 93
	−	5	89 ± 58	3	38 ± 64	5	55 ± 43	3	64 ± 60
B. thetaiotaomicron	+	4	399 ± 35	5	469 ± 113	2	463 ± 237	6	373 ± 103
	−	5	0	4	6 ± 26	7	41 ± 65	3	79 ± 68
B. ovatus	+	2	348 ± 69	2	541 ± 4	2	277 ± 47	2	570 ± 11
	−	3	0	3	0	3	0	3	0
B. ureolyticus	+	0		0		1	160	0	
	−	3	28 ± 31	3	8 ± 14	2	0	3	8 ± 14
Pseudomonas aeruginosa	+	0		1	269	0		0	
	−	4	55 ± 58	3	42 ± 73	4	4 ± 9	4	87 ± 25

[a] Number of positive (+) and negative (−) organisms tested. Negative were (the number of strains in parentheses) *B. vulgatus* (8), *B. distasonis* (2), *B. uniformis* (4), *B. melaninogenicus* (2), *B. bivius* (14), *B. disiens* (1), *Fusobacterium necrophorum* (3), *Fusobacterium nucleatum* (6), *Clostridium perfringens* (3), *Clostridium difficile* (3), *Escherichia coli* (4), *Salmonella typhi* (1), *Klebsiella pneumoniae* (4), *Proteus vulgaris* (4), *Yersinia enterocolitica* O:3 (4), *Haemophilus influenzae* (4), *Bordetella pertussis* (4), *Legionella pneumophila* (1), *Staphylococcus aureus* (4), *Staphylococcus epidermidis* (4), *Streptococcus faecalis* (4), β-*hemolytic streptococci* (4), *Streptococcus pyogenes* (3).

[b] The number and mean ± SD inhibition (decrease in OD_{405} × 1000) are given for positive and negative strains.

positive reaction with the same two strains. The decrease in OD_{405} values caused by positive strains in these species was consistently half that caused by *B. fragilis* itself. In view of what was said above about the excessive amount of bacteria used in the inhibition, this lower binding suggests only partial similarity between the target determinant of the MAb in *B. fragilis*, *B. thetaiotaomicron*, and *B. ovatus*.

All the other bacteria tested gave a negative result, except for a marginal reaction of BF6 with one *B. ureolyticus* strain, and BF5 with one *Pseudomonas aeruginosa* strain (Table I).

Twelve LPS preparations were tested by the inhibition EIA test. The only LPS preparation causing marked inhibition was that of *B. fragilis* (Table II).

C. Specificity of CPS MAbs

From the 12 monoclonals obtained by immunizing mice with whole *B. fragilis* organisms, two (2A4 and 2A5) with the highest titers in the primary EIA were selected for further studies. When these MAbs were tested in parallel with LPS MAbs as described above, they showed an unexpectedly restricted specificity; they yielded a positive reaction only with the prototype strain ATCC 23745 that was used for immunization (data not shown). Further studies were carried out with monoclonal 2A4.

TABLE II

Reaction of MAbs to *Bacteroides fragilis* LPS with LPSs Extracted from Different Organisms

	MAb			
LPS source	BF3	BF5	BF6	BF7
B. fragilis (ATCC 23745)	625[a]	643	596	568
Fusobacterium nucleatum	103	27	43	29
Salmonella re	145	26	145	106
Salmonella typhi	63	0	24	26
Salmonella typhimurium	128	69	54	52
Salmonella minnesota	79	13	32	72
Salmonella enteritidis	61	0	4	12
Salmonella abortus	87	0	44	60
Escherichia coli	65	0	76	28
Yersinia enterocolitica O:3	97	17	25	20
Klebsiella pneumoniae	100	0	0	0
Vibrio cholerae Inaba	70	0	33	0

[a] The values express the decrease in $OD_{405} \times 1000$ caused by LPS in inhibition EIA. Inhibitions caused by formalin-treated *B. fragilis* ATCC 23745 were 729, 707, 630, and 717 for clones BF3, BF5, BF6, and BF7, respectively.

D. Immunoblotting by LPS MAbs

A vertical sodium dodecyl sulfate–polyacrylamide gel electrophoresis (SDS–PAGE) slab gel with a gradient of 7 to 17.5%, according to the method of O'Farrell (38), transfer of antigens from the gel onto a nitrocellulose sheet as described by Towbin *et al.* (45) and modified by Gless *et al.* (10), was used (42) with purified *B. fragilis* LPS (Fig. 1A), the OM of strain ATCC 23745 (Fig. 1B), the OM of one inhibition EIA-positive *B. fragilis* strain (Fig. 1C), and one negative strain (Fig. 1D). In silver staining the LPS gave only one band (13,000–12,000 Da) (Fig. 1A, 1). In the corresponding gels from the prototype strain (Fig. 1B, 1) and the inhibition EIA-positive strain (Fig. 1D, 1), several heavy bands occurred in this molecular weight area, preventing the identification of any LPS bands. Silver staining of the inhibition EIA-negative strain (Fig. 1C, 1) showed 7–10 faint bands in the molecular weight area of 10,000 to 20,000. None of them was clearly identical with that of purified LPS. In addition to the bands in this range, several bands occurred in the higher molecular weight area of all silver-stained gels, except that of the purified LPS.

All four MAbs showed a very strong reaction in immunoblotting with purified *B. fragilis* LPS (Fig. 1A, 2–5). The reaction occurred in the molecular weight area of 8000 to 20,000 and was homogeneous. A strong and wide reaction was also observed in the immunoblotting of type strain ATCC 23745 (Fig. 1B, 2–5)

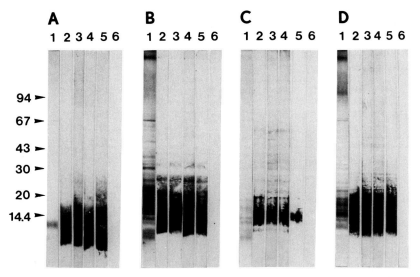

Fig. 1. Analysis of *B. fragilis* LPS (A), OM fraction of *B. fragilis* prototype strain ATCC 23745 (B), OM of an inhibition EIA-negative (C) and positive strain (D) by SDS–PAGE and immunoblotting. Silver-stained SDS–PAGE gel (1), immunoblotting with monoclonal BF3 (2), BF5 (3), BF6 (4), BF7 (5), and with a control MAb (6). Reprinted from reference (42) with permission of the publisher, American Society for Microbiology.

and the immunoassay-positive strain (Fig. 1D, 2–5). The reaction areas were even wider than that of purified LPS, with a range of l0,000 to 27,000 Da. The immunoblotting pattern of the inhibition EIA-negative strain (Fig. 1C, 2–5) differed from those obtained with the other OM preparations. The reaction was strikingly weaker and occurred in the molecular weight area of 12,000 to 20,000. One MAb (BF7, Fig. 1C, 5) gave a clearly narrower reaction with this strain than the other MAbs. The control MAb (a commercial MAb to myelin basic protein) did not react with purified LPS (Fig. 1A, 6). Various faint bands of larger molecular size than that of LPS occurred in immunoblotting both with MAbs to LPS and control MAb, (myelin basic protein) which indicated that these bands were probably due to anti-*B. fragilis* reactivity in the swine antiserum to rabbit IgG.

The inhibition EIA method may be more affinity-dependent than immunoblotting. This difference may explain the variable behavior of one *B. fragilis* strain in these tests. This organism, selected on the basis of its negative reaction in the inhibition EIA, showed a positive reaction in immunoblotting. The differences in staining intensities between the strains seemed to be due to different amounts of loaded LPS. The *B. fragilis* strain negative in the EIA consistently showed weaker reactions in silver staining and immunoblotting, although the protein load was made equal to that of the other strains.

Although molecular weight markers for proteins are not suitable for estimation of the size of LPS in SDS–gel electrophoresis (42), the estimated weight of purified LPS, 12,000–13,000, is very similar to that reported by Kasper (26) for the monomeric molecular weight of *B. fragilis* LPS, and by Goldman and Leive (11) for the lipid A – core oligosaccharide structure of *E. coli*. However, reliable particle size estimations can only be obtained with LPSs of known size as internal standards (42). The homogeneous staining patterns suggest that the LPS of *B. fragilis* does not contain long chains composed of repeating units. It thus closely resembles the rough-type LPSs of aerobic gram-negative bacteria.

There was a striking difference in the staining of LPS in silver-stained gel and in immunoblotting with MAbs. Immense and homogeneous staining occurred in immunoblotting in a very wide molecular weight range (8000–27,000). This difference may be due to washout of LPS during staining of the gel. This shows, however, that LPS can be transferred electrophoretically with great efficiency from the SDS gel to nitrocellulose. This is in agreement with the report by Bradbury *et al.* (3) on the efficiency of immunoblotting in the detection of the different components of LPS.

E. Nature and Localization of the Target Determinant of One LPS MAb

The reaction of one of the LPS MAbs (BF7) to LPS preparations extracted from 14 different *B. fragilis* strains was tested using both inhibition EIA and

TABLE III

Concentrations of Different *Bacteroides fragilis* LPS Preparations Causing 50% Inhibition in the Binding of the LPS-Specific Monoclonal (MAb BF7) and Polyclonal Antibodies to LPS Extracted from *B. fragilis* Strain NCTC 9343

	LPS from strain (μg/ml)																
	4361	9343	4117	E323	23745	Ic650	6059	6815	10584	2556	Tm4000	6851	6057	2554	2552	4225	5631
MAb	4.4	2.2	2.0	1.8	1.6	1.6	1.2	1.1	1.1	1.0	0.8	0.7	0.4	0.3	9.0	>100[a]	>100
Polyclonal antibody	0.1	0.3	5.0	0.1	0.4	0.04	0.3	0.1	0.1	0.1	0.03	0.3	0.2	0.7	7.5	>100	>100

[a] No significant inhibition was obtained even at the highest LPS concentration used.

immunoblotting (33). Two LPS preparations (4225,5631) gave a negative reaction, and the other 12 gave a positive reaction in both tests (Table III and Fig. 2). The two LPSs differed from the other preparations. One (5631) does not contain any D-galactose in its polysaccharide part. The second one (4225) contains D-galactose but in much lower quantities than the other preparations (46). This shows that the antigenic determinant of this MAb is located in the polysaccharide part of LPS and that D-Galactose is an essential part of it. When monomeric D-galactose was used in the inhibition EIA, no blocking was seen (data not shown). This observation suggests that this monosaccharide makes only a part of the determinant, and its absence significantly alters the antigenic specificity of the oligosaccharide.

The MAb BF7 and a polyclonal antiserum to *B. fragilis* LPS (27) yielded similar results in the inhibition EIA (Table III). This indicates that the determinant is of higher immunogenicity when compared to the other parts of LPS. This concept of immunodominancy was also supported by the finding that all clones obtained by immunizing mice with the OM preparation produced antibodies essentially equal to that selected for further characterization of the target determinant. Since the polyclonal antibody to this common determinant reacts with whole *B. fragilis* organisms in an indirect immunofluorescence assay (47), the

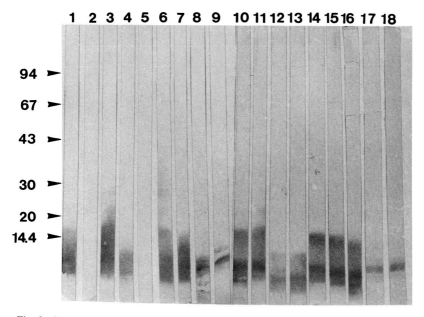

Fig. 2   Immunoblotting of 14 *B. fragilis* LPSs (1–14), prototype strains (ATCC 23745, NCTC 9343) (15,16), and two wild strains (17,18) with LPS MAb BF7. LPSs 2 and 5 were negative in EIA inhibition and did not contain D-galactose in their oligosaccharide moieties.

determinant has to be exposed on the surface of bacterial OM and thence available to antibodies. In our earlier study, the binding of LPS MAbs to their target on solid phase could also be inhibited by whole bacteria (Section III,B) (42). The exposed location of the galactose-containing determinant could be confirmed by electron microscopy–immunocytochemistry (EIC) (33). EIC labeling with the LPS MAb and protein A–gold and staining with ruthenium red (40) showed an intensive reaction on the surface of the OM (Fig. 3). In addition, some gold particles were bound to debris apparently detached from the bacteria. There was no binding in surface areas covered with capsule material.

Unexpectedly, only part (~10%) of organisms in the same culture yielded a positive reaction in the EIC (Fig. 3). This was not due to the capsule, since most of the negative bacteria in the EIC contained no visible capsule. The cells which gave a positive reaction in EIC were generally smaller than the organisms with-

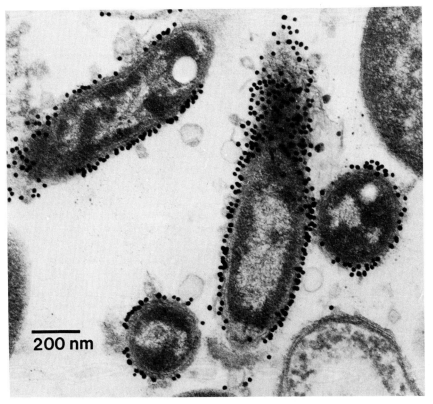

Fig. 3. EIC study of a *B. fragilis* strain isolated from a clinical specimen. Bacteria were incubated with one LPS MAb BF7 and protein A–gold (particle diameter 15 nm). Polysaccharide staining was with ruthenium red.

out any antibody binding (Fig. 3). It remains to be shown whether this heterogeneity is dependent on the growth phase of the organisms and whether it also occurs when the bacteria grow *in vivo*.

F. Immunoblotting by One CPS MAb

The reaction of one of the CPS MAbs (2A4) was studied by immunoblotting against the following antigens: whole cells of prototype strains ATCC 23745 and NCTC 9343, purified CPSs originating from these strains (27), whole cells of two clinical isolates recultured from our stock cultures (maintained in tryptone soya broth containing 20% glycerol at $-70°C$), and two fresh clinical isolates. The MAb yielded a clearly positive reaction with the whole cells of the prototype strains at a molecular weight area over 200,000 (Fig. 4). An unexpected finding was that only the CPS of NCTC 9343 strain gave a positive reaction in this test. The band was located in the same molecular weight area as that obtained with whole bacteria (Fig. 4). Thus, the CPS extracted from the strain used for immunization of the mice remained negative. Kasper *et al.* (27) showed that the CPSs of these reference strains differ from one another chemically and immunochemically. The present results, however, suggest that these CPSs must have a common antigenic determinant, but the determinant is more labile in the ATCC 23745 strain and does not resist the purification process. The labile nature of the determinant was further ascertained by the result of immunoblotting with clinical isolates. In agreement with the inhibition EIA results, none of the wild strains recultured from storage tubes yielded any reaction with the CPS MAb in immunoblotting (Fig. 4). However, when the same analysis was carried out on fresh clinical isolates (nine strains studied so far), bands equal to those with the prototype strains and the CPS of NCTC 9343 were obtained. This strongly suggests that the determinant of the MAb is lost during *in vitro* passages and storage of *B. fragilis*. The prototype strains were quite exceptional in this respect, since they remained positive after repeated culturing and storing. The cause–effect relationship of this phenomenon is an enigma. Have these strains adapted to continuous *in vitro* passages or were they originally selected for prototype strains because of their ability to retain their exopolysaccharides better than wild *B. fragilis* strains in general? These results further stress the caution that has to be used during *in vitro* studies of *B. fragilis*, and that strains isolated from clinical speciments should be used in conjunction with the reference strains.

G. Localization of the Target Determinant of One CPS MAb

To investigate whether the negative reactions in the inhibition EIA with the CPS MAbs were caused by a total absence of capsule or only the target determinant, ruthenium red-stained organisms were examined by electron microscopy. No difference was observed in the degree of capsulation between negative and

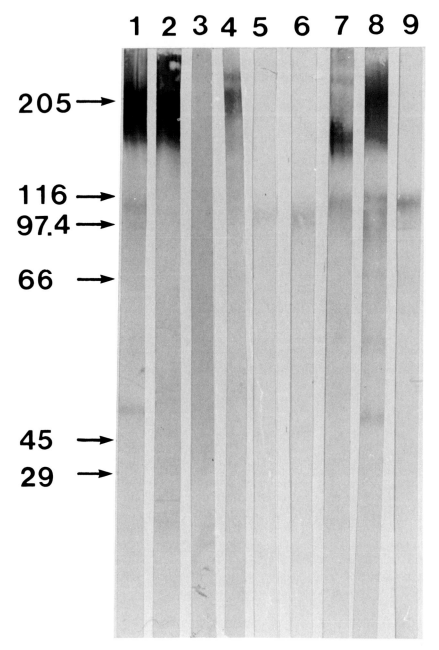

Fig. 4. Immunoblotting by one CPS MAb (2A4). Whole cells of prototype strains ATCC 23745 (1) and NCTC 9343 (2), CPSs prepared from these strains (3,4), whole cells of two *B. fragilis* strains taken from the stock culture (5,6), whole cells of two fresh clinical *B. fragilis* isolates (7,8), and a control (ATCC 23745 whole organisms) where the CPS MAb was omitted (9).

positive strains (data not shown). Encapsulated and unencapsulated organisms were seen among both positive and negative strains. This suggests that *B. fragilis* may lose the determinant and still retain the capsule.

That the determinant is actually located outside the bacterial cell, and possibly in the outermost areas of the capsule, was demonstrated by EIC with one CPS MAb (2A4) and protein A–gold (Fig. 5) (40). Gold particles (diameter 15 nm) were located at a distance of about 20 nm from the OM of the organism and attached to ruthenium red-positive projections. The length of these projections apparently reflects the original thickness of the capsule. In other areas of the cell surface the capsule had evidently collapsed because of dehydration, as shown by Lambe *et al.* (30). In contrast to the intensive binding pattern obtained with one LPS MAB, a much smaller amount of particles per one positive cell was observed in the EIC preparations with the CPS MAb. However, this does not mean that the original number of target determinants of the CPS MAb had been smaller, since a majority of determinants may have been destroyed or removed during the labeling process. When bacteria from the same culture were stained by indirect immunofluorescence method with the CPS MAb, an intensive staining

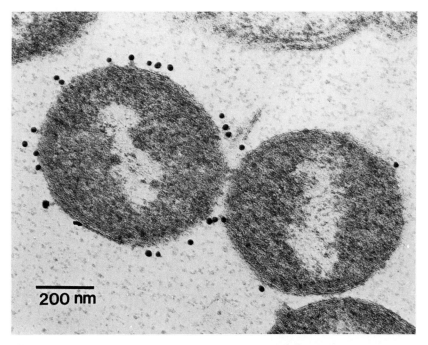

Fig. 5.   EIC study of a clinical *B. fragilis* isolate with a CPS MAb (2A4) and protein A–gold (particle diameter 15 nm). Polysaccharide staining was with ruthenium red.

of bacterial cell walls was observed (Fig. 6). This result apparently reflects much better the real density of the determinant on the surface of the organism than that obtained with EIC.

As with the LPS MAB, it was observed that only part of the bacteria was labeled with the CPS MAb. Again, it should be kept in mind that this result may also be artifactually low and does not show the original number of cells with the determinant. To find out the real amount and localization of the determinant of this MAb, the capsule had to be fixed by some method, for example, by cross-linking with polyclonal antibodies as described by Lambe *et al.* (30). Furthermore, the best possible estimation of the determinant characteristics can probably be obtained by studying bacterial vegetations in their original conformation in an infection focus. This can be attained by growing bacteria *in vivo* on synthetic or organic surfaces, and by fixing the exopolysaccharides on these surfaces before dehydration.

The localization and lability of the target structure of the CPS MAb have important implications. It seems to be one of the first structures recognized by the host's immune defense systems. By loosening this determinant when antibodies are bound to it, *B. fragilis* may interfere with the action of opsonizing antibodies. For this purpose, it is reasonable to think that the organism produces

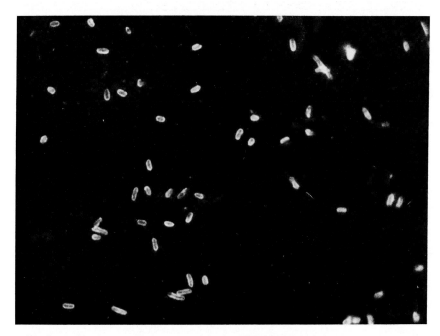

Fig. 6.   Indirect immunofluorescence staining by a CPS MAb (2A4) of the same *B. fragilis* strain as in Fig. 5. Magnification ×940.

this structure in large quantities in order to be able to neutralize as many anti-bodies as possible. If large amounts of this determinant are produced, it should be excreted in body fluids and urine in sufficient concentrations to be used as a diagnostic antigen. It remains to be shown whether this really is the case.

It is not possible to detect by polyclonal antibodies labile epitopes such as that recognized by the CPS MAb. When animals are immunized by purified CPSs or even infected with live bacteria, antibodies to the deep stable structures may far outnumber antibodies to the superficial labile determinants. These polyclonal antibodies yield a positive reaction even with capsular rudiments, as shown by Kasper *et al.* (24), and thus small changes in the fine structure of the capsule cannot be demonstrated by them.

IV. CONCLUSIONS

Hybridization of spleen cells of mice immunized with Triton X-100-treated OM preparation of *B. fragilis* leads to an exclusive formation of hybridomas producing antibodies to the LPS of *B. fragilis*. The conformation taken by LPS after treatment with Triton X-100 can be either reaggregations of plain LPS molecules, which is due to their amphipathic nature, or micelles formed in conjunction with some proteins detached from the OM of *B. fragilis.*

The monoclonals produced by these hybridomas recognize a galactose-con-taining determinant in the outer core of *B. fragilis* LPS. Monomeric galactose could not inhibit the binding of the LPS MAbs to their target. This observation suggests that this monosaccharide is only part of the determinant, and its absence drastically alters the antigenic specificity of the oligosaccharide.

EIC demonstrated that the determinant of the LPS MAbs is located on the surface of OM. This exposed location is the most plausible explanation for the higher immunogenicity of the determinant as compared with other parts of *B. fragilis* LPS.

The determinant appeared to be common to most *B. fragilis* isolates, which supports earlier observations on polyclonal antibodies (27,47). This and the absence of the heteropolysaccharide chain from *B. fragilis* LPS strongly suggest that the serovariation possibly occurring in *B. fragilis* cannot be based on varia-tion in the structure of LPS. The partial inhibition of the binding of the LPS MAbs caused by some *B. thetaiotaomicron* and *B. ovatus* strains suggests that a determinant similar but not identical to that in the LPS of *B. fragilis* occurs in these strains.

The galactose-containing determinant occurred only in part (10%) of the orga-nisms taken from the same *B. fragilis* culture. The bacterial cells labeled with the antibody were usually smaller than those remaining negative. This indicates that the expression of the determinant is dependent on the growth phase of bacteria.

By immunization of mice with air-exposed *B. fragilis*, hybridomas producing antibodies to the CPS of *B. fragilis* could be obtained. Since the bacteria were only transiently exposed to atmospheric oxygen during their manipulation, it is possible that live bacteria were injected into the mice. Although the animals showed no marked signs of peritoneal infection at the removal of their spleens, it is possible that the bacterium had started to regain its capsule but not to the extent that abscesses would have been produced.

The determinant of the MAbs to CPS could be demonstrated in the prototype strains used, and in the CPS extracted from the prototype strain NCTC 9343, but not in the CPS of strain ATCC 23745 that was used for immunizations. Furthermore, the antibodies did not react with clinical isolates recultured from storage tubes, whereas they yielded positive results in immunoblotting with fresh clinical isolates. This suggests that the determinant of the CPS MAbs is labile and cannot always resist purification, *in vitro* passages, or storage. The cause–effect relationship in the persistence of the determinant in the prototype strains subjected to several subculture and storage cycles remains an enigma. Have these strains adapted to continuous *in vitro* passages or were they originally selected as prototypes because they can retain their exopolysaccharides better than wild *B. fragilis* strains in general?

It could be demonstrated by EIC that the determinant of the CPS MAb is located at a distance of about 20 nm from the surface of *B. fragilis* OM. The association of the label with ruthenium red-positive projections indicated that the capsule had originally been 20 nm thick. The shrinkage of exopolysaccharides due to dehydration probably distorts the picture obtained by EIC. Therefore, it is not possible to draw conclusions about the amount of this determinant per organism. The intensive staining of bacteria in the immunofluorescence test suggests that the determinant is expressed in much larger amounts than those seen by EIC.

V. PROSPECTS FOR THE FUTURE

Further studies should be undertaken to explore the factors governing the expression of the target determinants of the MAbs described in this report. As the EIC results show, the determinants are expressed only in some of the bacteria in one culture. That the cells binding LPS MAbs were usually smaller than the negative ones suggests that the growth phase of the organism determines the appearance of the determinant. This has to be studied by EIC preparations of bacteria taken sequentially from broth cultures. Different culture conditions will also have to be tested for their ability to maintain the determinants.

The best way to obtain valid information about the occurrence and role of these determinants in clinical infections is to study experimental *B. fragilis* infections. For this purpose, bacteria could be grown on solid surfaces inserted into the peritoneal cavity or in tissues of experimental animals. The colonized surfaces could then be processed for immunohistochemical observation, carefully avoiding the collapse and washout of loose exopolysaccharides. In such an experimental procedure the effect of antibodies, including the present MAbs, and antibiotics on the production of the capsule and other extracellular structures and on the attachment of bacteria can also be studied.

Experimental infections also provide data on the occurrence of the antigens of these MAbs in different body fluids in standardized conditions. However, the final confirmation of the usefulness of these MAbs in the rapid diagnosis of infections with *B. fragilis* can only be obtained from clinical specimens. Experiments are under way to test the specificity and sensitivity of the immunofluorescence technique and different modifications of the EIA with MAbs in the detection of *B. fragilis* organisms and detached LPS and CPS in specimens taken directly from the infection focus and in specimens of body fluids. One of the major advantages of antigen detection methods is their independence of the occurrence of live bacteria in the specimens. This has the implication that culture alone is not a sufficient reference method in these comparative studies. It has to be supported by the demonstration of bacterial metabolites in the specimens by high-performance liquid chromatography or gas–liquid chromatography. The present MAbs can well be used in the rapid identification of suspected *B. fragilis* isolates

VI. SUMMARY

Monoclonal antibodies (MAbs) were produced against *B. fragilis* lipopolysaccharide (LPS) and capsular polysaccharide (CPS) by immunizing mice before hybridization with air-exposed whole organisms or Triton X-100-treated outer membranes (OM) of *B. fragilis*, respectively. The LPS MAbs appeared to react with a determinant located in the oligosaccharide part of LPS and containing D-galactose. This determinant was common to most (96%) *B. fragilis* isolates. A determinant closely resembling it also occurred in some *B. thetaiotaomicron* and *B. ovatus* strains, but not in the other anaerobic and aerobic bacteria tested. Electron microscopy–immunocytochemistry (EIC) studies showed that the determinant was located on the surface of OM, but it was expressed only on about 10% of bacterial cells taken from the same culture. This suggests that the occurrence of this determinant depends on the growth phase of the organism. The target determinant of the CPS MAbs appeared to be very labile. It could usually be demonstrated only in fresh *B. fragilis* isolates. It was shown by EIC that the determinant was located in the outer part of the *B. fragilis* capsule.

ACKNOWLEDGMENTS

This work was supported by the Academy of Finland.

REFERENCES

1. Abshire, R. L., Dowell, V. R., Jr., and Lombard, G. L. (1979). Serologic study of tri-chloroacetic acid extracts of *Bacteroides fragilis*. *J. Clin. Microbiol.* **9**, 274– 279.
2. Baltimore, R. S., and Mitchell, M (1980). Immunologic investigations of mucoid strains of *Pseudomonas aeruginosa:* Comparison of susceptibility to opsonic antibody in mucoid and nonmucoid strains. *J. Infect. Dis.* **141**, 238–247.
3. Bradbury, W. C., Mills, S. D., Preston, M. A., Barton, L. J., and Penner, J. L. (1984). Detection of lipopolysaccharides in polyacrylamide gels by transfer to nitrocellulose followed by immunoautoradiography with antibody and ^{125}I-protein A: "LPS blotting". *Anal. Biochem.* **137**, 129–133.
4. Cherniak, R., Lombard, G. L., and Dowell, V. R., Jr. (1979). Immunochemical evidence for multiple serotypes of *Bacteroides fragilis*. *J. Clin. Microbiol.* **9**, 699–704.
5. Elhag, K. M., and Tabaqchali, S. (1978). A study of somatic antigens of *Bacteroides fragilis*. *J. Hyg.* **80**, 439–449.
6. Elhag, K. M., Bettelheim, K. A., and Tabaqchali, S (1977). Serological studies of *Bacteroides fragilis*. *J. Hyg.* **79**, 233–241.
7. Felton, L. D., Prescott, B., Kauffman, G., and Ottinger, B. (1955). Pneumococcal antigenic substances from animal tissues. *J. Immunol.* **74**, 205–213.
8. Fletcher, M., and Floodgate, G. D. (1973). An electron-microscopic demonstration of an acidic polysaccharide involved in the adhesion of a marine bacterium to solid surfaces. *J. Gen. Microbiol.* **74**, 325–334.
9. Gankema, H., Wensink, J., Guinee, P. A. M., Jansen, W. H., and Withol, B. (1980). Some characteristics of the outer membrane material released by growing enterotoxigenic *Eschericia coli*. *Infect. Immun.* **29**, 704–713.
10. Gless, W. F., Briggs, R. C., and Hnilica, L. S. (1981). Use of lectins for detection of elec-trophorectically separated glycoproteins transferred onto nitrocellulose sheets. *Anal. Biochem.* **115**, 219–224.
11. Goldman, R. C., and Leive, L. (1980), Heterogeneity of antigenic side-chain length in lipopolysaccharide from *Escherichia coli* 0111 and *Salmonella typhimurium* LT2. *Eur. J. Bio-chem.* **107**, 145–153.
12. Gorbach, S. L., and Bartlett, J. G. (1974). Anaerobic infections (second of three parts). *N. Engl. J. Med.* **290**, 1237–1245.
13. Govan, J. R. W. (1975). Mucoid strains of *Pseudomonas aeruginosa:* The influence of culture medium on the stability of mucus production. *J. Med. Microbiol.* **8**, 513–522.
14. Govan, J. R. W., and Fyfe, J. A. M. (1978). Mucoid *Pseudomonas aeruginosa* and cystic fibrosis: Resistance of the mucoid form to carbenicillin, flucloxacillin, and tobramycin and the isolation of mucoid variants *in vitro*. *J. Antimicrob. Chemother.* **4**, 233–240.
15. Guerrant, G. O., Lambert, M. A., and Moss, C. W. (1982). Analysis of short-chain acids from anaerobic bacteria by high-performance liquid chromatography. *J. Clin. Microbiol.* **16**, 355–360.
16. Helenius, A., McCaslin, D. R., Fries, E., and Tanford, C. (1979). Properties of detergents. *In* "Biomembranes," Part G (S. Fleischer and L. Packer, eds.), Methods in Enzymology, Vol. 56, pp. 734–749. Academic Press, New York.

17. Hill, H. R., Ritel, M. E., Menge, S. K., Johnson, D. R., and Matsen, J.M. (1975). Rapid identification of group B streptococci by counterimmunoelectrophoresis. *J. Clin. Microbiol.* **1**, 188–191.

18. Hofstad, T., and Kristoffersen, T. (1970). Chemical characteristics of endotoxin from *Bacteroides fragilis* NCTC 9343. *J. Gen. Microbiol.* **61**, 15–19.

19. Hofstad, T. (1977). Cross-reactivity of *Bacteroides fragilis* O-antigens. *Acta Pathol. Microbiol. Scand., Sect. B* **85B**, 9–13.

20. Howard, J. G., Christie, C. H., Jacob, M. J., and Elson, J. (1970). Studies on immunological paralysis. III. Recirculation and antibody neutralizing activity of ^{14}C-labeled type III pneumococcal polysaccharide in paralyzed mice. *Clin. Exp. Immunol.* **7**, 583–596.

21. Joiner, K. A., McAdam, K. P., and Kasper, D. L. (1982). Lipopolysaccharides from *Bacteroides fragilis* are mitogenic for spleen cells from endotoxin responder and nonresponder mice. *Infect. Immun.* **36**, 1139–1145.

22. Kasper, D. L. (1976). The polysaccharide capsule of *Bacteroides fragilis* subspecies *fragilis:* Immunochemical and morphologic definition. *J. Infect. Dis.* **133**, 79–87.

23. Kasper, D. L., Eschenbach, D. A., Haynes, M. E., and Holmess, K. K. (1978). Quantitative determination of serum antibody response to the capsular polysaccharide of *Bacteroides fragilis* subspecies *fragilis* in women with pelvic inflammatory disease. *J. Infect. Dis.* **138**, 74–80.

24. Kasper, D. L., Onderdonk, A. B., Reinap, B. G., and Lindberg, A. A. (1980). Variations of *Bacteroides fragilis* with *in vitro* passage: Presence of an outer membrane-associated glycan and loss of capsular antigen. *J. Infect. Dis.* **142**, 750–756.

25. Kasper, D. L., Onderdon, A. B., Polk, A. F., and Bartlett, J. G. (1979). Surface antigens as virulence factors in infection with *Bacteroides fragilis*. *Rev. Infect. Dis.* **1**, 278–290.

26. Kasper, D. L. (1976). Chemical and biological characterization of the lipopolysaccharide of *Bacteroides fragilis* subspecies *fragilis*. *J. Infect. Dis.* **134**, 59–66.

27. Kasper, D. L., Weintraub, A., Lindbert, A. A., and Lnngren, A. A. (1983). Capsular polysaccharides from two *Bacteroides fragilis* reference strains: Chemical and immunochemical characterization. *J. Bacteriol.* **153**, 991–997.

28. Kasper, D. L., and Seiler, M. W. (1975). Immunochemical characterization of the outer membrane complex of *Bacteroides fragilis* subspecies *fragilis*. *J. Infect. Dis.* **132**, 440–450.

29. Kuusi, N., Nurminen, M., and Sarvas, M. (1981). Immunochemical characterization of major outer membrane components from *Salmonella typhimurium*. *Infect. Immun.* **33**, 750–757.

30. Lambe, D. W., Jr., Mayberry-Carson, K. J., and Ferguson, K. P. (1984). Morphological stabilization of the glycocalyces of 23 strains of five *Bacteroides* species using specific antisera. *Can. J. Microbiol.* **30**, 809–819.

31. Lambe, D. W. Jr., and Moroz, D. A. (1976). Serogrouping of *Bacteroides fragilis* subspecies *fragilis* by agglutination test. *J. Clin. Microbiol.* **3**, 586–592.

32. Linko-Kettunen, L., Arstila, P., Jalkanen, M., Jousimies-Somer, H., Lassila, O., Lehtonen, O.-P., Weintraub, A., and Viljanen, M. K. (1984). Monoclonal antibodies to *Bacteroides fragilis* lipopolysaccharide. *J. Clin. Microbiol.* **20**, 519–524.

33. Linko-Kettunen, L., Weintraub, A., Arstila, P., Pelliniemi, L. J., and Viljanen, M. K. (1986). Characterization of the antigenic determinant of the monoclonal antibody to *B. fragilis* lipopolysaccharide. Submitted for publication.

34. Lüderitz, O., Freudenberger, M. A., Galanos, C., Lehmann, V., Rietschel, E. T., and Shaw, D. W. (1982). Lipopolysaccharides of gram-negative bacteria. *In* "Microbial Membrane Lipids" (C. S. Razin, and S. Rottem, eds.), Vol. 17, pp. 79–151. Academic Press, New York.

35. Miller, J., Sande, M. A., Gwaltney, J. M., Jr., and Hendley, J. O. (1978). Diagnosis of pneumococcal pneumonia by antigen detection in sputum. *J. Clin. Microbiol.* **7**, 459–462.

36. Nelles, M. J., and Niswander, C. A. (1984). Mouse monoclonal antibodies reactive with J5 lipopolysaccharide exhibit extensive serological cross-reactivity with a variety of gram-negative bacteria. *Infect. Immun.* **46**, 677–681.

37. Nieburg, P. I., Rabinowitz, R. C., and Weiner, L.B. (1977). Diagnosis of pneumococcal peritonitis by countercurrent immuneolectrophoresis (CIE). *Scand. J. Infect. Dis.* **9**, 57–58.
38. O'Farrell, P. H. (1975). High resolution two-dimensional electrophoresis. *J. Biol. Chem.* **250**, 4007–4021.
39. Rissing, J. P., Buxton, T. B., Harris, R., and Moore, W. (1981). Assessment of lipopolysaccharide and outer membrane of *Bacteroides fragilis* by an antibody-inhibition enzyme-linked immunosorbent assay in physiological fluids and infected animals. *J. Lab. Clin. Med.* **98**, 784–794.
40. Robinson, E. N., Jr., McGee, Z. A., Kaplan, J., Hammond, M. E., Larson, J. K., Buchanan, T. M., and Schoolnik, G. K. (1984). Ultrastructural location of specific gonococcal macromolecules with antibody–gold sphere immunological probes. *Infect. Immun.* **46**, 361–366.
41. Rotfield, L., and Perlan-Kothencz, M. (1969). Synthesis and assembly of bacterial membrane components. A lipopolysaccharide–phospholipid–protein complex excreted by living bacteria. *J. Mol. Biol.* **44**, 477–492.
42. Russell, R., and Johnson, K. (1975). SDS–polyacrylamide gel electrophoresis of lipopolysaccharides. *Can. J. Microbiol.* **21**, 2013–2018.
43. Schwartzmann, S., and Boring, J. R., III (1971). Anti-phagocytic effect of slime from a mucoid strain of *Pseudomonas aeruginosa*. *Infect. Immun.* **3**, 762–767.
44. Sutherland, I. W. (1977). Bacterial exopolysaccharides: Their nature and production. *In* "Surface Carbohydrates of the Prokaryotic Cell" (I. W. Sutherland, ed.), pp. 27–96. Academic Press, New York.
45. Towbin, H., Staehelin, T., and Gordon, J. (1981). Electrophoretic transfer of proteins from polyacrylamide gels to nitrocellulose sheets: Procedure and some applications. *Proc. Natl. Acad. Sci. U.S.A.* **126**, 103–109.
46. Weintraub, A., Larsson, B., and Lindberg, A. A. (1985). Chemical and immunochemical analyses of *Bacteroides fragilis* lipopolysaccharides. *Infect. Immun.* **49**, 197–201.
47. Weintraub, A., Lindberg, A. A., and Kasper, D. L. (1983). Characterization of *Bacteroides fragilis* strains based on antigen-specific immunofluorescence. *J. Infec. Dis.* **147**, 780.
48. Weintraub, A., Zähninger, U., and Lindberg A. A. (1985). Structural studies of the polysaccharide part of the cell wall lipopolysaccharide from *Bacteroides fragilis* NCTC 9343. *Eur. J. Biochem.* **151**, 657–661.
49. Wollenweber, H.-W., Rietschel, E. T., Hofstad, T., Weintraub, A., and Lindberg, A. A. (1980). Nature, type of linkage, quantity, and absolute configuration of (3-hydroxy) fatty acids in lipopolysaccharides from *Bacteroides fragilis* NCTC 9343 and related strains. *J. Bacteriol.* **144**, 898–903.
50. Wood, W. B. (1960). Phagocytosis, with particular reference to encapsulated bacteria. *Bacteriol. Rev.* **24**, 41–49.
51. Yamada, H., and Mizushima, S. (1980). Interaction between major outer membrane protein (O-8) and lipopolysaccharide in *Escherichia coli* K12. *Eur. J. Biochem.* **103**, 209–218.

6

Monoclonal Antibodies against Surface Components of *Streptococcus pneumoniae*

LARRY S. MCDANIEL AND DAVID E. BRILES

The Cellular Immunobiology Unit of the Tumor Institute
Departments of Microbiology and Pediatrics, and
The Comprehensive Cancer Center
University of Alabama at Birmingham
Birmingham, Alabama

I. INTRODUCTION

It is generally accepted that a major virulence factor of *Streptococcus pneumoniae* is its capsular polysaccharide (36,42,53,74,75). It has been shown that pneumococcal virulence is related, at least in part, to the amount of capsule

143

covering the organism (42,49). In order to be maximally protected against pneumococcal infection, the host must possess anticapsular antibodies (52). These antibodies are usually type-specific and play an important role in facilitating complement-mediated phagocytosis (20).

Some reports had indicated that antibodies to cell wall components of the pneumococcus were not opsonic and would not be protective (3,20,37). However, it has recently been demonstrated that mice can be protected from fatal *S. pneumoniae* infections using monoclonal antibodies against phosphocholine (PC) (13,14,17), cell surface protein (54,56,57), and an as yet undescribed non-PC determinant of the cell wall polysaccharide (L. S. McDaniel and D. E. Briles, manuscript in preparation).

The existence of pneumococcal surface components, in addition to the capsule, that are necessary for virulence could account for the early observations that the most protective horse antipneumococcal sera were made against highly virulent pneumococci (73), and that the presence of anticapsular antibody in the sera did not necessarily mean that they would be highly protective (50). Although there have been a number of early reports of protective antibodies directed against antigens other than the capsular polysaccharide (28,29,40,64,72), the subject ceased to be a major topic of investigation after Avery and Goebel demonstrated in 1933 that the protective properties of an immune serum from a horse could be completely removed by absorption with isolated type 1 polysaccharide (4).

The exploration of the pneumococcal cell wall with monoclonal antibodies has begun to identify surface components other than the capsule which may affect the outcome of host–parasite interaction involving *S. pneumoniae*. Some of these monoclonal antibodies may prove useful in the form of diagnostic reagents, in the identification of potential vaccine components, and possibly for antipneumococcal therapy.

We have chosen to identify cell wall antigens of the pneumococcus using monoclonal anti-cell wall antibodies that can protect mice against pneumococcal infection. One reason for taking this approach is that it allows us to focus our study directly on those surface components that can elicit protection. Furthermore, antigens that are minor components of the cell wall might easily escape investigation using procedures in which cells are first fractionated, and the various components are then tested for their ability to elicit protection.

We have produced a panel of hybridoma antibodies reactive with surface components of the pneumococcus. Two of the antibodies, Xi64 and Xi126, recognize a pneumococcal surface protein (Psp) and are able to protect mice against infection with certain strains of pneumococci (55,56). This panel of antibodies appears to recognize several different molecular species. We are characterizing these molecules and have already described our observations on an initial molecule designated PspA (57).

II. BACKGROUND

A. Antibodies to Phosphocholine

When mice are immunized with *S. pneumoniae* one of the most prominent antibody responses is to the PC determinants (24–26) found in the teichoic acids, and lipoteichoic acids of the pneumococcus (19,21,73). Both humans and mice have at least several micrograms per milliliter of anti-PC antibody in their normal serum at all times (15,17,34). Although both the mouse and human anti-PC antibodies are able to enhance the resistance of mice to pneumococcal infection (11,15,17,54), it is not clear whether or not the pneumococcus is the bacterium that elicits the bulk of the naturally occurring anti-PC antibody in mouse and human sera (15). Although antisera reactive with pneumococcal cell wall antigens have been produced since the earliest days of pneumococcal studies, the realization that anti-PC antibodies could be a predominant part of this response was not apparent until 1969 (26,68). One of the reasons for the late recognition of anti-PC antibodies undoubtedly was the fact that most experimental antibodies were made in the rabbit and that the rabbit is unique in its inability to respond to pneumococcal PC. When immunized with nonencapsulated pneumococci the bulk of the antibody to teichoic acid is not directed against the PC determinant, and that anti-PC antibody which is made never reaches serum levels above 1 to 10 µg/ml (J. L. Claflin, personal communication).

Anti-PC antibodies first came to prominence with the discovery that a myeloma antibody produced by a BALB/c mouse reacted specifically with pneumococcal C-polysaccharide and that this reaction could be specifically inhibited with free PC (26). This anti-PC binding myeloma protein was the very first example of a myeloma antibody showing specificity for a known antigen (62). As additional antibodies were tested it turned out that anti-PC myeloma antibodies had an unusually high frequency and many different PC-binding mouse myeloma antibodies were discovered (61,62).

The anti-PC myeloma antibodies were classified into three families, T15, M603, and M511, based on the variable-region family of the light chains (24,61). Each of the three families of antibodies could also be shown to have different cross-reactive idiotypes (24). One of the most interesting things about these anti-PC antibodies is that they all have almost indistinguishable heavy-chain variable regions, and are all coded for by the same germ line V_H gene (61).

Shortly after myeloma anti-PC antibodies were shown to bind pneumococcal C-carbohydrate, it was shown that if mice were immunized with heat-killed rough pneumococci they produced antibodies to PC, and the idiotype and specificity of the antibodies were essentially the same as the anti-PC binding monoclonal antibodies (24,26,68). When most strains were immunized with nonencapsulated *S. pneumoniae*, a roughly 1:1 ratio of anti-PC antibodies of the T15 and M511 families were produced, with very little of the anti-PC antibody being of the M603 family (24). The BALB/c strain was unusual in that its anti-PC antibody response was almost exclusively of the T15 family (24,68).

By pretreating mice with monoclonal or polyclonal antibodies directed to the T15 idiotype, it has been possible to enhance or suppress the production of T15 anti-PC antibodies. When the anti-PC response of BALB/c mice was suppressed, the mice were rendered more susceptible to pneumococcal infection (17). When antiidiotypes were used to enhance the T15 antibody response to PC, the treated mice became more resistant to pneumococcal infection (58).

By using IgM and IgG_1 antibodies of the T15, M603, and M511 idiotypes, it became apparent that all IgG_1 and IgM T15 anti-PC antibodies were protective against intravenous (iv) pneumococcal infection. However, M603 and M511 antibodies of the same isotypes were not protective (12,14).

Further studies of the T15 antibodies showed that IgG antibodies were more protective that IgM antibodies, and IgA antibodies were not protective at all (11). In a comparison of antibodies of the IgG_1, IgG_{2b}, and IgG_3 isotypes, no significant difference in protective capacity was observed.

B. Monoclonal Antibodies to Capsular Antigens of *Streptococcus pneumoniae*

The development of monoclonal anticapsular antibodies has been handicapped by the relatively poor immune responses that mice make to these antigens. Several years ago however, Kenneth Schroer and Philip Baker succeeded in making a panel of different monoclonal antibodies to the type 3 polysaccharide by using cells from mice that had been not only immunized with the type 3 polysaccharide, but also pretreated with the mitogen concanavalin A (66,67). It has been determined that both the IgG_3 and the IgM anti-type 3 antibodies are able to protect against death by the iv inoculation of mice with type 3 *S. pneumoniae* (11). As in the case of the anti-PC antibodies, the IgG_3 antibodies were much more protective than the IgM antibodies (11).

We have recently prepared an anti-type 5 monoclonal antibody that is protective against mouse infections with an extremely virulent type 5 pneumococcal strain (L. S. McDaniel and D. E. Briles, unpublished observations). Another group of recent studies have yielded monoclonal antibodies to the type 14 capsular polysaccharides (M. Egan, D. Pritchard, and B. Gray, University of Alabama at Birmingham, unpublished observations).

III. RESULTS AND DISCUSSION

A. Production of Monoclonal Antipneumococcal Antibodies

To obtain monoclonal antibodies against noncarbohydrate surface components of the pneumococcus, we chose to immunize mice with the nonencapsulated pneumococcal strain R36A. When mice are immunized with R36A, much of the antibody response is directed toward PC (24,26). In an attempt to optimize the generation of antiprotein antibodies, we immunized X-linked immunodeficient mice (*xid*), which respond poorly to carbohydrate antigens (16,63,65) and to PC (59) but make relatively normal responses to protein antigens (65).

Spleen cells from immunized mice were fused with the non-Ig producing mouse myeloma line P3-X63-Ag.8.653 using polyethylene glycol 4000 as described previously (41,56). Hybridoma antibodies were used as unfractionated tissue culture supernatants or isolated by precipitation from mouse ascites fluid with 48% saturated ammonium sulfate. Antibodies were quantitated by isotype-specific radioimmunoassay (RIA) (18).

In a single fusion, 17 of the 42 hybrids producing antibody that reacted with R36A did not bind PC. Three of these hybrids were recloned and designated Xi64 (IgM_k), Xi69 (IgM_k), and Xi126 ($IgG_{2b,k}$). It seemed likely that the antibodies secreted by these hybrids were reacting with protein antigens, since they bound readily to R36A but not to R36A that had been treated with proteases (56).

We have used this same immunization protocol to produce hybridoma antibodies to heat-killed encapsulated pneumococci. In those fusions, we have been able to produce monoclonal antibodies against pneumococcal protein and carbohydrate surface antigens. Table I lists a number of the antipneumococcal hybrids we have produced, and some of their properties. The main emphasis of this review will focus on the first four hybrids in Table I, since the fine specificity of those antibodies and the identity of the antigens they recognize has been extensively characterized.

B. Antigen Characterization

1. Extraction of Soluble Antigens

We have investigated several approaches to obtain cell-free soluble antigen preparations from the pneumococcus. Two procedures we have utilized are the preparation of a total-cell lysate (TCL) (56) and a cell wall extract (CWE) (57). Both procedures take advantage of the fact that the pneumococcus contains an autolytic enzyme (48) which can be induced by incubation of the bacterium in the presence of low concentrations of detergents.

To prepare TCL, pneumococci were suspended in a lysis buffer of 0.1% sodium deoxycholate, 0.01% sodium dodecyl sulfate, and 0.15 M sodium citrate

TABLE I

Antipneumococcal Cell Surface Hybridomas

Hybrid	Isotype	Immunizing Pneumococcus	Nature of antigen	Molecular weight of protein	Protect against
Xi64	u,k	R36A	PspA[a]	84,000, 76,000	Type 2 and 3
Xi69	u,k	R36A	PspA	84,000, 76,000	N[b]
Xi126	γ2b,k	R36A	PspA	84,000, 76,000	Type 2 and 3
HPR36A	u,k	R36A	PspA	84,000, 76,000	N
T4A49	γ2a,k	Type 4	Protein	63,000	N
T5V3	γ2b,k	Type 5	Protein	84,000	N
SR4H1	γ2b,k	Type 4	Protein	56,000	C[c]
SR4H2	u,k	Type 4	Protein	70,000	C
SR4W1	γ2a,k	Type 4	Protein	96,000	C
T5V30	u,k	Type 5	Capsule	—	Type 5
D3114/63	u,k	Type 6A	C-carbohydrate	—	Type 3

[a] PspA is pneumococcal surface protein A, which is our designation of the protein antigen detected by our antibodies.

[b] Antibody failed to protect against *Streptococcus pneumoniae* isolates tested to date.

[c] Antibody is currently being evaluated for its protective ability.

for 5 min at 37°C. To prepare CWE, we have used a modification (57) of an autoplast formation procedure described by Lacks and Neuberger (46) in which pneumococci are incubated at room temperature overnight in 20% sucrose and 0.05 M MgCl$_2$ to allow digestion of the cell wall by the autolytic enzyme. The protoplasts were removed by centrifugation and discarded. Both the TCL and CWE preparations are finally dialyzed against phosphate-buffered saline (PBS) and, following protein determinations, they were stored at −20°C.

2. Inhibition of Antipneumococcal Antibodies

We have previously described an enzyme-linked immunosorbent assay (ELISA) procedure in which we have assayed the ability of various pneumococcal cell components to block the binding of hybridoma antibodies to heat-killed pneumococci that are coated on microtitration plates (56). In this procedure, flat-bottom polystyrene microtitration plates were coated by adding 100 μl of 10^8 pneumococci per milliliter which had been heat-killed at 60°C for 30 min. The use of heat-killing is important for two reasons: (a) it inactivates the autolytic enzyme thus preventing subsequent autolysis and (b) for unknown reasons, it causes the pneumococci to adhere to the microtitration plates. This latter property of heat-killed pneumococci makes it unnecessary to use binding enhancers such as 0.1% glutaraldehyde.

Table II presents representative data obtained from an experiment where TCL

TABLE II

Inhibition of Binding of Xi126 and 59.6C5 to Heat-Killed R36A[a]

Hybridoma	Amount of inhibitor required for 50% inhibition[b]		
	TCL	CWE	Trypsin-treated TCL
Xi126	80	15	>1000
59.6C5	150	32	110

[a] Individual wells of microtiter plates were coated using 100 μl of a PBS solution containing 10^7 heat-killed R36A organisms. The inhibitors were titered in the wells, and 50 μl of a dilution of monoclonal antibody which would give approximately 70% of total binding was added to the wells. Following incubation, the plates were developed using a goat antimouse alkaline phosphatase second antibody in a typical ELISA procedure.

[b] The concentration of the inhibitor is based on the total proteins in the preparation. CWE, Cell wall extract; TCL, total-cell lysate.

or CWE preparations were used as inhibitors. In this experiment, both of these preparations were able to inhibit the binding of hybridoma antibody Xi126 to the intact nonencapsulated pneumococcus strain R36A. However, based on total protein, one-fifth as much CWE as TCL was required to inhibit the binding of Xi126 to R36A. Thus it appears that there is a significant enrichment of the Psp detected by Xi126 in CWE as compared to TCL.

We were also able to use this assay to assess the biochemical nature of the antigenic epitope recognized by our monoclonal antibodies. Treatment of the crude lysate with protease prior to use in the inhibition assay essentially destroyed the ability of the lysate to inhibit the binding of Xi126 to R36A (Table II), indicating that the target of this antibody is a protein and not simply a carbohydrate attached to the bacterial wall by a polypeptide.

We have been able to use this same assay to demonstrate a lack of reactivity of our antibodies with other cell wall antigens and capsular polysaccharide from the pneumococcus. In these experiments, free PC, C-polysaccharide, or type 3 pneumococcal polysaccharide failed to inhibit the binding of Xi64, Xi69, or Xi126 to R36A (56).

Since the antigen recognized by our antibodies is at least in part protein, it seemed likely that even as a component of CWE it could be used to coat microtitration plates. This procedure works and has eliminated much of the well-to-well variation seen when the wells are coated with whole R36A.

To coat microtitration plates with CWE, we use a 10-μg/ml solution of total proteins in the CWE diluted in PBS. Wells are coated by incubating 100 μl of the diluted CWE in them overnight at 4°C. This increases the sensitivity of our assay so that we can now use this inhibition assay as an ELISA or RIA to test serum

samples for the presence of antibodies with the same specificity as our monoclonal antibodies (L. S. McDaniel, K. Widenhofer, and D. E. Briles, manuscript
in preparation).

C. Binding of Hybridoma Antibodies to Pneumococcal Strains

The fact that antibodies reactive with particular antigens are able to protect
against pneumococcal infection provides good evidence that those antigens can
elicit protective antibodies. To understand how these antibodies function and to
identify those Psp variants that might best be used in vaccines, it has been
necessary to develop an assay that would allow us to screen different pneumococcal isolates for their ability to be bound by each antiprotein monoclonal
antibody we produce.

1. Quantitative Measurement of the Ability of ^{125}I-Labeled Antibodies to Bind Whole Pneumococci

This procedure allows us quantitatively to compare the binding of a particular
^{125}I-labeled antipneumococcal antibody to different isolates of living (or killed)
pneumococci (56,76). Hybridoma antibodies purified from ascites fluid by ammonium sulfate precipitation are radiolabeled with ^{125}I using chloramine T (35).
We have described the procedure in detail previously (56). The pneumococci
(usually 10^8) are incubated in a 0.3-ml volume for 30 min at 37°C with the ^{125}I-
labeled monoclonal antibody. The incubation mixture also contains chelated
$^{57}CoCl_3$ as a volume marker. Following centrifugation the majority of the supernatant is aspirated. By counting the pellet in a two-channel γ counter, it is
possible to determine the percentage of the ^{125}I-labeled monoclonal antibody that
is bound to the bacteria. This procedure avoids having to wash the bacteria
repeatedly or accurately measure the amount of supernatant removed.

Table III shows representative data obtained using three different anti-Psp
monoclonal antibodies. The different antibodies gave very different patterns of
reactivity, indicating that there may be a number of distinct Psps on different
serotypes of pneumococci.

The failure of monoclonal antibodies to bind to pneumococci in this assay
indicates that the antigen detected by the antibody is not exposed on the bacterial
surface. Failure of a monoclonal antibody to bind a particular strain of pneumococci cannot rule out the possibility that antigen is produced but not exposed
on the surface. To determine whether or not nonreactive pneumococci might
actually carry a sequestered form of the antigen, it is necessary to use either the
assay described above, where total bacterial lysates are used in inhibition assays,
or the colony blot assay described below, where unavoidable lysis of the bacteria

TABLE III

**Reactivity of Monoclonal Antibodies
with Different Pneumococcal Serotypes
in the Quantitative Binding Assay**[a]

Serotype	T4A49	T5V3	Xi69
1	<1	1	5
2	1	<1	20
3	<1	2	4
4	23	1	6
5	<1	40	7
6A	1	2	5
8	17	1	3
9V	16	1	3
10	1	1	3
14	1	1	1
19F	2	<1	2
23F	2	1	3
R	1	<1	10

[a] The percentage binding to approximately 5×10^7 viable pneumococci by 20,000 cpm of ^{125}I-labeled hybridoma antibody at 37°C for 30 min as previously described (56).

takes place when bacterial colonies are bound to the nitrocellulose membrane (57).

We have also used the quantitative binding assay to examine the susceptibility of pneumococcal surface antigens to protease. In these experiments heat-killed R36A were treated with either pepsin or trypsin prior to assaying their ability to bind radiolabeled hybridoma antibodies. We found that such treatment essentially abolished the ability of Xi64, Xi69, Xi126, and HPR36A to bind to R36A (56).

2. Colony Blot Assay

We have used a colony blot procedure to assay various pneumococcal isolates for the presence of antigen reactive with our monoclonal antibodies. Although this assay is not quantitative, it allows us rapidly to screen a large number of pneumococcal isolates. Thus, this assay allows serotyping of pneumococci based on their protein antigens and facilitates screening of large numbers of isolates in order to identify those antibodies that appear to recognize the most cross-reactive epitopes on the pneumococcal proteins. Pneumococci carrying these cross-reactive epitopes would be those isolates from which the cross-reactive protein, or the gene producing it, could be isolated for eventual use in vaccine production.

In the colony blot assay (57), pneumococcal isolates are spotted in patches on blood agar plates and allowed to grow overnight. A portion of the bacteria in each patch are transferred to a nitrocellulose membrane by placing the membrane in contact with the agar surface and then gently lifting it off. Following blocking of the unreacted sites on the membrane with a 1% solution of bovine serum albumin (BSA), individual membranes are sequentially incubated with antibody, alkaline phosphatase conjugated goat antimouse antibody, and the phosphatase substrate 5-bromo-4-chloro-3-indolyl phosphate (BCIP) (Sigma).

In this assay, any colonies producing an antigen detected by the primary antibody appear as blue spots on the membrane. A control is included to rule out the possibility of any cross-reactive antibodies in the secondary alkaline phosphatase conjugate. Although it is possible that some organisms could have endogenous phosphatase which may interfere with the assay, we have not encountered such problems with the pneumococcus or other streptococci.

We have found that the colony blot assay provides a reliable means of identifying isolates carrying pneumococcal proteins detected by the individual monoclonal antibodies. One particularly desirable property of the colony blot assay is that strains with weakly cross-reactive antigens (as determined by the quantitative binding assay) are not detected.

D. Competitive Inhibition Assay

Using the quantitative binding assay described above, we have tested competitive binding among our four hybridoma antibodies to determine if they recognize the same or different epitopes. In this case the target organism was 10^7 heat-killed R36A pneumococci. We used each of the four monoclonal antibodies at concentrations ranging from 3 to 1000 μg/ml to inhibit the binding of 20,000 cpm of labeled monoclonal antibody to the bacterial surface. A series of experiments were carried out in which each of our four antibodies along with a control anti-PC antibody were labeled and inhibited by the corresponding unlabeled antibodies. Table IV presents representative data obtained in these experiments. The anti-PC antibody failed to inhibit the binding of the four antiprotein antibodies, and the four antiprotein antibodies failed to inhibit the binding of the anti-PC antibody to R36A. Among the four antiprotein antibodies, however, differences in their ability to inhibit each other were observed. A hierarchy of the ability of each these four antibodies to inhibit the binding of each other to heat-killed R36A was observed and is depicted in Table V.

E. Characterization of PspA

As an additional biochemical characterization of the antigens detected by our monoclonal antibodies, we have used gel electrophoresis. One useful protocol

TABLE IV

Inhibition of ^{125}I-Labeled Xi126 Binding to Surface Epitopes on R36A with Nonlabeled Monoclonal Antibodies[a]

Antibody concentration (μg/ml)	% Inhibition of ^{125}I-labeled Xi126 by				
	Xi64	Xi69	Xi126	HPR36A	22.1A4
10	NT[b]	0	63	41	0
30	NT	0	83	41	0
100	22	0	75	63	0
300	31	10	94	70	0
1000	19	17	96	84	18

[a] The binding of ^{125}I-labeled Xi126 to 10^7 heat-killed R36A cells was carried out in the presence of varying concentrations of nonlabeled individual antibodies as described in Table III.

[b] NT, Not tested.

has been electrophoresis of immunoprecipitated antigens of pneumococci surface-labeled with [125]I. Another is the use of an immunoblot procedure to allow monoclonal antibodies to identify reactive antigens when solubilized whole pneumococci or CWEs are electrophoresed. Using both of these procedures, we have been able to identify a protein molecule reactive with all four monoclonal antibodies. This molecule has been designated PspA for pneumococcal surface protein 1 (57).

1. Immunoprecipitation of Surface-Labeled Molecules

Immunoisolation of surface-labeled protein antigens is very useful for obtaining molecular weight estimates of such molecules and offers further evidence for

TABLE V

Ranking of Antipneumococcal Protein Antibodies by Their Ability to Compete for Binding Sites on the Surface of R36A

Inhibition of binding of	Rank of inhibitors
Xi64	Xi64 > (Xi69, Xi126) > HPR36A
Xi69	(Xi69, HPR36A) > Xi64 > Xi126
Xi126	Xi126 > HPR36A > Xi64 > Xi69
HPR36A	(HPR36A, Xi126) > Xi69 > Xi64

the exposure of these molecules to the external environment. We have surface-labeled intact viable R36A pneumococci with ^{125}I (57) by a lactoperoxidase procedure previously described for the labeling of lymphocyte surface antigens (31). We used exponentially growing cells concentrated to approximately 1 × 10^{11} colony-forming units (CFU). Following labeling and washing of cells to remove unbound ^{125}I, the pneumococci were lysed using the same lysis buffer described earlier in this chapter for the preparation of crude lysates. The lysate was centrifuged and the supernatant was collected for use in the immunoprecipitation procedure.

Immunoisolation of the radiolabeled cell surface components was carried out using a solid-phase immunoadsorption technique (SPIT) (9,23,24,57). In this procedure, wells of a polyvinyl microtiter plate were coated with antibody, and following blocking of unreacted sites with BSA, label lysate was added to the wells. After washing away unbound material, the immunoisolated components were eluted from the wells with sodium dodecyl sulfate–polyacrylamide gel electrophoresis (SDS–PAGE) sample buffer (47) prior to being resolved by SDS–PAGE.

Using this procedure, we have observed that all four of our antibodies will precipitate two molecules with an estimated molecular weight of 84,000 and 76,000 from the nonencapsulated strain R36A against which they were made (57).

2. Immunoblot Analysis of Pneumococcal Antigens

Another approach to identifying immunoreactive SDS–PAGE separated molecules is through immunoblot (''Western'') analysis (22). The immunoblot procedure we utilize has the added advantage of no hazards from radioactive material because the immune complex on the membrane is visualized using a secondary goat antimouse antibody conjugated to alkaline phosphatase (10,45,57).

Figure 1 shows the results of an immunoblot of CWE prepared from several different pneumococcal isolates probed with antibody Xi64. We have obtained comparable results using our other antibodies.

These data, along with results from the immunoprecipitation and competitive inhibition experiments, suggested that all four antibodies react with the same cell wall molecule. To test this possibility further, we absorbed CWE from R36A with Xi64. The absorbed CWE was electrophoresed, electroblotted onto nitrocellulose, and individual strips probed with all four antibodies (57). Table VI depicts the results from this cross-absorption experiment. Xi64 removed the antigen detected by itself and our three other antibodies from the CWE. On the other hand, anti-type 3 hybridoma antibody, CA3-1, used as a control failed to absorb out the antigen. The results of this experiment indicated that all four antibodies recognize the same molecule.

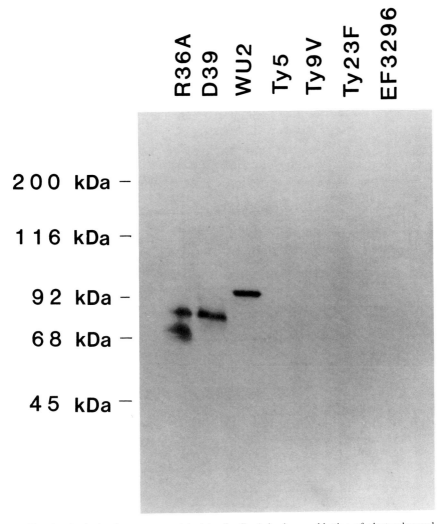

Fig. 1. Analysis of pneumococcal isolates for PspA by immunoblotting of electrophoresed CWE. SDS–PAGE was carried out using 20 µg total proteins of CWE prepared from the different isolates. R36A is a nonencapsulated variant of D39; strain D39 is a type 2; strain WU2 is a type 3; and EF3296 is a type 4. Other isolates included are serotypes 5 (Ty5), 9V (Ty9V), and 23F (Ty23F). Following transfer to nitrocellulose, the blotted antigens were reacted with Xi64 to detect PSP1.

TABLE VI

Reactivity of Absorbed CWE with Antipneumococcal Protein Antibodies in an Immunoblot Analysis

CWE absorbed with	Reactivity with			
	Xi64	Xi69	Xi126	HPR36A
Xi64	−	−	−	−
CA3-1[a]	+	+	+	+
None	+	+	+	+

[a] An isotype-matched anti-type 3 polysaccharide monoclonal antibody.

F. Antibody-Mediated Protection against Pneumococcal Infection

We have conducted experiments using different pneumococcal isolates to assess the protective ability of our monoclonal antibodies in mice. In these experiments, mice are injected ip with the test antibody in diluted ascites fluid 1 hr prior to an iv challenge with a lethal dose of virulent pneumococci. The mice are then observed for 10 days to determine their ability to survive. We have found that two of our antibodies, Xi64 and Xi126, protect mice against challenge with pneumococci (55,56). The results from these experiments are summarized in Table VII.

TABLE VII

Protection of CBA/N (*xid*) Mice from Fatal Pneumococcal Infection

Hybridoma antibody	Specificity of antibody	% Mice alive 10 days after challenge with		
		D39	WU2	A66
Xi64	Protein	100	100	100
Xi126	Protein	50	100	100
Xi69	Protein	0	0[a]	0
HPR36A	Protein	ND[b]	0	0
22.1A4	PC	0	100	100
159.4D5	PC	100	100	ND
None	—	0	0	0

[a] At 5 days 50% were alive; all controls died within 36 hr of challenge.
[b] ND, Not determined.

IV. CONCLUSIONS

We and others have shown that monoclonal antibodies directed against cell surface components other than the capsule can protect mice against fatal iv challenge with pneumococci. This includes antibodies against PC (13,14,17,54,71), antibodies to a non-PC nonprotein determinant of the cell wall polysaccharide (L. S. McDaniel and D. E. Briles, manuscript in preparation), and cell surface protein (55–57). The discovery of protective antiprotein antibodies could prove to be important in the development of a childhood vaccine, as discussed in Section V.

The fact that antibodies to components other than the capsule can protect mice, suggests that the capsule does not completely obscure all underlying antigens. It may be that these antigens somehow project through the capsule or that there are gaps in the capsule. It is possible that antibodies to such cell surface components may contribute to the nonspecific immunity to pneumococci that is seen in the absence of type-specific antibody (70).

We have suggested that one reason protective antibodies to protein components of the pneumococcus may have been difficult to detect in the past is that the cell wall and capsular polysaccharide may dominate the immune responses to the pneumococcus (55,56). There was an early interest in protein antigens from the pneumococcus (5–8,38). However, to our knowledge, the last investigation of pneumococcal protein antigens was in 1949 when a single rabbit antiserum to boiled pneumococcal "M" protein failed to protect mice against pneumococcal infection (3). This study long preceded the advent of monoclonal antibody technology. It is possible that by using this technology, we have amplified lymphocyte clones which would normally be overshadowed in an immune response to whole pneumococci.

In this chapter we have reviewed our current understanding of the development and action of anti-PC antibodies against the pneumococcus. Our primary focus, however, has been to describe our studies with the polymorphic PspA antigen detected by some of our antiprotein antibodies.

Our competitive binding study (56) demonstrated that the four anti-PspA antibodies reacted with four different but closely associated epitopes. Confirmation that these epitopes were expressed on the same molecule came from our cross-absorption experiments (57), in which Xi64 was able to absorb out PspA so that the other antibodies could no longer react with it. We have also observed in different pneumococcal strains that PspA does not always bind all four of our antibodies, indicating a difference in the expression of epitopes in these strains (57).

There is also diversity in the banding pattern observed in immunoblot analysis of PspA from different strains (57). As shown in Fig. 1, of three strains which possess PspA, R36A gives an 84- and 76-kDa band, D39 only an 84-kDa band, and WU2 a 92-kDa band.

V. PROSPECTS FOR THE FUTURE

The pneumococcus results in more visits to pediatricians and in more hospitalizations than any other infectious disease. As such, control of infections caused by pneumococci is an important part of pediatric medicine. In most cases, antibiotics offer an effective treatment and the current capsular vaccine offers effective protection in adults (2). It may therefore be asked why there should be concern for better control of an already controlled pathogen. As was pointed out in the first volume of this treatise (39), there are populations at risk of infection that are not adequately protected by these treatments. Also, there is a growing threat of increased drug resistance in the pneumococcus (51).

The populations at risk are the elderly, very young children, and expectant mothers. In the United States, pneumococcal disease in the elderly is the second leading cause of death by infectious agents (30). It also accounts for a large part of the otitis media and meningitis infections in young children (33,43). The present pneumococcal vaccine consists of a mixture of the capsular polysaccharides from the pneumococcal types most commonly associated with infection (2). Although this vaccine affords good immunity in adults, it is not effective in young children because they do not develop the ability to respond to polysaccharides until they are 6 months to 2 years of age (1,27,32,44), which is the time they are most at risk. Additionally, since the induced antibodies are specific for particular polysaccharide types, infections with serotypes not included in the vaccine are generally not prevented by vaccination (2). While pneumococcal infections respond to treatment with antibiotics in the elderly and in immunodeficient or immunosuppressed patients, the responses are frequently too late to reverse the disease before fatal damage has been done.

Thus, it is important to continue to develop a better understanding of the diseases caused by pneumococci and possible means of control. At least two improvements in the control of pneumococcal disease would be (a) an improved vaccine for the populations at risk, and (b) antibody-mediated therapy for those who may fail to respond to a vaccine.

In the first case, young children and infants would stand to benefit the most from a vaccine containing components that would stimulate protective immunity against pneumococcal infection in that age group. Our recent success of developing protective antibodies against Psp provides preliminary evidence for such a potential protein vaccine. Infants mount nearly normal responses to protein antigens (69), as is well established by use of protein-containing vaccines such as DPT (diptheria, pertussis, and tetanus).

In the second case, along with infants, the elderly and immunocompromised individuals would benefit from antibody-mediated therapy and prophylaxis. Long before the antibiotic era, therapy for pneumococcal pneumoniae involved passive antibody treatment (74). Even today, immunocompromised patients with pneumococcal pneumoniae respond to treatment with immune globulins (39). It has been suggested that future development of human hybridoma antibodies against pneumococcal capsular polysaccharides could be used in the treatment of this disease (39). Given the current state of human hybridoma production, and the obvious problem of trying to treat infections with more than 80 capsular serotypes, such an approach to therapy has limitations. We would propose that antibodies directed against species-specific antigens such as PC or cross-reactive Psp could possibly be useful as prophylaxis agents.

Recent molecular manipulations have allowed the attachment of mouse variable-region genes against PC to be coupled to human genes encoding immunoglobulin constant regions (60). The resultant antibody molecules have mouse anti-PC antigen-binding sites and human Fc. Such a molecule could be used in the treatment of human pneumococcal infection with potentially limited deleterious side effects.

Our results indicate that a particular anti-Psp monoclonal antibody may react with some but not all pneumococcal isolates of a given capsular serotype. Therefore, as a means to understand better the diseases caused by pneumococci, such anti-Psp antibodies may provide an epidemiological typing system which could distinguish among pneumococci of the same capsular serotype.

Finally, the identification of cell wall species-specific antigens such as PC or the antigen detected by monoclonal antibody D3114/63 could have important diagnostic benefits. Antibodies directed against these antigens may allow for the diagnosis of the infecting organism by the detection of degraded cell wall products.

VI. SUMMARY

Monoclonal antibodies were produced to surface components of *S. pneumoniae*. We have described our studies using four of these antibodies to characterize PspA, a polymorphic surface protein detected on some but not all pneumococcal isolates. Two of these four antibodies protected mice against fatal pneumococcal challenge, indicating that such protein molecules might be potential components of a vaccine for eliciting protective antibodies in children too young to respond to polysaccharide antigens.

We have described a number of assays used in the characterization of antigens from the pneumococcus. The colony blot assay was found to be a reliable and rapid means of screening large numbers of pneumococcal isolates for antigens reactive with specific antibodies, which may allow for better serotyping of the pneumococcus based on protein antigens. The molecular weight of antigens was estimated by sodium dodecyl sulfate–gel electrophoresis of immunoprecipitated molecules and by immunoblot analysis of electrophoresed molecules. Topological relationships of the epitopes recognized by these antibodies are investigated by competitive binding of antibodies to antigen and by immunoabsorption of antigen.

ACKNOWLEDGMENTS

This work was supported by grants CA 16673 and CA 13148 awarded by the National Cancer Institute, and grants AI 18557 and AI 21548 awarded by the National Institute of Allergy and Infectious Diseases. David E. Briles is recipient of a Research Career Development Award, AI 00498.

Our thanks are due to Colynn Forman, Geraldine Scott, and Karen Widenhofer for skillful technical assistance and to Carol McNeeley for preparation of the manuscript.

REFERENCES

1. Anderson, P., Smith, D. H., Ingram, D. L., Wilkins, J., Wehrle, P. F., and Howie, V. M. (1977). Antibody to polyribophosphate of *Haemophilus influenzae* type b in infants and children. *J. Infect. Dis.* **136**, S57–S62.
2. Austrian, R. (1979). Pneumococcal vaccine: Development and prospects. *Am. J. Med.* **67**, 547–549.
3. Austrian, R., and MacLeod, C. M. (1949). A type-specific protein from pneumococcus. *J. Exp. Med.* **89**, 439–450.
4. Avery, O. T., and Goebel, W. F. (1933). Chemoimmunological studies on the soluble specific substance of pneumococcus. I. The isolation and properties of the acetyl polysaccharide of pneumococcus type I. *J. Exp. Med.* **58**, 731–755.
5. Avery, O. T., and Heidelberger, M. (1923). Immunological relationships of cell constituents of pneumococcus. *J. Exp. Med.* **38**, 81–85.
6. Avery, O. T., and Heidelberger, M. (1925). Immunological relationships of cell constituents of pneumococcus. Second paper. *J. Exp. Med.* **42**, 367–376.
7. Avery, O. T., and Morgan, H. J. (1925). Immunological reactions of the isolated carbohydrate and protein of pneumococcus. *J. Exp. Med.* **42**, 347–353.
8. Avery, O. T., and Neill, J. M. (1925). The antigenic properties of solutions of pneumococcus. *J. Exp. Med.* **42**, 355–365.
9. Basta, P., Kubagawa, H., Kearney, J. F., and Briles, D. E. (1983). Ten percent of normal B cells and plasma cells share a V_H determinant(s) (J606-GAC) with a distinct subset of murine V_HIII plasmacytomas. *J. Immunol.* **130**, 2423–2428.
10. Blake, M. S., Johnston, K. H., Russell-Jones, G. H., and Gotschlich, E. C. (1984). A rapid, sensitive method for detection of alkaline phosphotase-conjugated anti-antibody on Western blots. *Anal. Biochem.* **136**, 175–179.
11. Briles, D. E., Claflin, J. L., Schroer, K., and Forman, C. (1981). Mouse IgG_3 antibodies are highly protective against infection with *Streptococcus pneumoniae*. *Nature (London)* **294**, 88–90.
12. Briles, D. E., Forman, C., Hudak, S., and Claflin, J. L. (1982). Anti-PC antibodies of the T15 idiotype are optimally protective against *Streptococcus pneumoniae*. *J. Exp. Med.* **156**, 1177–1185.

13. Briles, D. E., Forman, C., Hudak, S., and Claflin, J. L. (1984). The effects of subclass on the ability of IgG anti-phosphocholine antibodies to protect mice from fatal infection with *Streptococcus pneumoniae*. *J. Mol. Cell. Immunol.* **1**, 305–309.

14. Briles, D. E., Forman, C., Hudak, S., and Claflin, J. F. (1984). The effects of idiotype on the ability of IgG1 anti-phosphocholine antibodies to protect mice from fatal infection with *Streptococcus pneumoniae*. *Eur. J. Immunol.* **14**, 1029–1030.

15. Briles, D., Horowitz, J., McDaniel, L. S., Benjamin, W. H., Jr., Claflin, J. L., Booker, C. L., Scott, G., and Forman, C. (1986). Genetic control of susceptibility to pneumococcal infection. *In* "Current Topics in Microbiology and Immunology: Genetic Control of the Susceptibility to Bacterial Infection" (D. E. Briles and M. D. Cooper, eds.), Vol. 124, pp. 103–120. Springer-Verlag, Berlin and New York.

16. Briles, D.E., Nahm, M., Marion, T. N., Perlmutter, R. M., and Davie, J. M. (1982). Streptococcal group-A carbohydrate has properties of both a thymus-independent (TI-2) and a thymus-dependent antigen. *J. Immunol.* **128**, 2032–2035.

17. Briles, D. E., Nahm, M., Schroer, K., Davie, J., Baker, P., Kearney, J., and Barletta, R. (1981). Antiphosphocholine antibodies found in normal mouse serum are protective against intravenous infection with type 3 *Streptococcus pneumoniae*. *J. Exp. Med.* **153**, 694–705.

18. Briles, D. E., Perlmutter, R. M., Hansburg, D., Little, J. R., and Davie, J. M. (1979). Immune response deficiency of BSVS mice. II. Generalized deficiency to thymus-dependent antigens. *Eur. J. Immunol.* **9**, 255–261.

19. Briles, E. B., and Tomasz, A. (1973). Pneumococcal Forssman antigen: A choline-containing lipoteichoic acid. *J. Biol. Chem.* **248**, 6394–6397.

20. Brown, E. J., Hosea, S. W., Hammer, C. H., Burch, C. G., and Frank, M. M. (1982). A quantitative analysis of the interactions of antipneumococcal antibody and complement in experimental pneumococcal bacteremia. *J. Clin. Invest.* **69**, 85–98.

21. Brundish, D. E., and Baddiley, J. (1968). Pneumococcal C-substance, a ribitol teichoic acid containing choline phosphate. *Biochem. J.* **110**, 573–582.

22. Burnette, W. N. (1981). Western blotting: Electrophoretic transfer of proteins from sodium dodecyl sulfate–polyacrylamide gels to unmodified nitrocellulose and radiographic detection with antibody and radioiodinated protein A. *Anal. Biochem.* **112**, 195–203.

23. Chen, C. H., Chanh, T. C., and Cooper, M. D. (1984). Chicken thymocyte-specific antigen identified by monoclonal antibodies: Ontogeny, tissue distribution and biochemical characterization. *Eur. J. Immunol.* **14**, 385–391.

24. Claflin, J. L. (1976). Uniformity in the clonal repertoire for the immune response to phosphorylcholine in mice. *Eur. J. Immunol.* **6**, 669–674.

25. Claflin, J. L., and Davie, J. M. (1974). Clonal nature of the immune response to phosphorylcholine. III. Species-specific characteristics of rodent anti-phosphorylcholine antibodies. *J. Immunol.* **113**, 1678–1684.

26. Cohn, M., Notani, G., and Rice, S. (1969). Characterization of the antibody to the C-carbohydrate produced by a transplantable mouse plasmacytoma. *Immunochemistry* **6**, 111–123.

27. Cowan, M. J., Ammann, A. J., Wara, D. W., Howie, V. M., Schultz, L., Doyle, N., and Kaplan, M. (1978). Pneumococcal polysaccharide immunization in infants and children. *Pediatrics* **62**, 721–727.

28. Day, H. B. (1934). Preparation of pneumococcal species antigen. *J. Pathol. Bacteriol.* **38**, 171–173.

29. Dubos, R. J. (1938). Immunization of experimental animals with a soluble antigen extracted from pneumococci. *J. Exp. Med.* **67**, 799–808.

30. Fraser, D. W. (1982). What are our bacterial disease problems. *In* "Seminars in Infectious Diseases. Vol. IV: Bacterial Vaccines" (J. B. Robbins, J. C. Hill, and J. C. Sadoff, eds.), p. xix. Thieme-Stratton, New York.

31. Goding, J. W. (1980). Structural studies of murine lymphocyte surface IgD. *J. Immunol.* **124**, 2082–2088.
32. Gotschlich, E. C., Goldschneider, I., Lepow, M. L., and Gold, R. (1977). The immune response to bacterial polysaccharides in man. *In* "Antibodies in Human Diagnosis and Therapy" (E. Haber and R. Krause, eds.), p. 391. Raven, New York.
33. Gray, B. M., Converse, G. M., III, and Dillon, H., Jr. (1979). Serotypes of *Streptococcus pneumoniae* causing disease. *J. Infect. Dis.* **140**, 979–983.
34. Gray, B. M., Dillon, H. C., and Briles, D. E. (1983). Epidemiological studies of *Streptococcus pneumoniae* in infants: Development of antibody to phosphocholine. *J. Clin. Microbiol.* **18**, 1102–1107.
35. Greenwood, F. C., Hunter, W. M., and Glover, J. S. (1963). The preparation of ^{131}I-labeled human growth hormone of high specific radioactivity. *Biochem. J.* **89**, 114–123.
36. Griffth, F. (1928). The significance of pneumococcal types. *J. Hyg.* **27**, 113–159.
37. Heffron, R. (1979). "Pneumonia, With Special Reference to Pneumococcus Lobar Pneumonia," p. 805. Harvard Univ. Press, Cambridge, Massachusetts.
38. Heidelberger, M., and Kabat, E. A. (1938). Chemical studies on bacterial agglutination. IV. Quantitative data on pneumococcus R (Dawson S)-anti-R(S) systems. *J. Exp. Med.* **67**, 545–550.
39. Hunter, K. W., Jr. (1985). Human monoclonal antibodies for prophylaxis and therapy of bacterial infections. *In* "Monoclonal Antibodies against Bacteria" Volume I (A. J. L. Macario and E. Conway de Macario, eds.), Vol. I, pp. 207–231. Academic Press, Orlando, Florida.
40. Julianelle, L. A. (1930). Reactions of rabbits to intracutaneous injections of pneumococci and their products. II. Resistance to infection. *J. Exp. Med.* **52**, 895–900.
41. Kearney, J. F., Radbuch, A., Liesegang, B., and Rajewsky, K. (1979). A new mouse myeloma cell line that has lost immunoglobulin expression but permits the construction of antibody-secreting hybrid cell lines. *J. Immunol.* **123**, 1548–1550.
42. Klainer, A. S. (1982). Pneumococcal pneumoniae. *In* "Seminars in Infectious Diseases, Vol. IV: Bacterial Vaccines" (J. B. Robbins, J. C. Hill, and J. C. Sadoff, eds.), pp. 3–9. Thieme-Stratton, New York.
43. Klein, J. O. (1981). The epidemiology of pneumococcal diseases in infants and children. *Rev. Infect. Dis.* **3**, 246–253.
44. Klein, J. O., Toele, D. W., Sloyer, J. L., Jr., Ploussard, J. H., Howie, V., Makela, P. H., and Karma, P. (1982). Use of pneumococcal vaccine for prevention of recurrent episodes of otitis media. *In* "Seminars in Infectious Diseases. Vol. IV: Bacterial Vaccines" (J. B. Robbins, J. C. Hill, and J. C. Sadoff, eds.), pp. 305–310. Thieme-Stratton, New York.
45. Knecht, D. A., and Dimond, R. L. (1984). Visualization of antigenic proteins on western blots. *Anal. Biochem.* **136**, 180–184.
46. Lacks, S., and Neuberger, M. (1975). Membrane localization of a deoxyribonuclease implicated in the genetic transformation of *Diplococcus pneumoniae*. *J. Bacteriol.* **124**, 1321–1329.
47. Laemmli, U. K. (1970). Cleavage of structural proteins during the assembly of the head of the bacteriophage T4. *Nature (London)* **227**, 680–685.
48. Lee, C. J., and Liu, T. Y. (1977). The autolytic enzyme activity upon pneumococcal cell wall. *Int. J. Biochem.* **8**, 573–580.
49. Lentnek, A., LeFrock, J. L., and Molavi, A. (1984). *Streptococcus pneumoniae*. *In* "The Pneumonias: Clinical Approaches to Infectious Diseases of the Lower Respiratory Tract" (M. E. Levison, ed.), pp. 261–271. Wright, Boston, Massachusetts.
50. Levy-Bruhl, M., and Borin, P. (1925). Mise en exidence des capsules due pneumocoque III (*Pneumococcus mucosus*) en milieux liquides ou albumineux. *Seances Soc. Biol. Ses Fil.* **92**, 1343.
51. Liu, H. H., and Tomasz, A. (1985). Penicillin tolerance in multiply drug-resistant natural isolates of *Streptococcus pneumoniae*. *J. Infect. Dis.* **152**, 365–372.

52. MacLeod, C. M., Hodge, R. G., Heidelberger, M., and Bernhard, W. G. (1945). Prevention of pneumococcal pneumonia by immunization with specific capsular polysaccharides. *J. Exp. Med.* **82,** 445–465.
53. MacLeod, C. M., and Krauss, M. R. (1950). Relation of virulence of pneumococcal strains for mice to the quality of capsular polysaccharide formed in vitro. *J. Exp. Med.* **92,** 1–9.
54. McDaniel, L. S., Benjamin, W. H., Jr., Forman, C., and Briles, D. E. (1984). Blood clearance by anti-phosphocholine antibodies as a mechanism of protection in experimental pneumococcal bacteremia. *J. Immunol.* **133,** 3308–3312.
55. McDaniel, L. S., and Briles, D. E. (1985). Protective effects of antibodies to pneumococcal cell wall proteins. *In* "Microbiology—1985" (L. Leive, ed.), pp. 103–105. Am. Soc. Microbiol., Washington, D.C.
56. McDaniel, L. S., Scott, G., Kearney, J. F., and Briles, D. E. (1984). Monoclonal antibodies against protease-sensitive pneumococcal antigens can protect mice from fatal infection with *Streptococcus pneumoniae. J. Exp. Med.* **160,** 386–397.
57. McDaniel, L. S., Scott, G., Widenhofer, K., Carroll, J., and Briles, D. E. (1986). Analysis of a surface protein of *Streptococcus pneumoniae* recognized by protective monoclonal antibodies. *Microb. Pathog.* In press.
58. McNamara, M. K., Ward, R. E., and Kohler, H. (1984). Monoclonal idiotype vaccine against *Streptococcus pneumoniae* infection. *Science* **226,** 1325–1326.
59. Mond, J. J., Lieberman, R., Inman, J. K., Mosier, D. E., and Paul, W. E. (1977). Inability of mice with defect in B-lymphocyte maturation to respond to phosphocholine on immunogenic carriers. *J. Exp. Med.* **146,** 1138–1142.
60. Morrison, S. L. (1985). Transfectomas provide novel chimeric antibodies. *Science* **229,** 1202–1207.
61. Perlmutter, R. M., Crews, S. T., Douglas, R., Sorensen, G., Johnson, N., Nivera, N., Gearhart, P. J., and Hood, L. (1984). The generation of diversity in phospholylcholine-binding antibodies. *Adv. Immunol.* **35,** 1–59.
62. Potter, M. (1972). Immunoglobulin-producing tumors and myeloma proteins of mice. *Physiol. Rev.* **52,** 631–719.
63. Quintans, J. (1977). The "patchy" immunodeficiency of CBA/N mice. *Eur. J. Immunol.* **7,** 749–751.
64. Sabin, A. B. (1932). On the presence in anti-pneumococcus serum of type-specific protective antibody not neutralized by homologous specific soluble substance. *J. Exp. Med.* **53,** 93–107.
65. Scher, I. (1982). The CBA/N mouse strain: An experimental model illustrating influences of the X-chromosome on immunity. *Adv. Immunol.* **33,** 1–71.
66. Schroer, K. R., Kim, K. J., Prescott, B., and Baker, P. J. (1979). Generation of anti-type IV pneumococcal polysaccharide hybridomas from mice with an X-linked B-lymphocyte defect. *J. Exp. Med.* **150,** 698–702.
67. Schroer, K. R., Kim, K. J., Amsbaugh, D. F., Stashak, P. W., and Baker, P. J. (1980). Lymphocyte hybridomas which secrete antibodies to the type III pneumococcal polysaccharide: Idiotypic characterization. *In* "Microbiology" (D. Schlesinger, ed.), pp. 178–180. Am. Soc. Microbiol., Washington, D.C.
68. Sher, A., and Cohn, M. (1972). Inheritance of an idiotype associated with the immune response of inbred mice to phosphorylcholine. *Eur. J. Immunol.* **2,** 319–326.
69. Smith, R. T., Eitzman, D. V., Catlin, M. E., Wirtz, E. O., and Miller, B. E. (1964). The development of the immune response. Characterization to the response of the human infant and adult to immunization with *salmonella* vaccines. *Pediatrics* **33,** 163–183.
70. Smith, M. R., and Wood, B. (1958). Surface phagocytosis: Further evidence of its destructive action upon fully encapsulated pneumococci in the absence of type specific antibody. *J. Exp. Med.* **107,** 1–12.
71. Szu, S. C., Clarke, S., and Robbins, J. B. (1983). Protection against pneumococcal infection in

mice conferred by phosphocholine binding antibodies: Specificity of the phosphocholine binding and relation to several types. *Infect. Immun.* **39**, 993–999.

72. Tillett, W. S. (1928). Active and passive immunity to pneumococcus infection induced in rabbits by immunization with R pneumococci. *J. Exp. Med.* **48**, 791–804.

73. Tomasz, A. (1967). Choline in the cell wall of a bacterium: Novel type of polymer-linked choline in pneumococcus. *Science* **157**, 694–697.

74. White, B. (1938). "The Biology of the Pneumococcus." Oxford Univ. Press, London and New York.

75. Wood, B., and Smith, M. R. (1949). The inhibition of surface phagocytosis by the capsular slime layer of pneumococcus type III. *J. Exp. Med.* **90**, 85–96.

76. Wood, B., and Smith, M. R. (1958). Host-parasite relationships in experimental pneumoniae due to pneumococcus type III. *J. Exp. Med.* **90**, 85–96.

7

Monoclonal Antibodies
to *Bordetella pertussis*

CHARLOTTE D. PARKER

Department of Microbiology
School of Medicine
University of Missouri
Columbia, Missouri

I. INTRODUCTION

Bordetella pertussis, a small gram-negative coccobacillus which causes whooping cough, undergoes frequent antigenic variations. The nature of these variations has fascinated researchers since the time of Bordet (25). Cells and products of *Bordetella* species have several almost unique biological activities, such as immune adjuvant properties and sensitization of animals to histamine lethality (both reviewed by Munoz and Bergman (29), and production of ana-denylate cyclase (AC) enzyme which is active within human phagocytes (4). Monoclonal antibodies offer a precise method for studying the antigenic mosaic

165

MONOCLONAL ANTIBODIES
AGAINST BACTERIA
Volume III

of bacterial cells (9). Recently, monoclonal antibodies have been prepared which react with *B. pertussis* and its components. The utility of such antibodies for investigation of relevant *B. pertussis* antigens will be discussed in this chapter.

II. BACKGROUND

A. Growth

Bordetella pertussis is an obligately aerobic, slow-growing, gram-negative bacterium which oxidizes amino acids as its carbon, nitrogen, and energy sources (17). Growth of this organism is inhibited by small amounts of fatty acids, agar, peroxides, heavy metals, autoclaved cysteine, or other trace substances (37). Nicotinamide and cysteine are required growth factors, while iron, glutathione, and ascorbic acid stimulate growth and substances such as charcoal, albumin, starch, ion exchange resins, or cyclodextrins are frequently incorporated into agar media to neutralize inhibitors (15,30). A defined liquid medium supports good growth (43), but requires heavy inoculation and up to 5 days of incubation. These bacteria have a minimum replication time of about 6 hr. The closely related species *B. parapertussis* and *B. bronchiseptica* have similar properties, although they grow somewhat more rapidly and are less fastidious.

B. Pathogenesis

Bordetella pertussis is a noninvasive parasite of the respiratory mucosa, which causes whooping cough in humans. Bacteria adhere to the cilia of ciliated nasopharyngeal and tracheal cells, resulting in death of the ciliated cells. Dead epithelial cells are extruded from the epithelium, leaving a denuded mucosa lacking cilia. Both the lack of ciliated cells in the respiratory tract and toxic moieties may contribute to whooping cough symptoms. *Bordetella parapertussis* can cause a similar disease in humans, and *B. bronchiseptica* causes respiratory infections of animals.

Bordetella pertussis makes a variety of substances which are important in pathogenesis and immunity (see Table I). A recent review (51) discusses the toxins of *B. pertussis*. Production of these substances is regulated coordinately, that is, all are produced or none are produced (see below).

The most studied virulence factor of *B. pertussis* is pertussis toxin (PT), which has also been called pertussigen, histamine-sensitizing factor, lymphocytosis-promoting factor, and islet-activating protein. This toxin is believed to be responsible for most, if not all, of the generalized symptoms of the disease, including lymphocytosis and elevated plasma insulin. PT is also a hemagglutinin (2) and has recently been shown to be an adhesin (49) which works in concert

TABLE I

Antigenic Variation of *Bordetella pertussis*[a]

Antigen	Phase I	Phase III	Modulated	Reference
Agglutinogens	+	−	−	25,27
AC	+	−	−	13,27,31
FHA	+	−	−	Armstrong, S. K., D. W. Frank, and C. D. Parker (unpublished)
HLT	+	−	−	26
Hemolysin	+	−	?	56
OMP pattern	X Mode	C Mode	C Mode	52
PT	+	−	−	32,33,52
TCT	+	?	?	11

[a] +, Positive; −, negative; ?, unknown; AC, adenylate cyclase; FHA, filamentous hemagglutinin; HLT, heat-labile toxin; OMP, outer-membrane protein; PT, pertussis toxin; TCT, tracheal cytotoxin.

with the filamentous hemagglutinin (FHA) to mediate adherence to ciliated human respiratory cells.

PT is a hexameric protein which contains five nonidentical subunits (47). It conforms to the A : B model of bacterial toxins consisting of both an enzymatically "active" and a tissue "binding" portion, as described by Gill (10). The toxic activity of PT is due to ADP-ribosyltransferase activity of subunit 1 (S1) (20). S1 ADP-ribosylates the eukaryotic cell membrane protein N_i (50), which is part of the receptor–AC system. Modification of N_i produces cells which are refractory to hormone signals which would decrease the intracellular cyclic adenosine monophosphate (cAMP) level. The result of PT action is elevation of intracellular cAMP. The elevation may not occur for many hours, but it then persists for weeks.

Another important property of PT is its mitogenic effect on lymphocytes. The A-protomer is not a mitogen, probably because it does not bind to cells. The B-oligomer lacks toxicity but shows mitogenic effects equivalent to intact PT (48). Mitogenicity is characteristic of immune adjuvants, and PT is an excellent adjuvant (29). The adjuvant effect of PT has stirred questions as to which antigens induce protective levels of antibody to *B. pertussis*, since traces of PT enhance antibody production to weak antigens.

Pittman in 1979 hypothesized that PT is the cause of both disease and of immunity to disease (34). Passive protection tests done in mice showed that antibody to PT protected infant mice from aerosol challenge with *B. pertussis* (39). This hypothesis is increasingly being accepted, although there is evidence which suggests that virulence is multifactorial.

The FHA has also been studied extensively. FHA is a surface protein of *B.*

pertussis (see Section III,A). It forms characteristic fibrils when purified (2), and has been shown to be an adhesin for human ciliated respiratory cells (49). PT interacts with FHA in a synergistic manner to mediate bacterial attachment to cilia. Antibodies to FHA protected infant mice in passive protection tests against respiratory challenge (39).

The AC has been purified in an enzymatically active form (14) but not in a biologically active form. However, AC appears to be taken up by phagocytes, and to elevate their cAMP levels (4). Studies of mutants suggest that AC plays an important role in disease (57). The AC enzymatic activity is stimulated by calmodulin (58). Thus, both PT and AC lead to elevations of cAMP in eukaryotic cells. The stimulation of pertussis AC by calmodulin may be important in the pathogenesis of whooping cough.

Tracheal cytotoxin (TCT) was reported by Goldman *et al,* in 1982 (11). This peptide contains diaminopimelic acid and sugars. TCT kills ciliated hamster tracheal cells in organ culture by inhibiting DNA synthesis. TCT is of low molecular weight, and may act during natural infections.

Heat-labile toxin (HLT), also called dermonecrotic toxin, is poorly characterized (20a). HLT is found in the cytoplasm and is not thought to play a role in whooping cough because no antibodies to HLT appear following natural infection. However, HLT must be toxoided or destroyed in current pertussis vaccines. HLT induces sudden death in rodents.

The lipopolysaccharide (LPS) of *B. pertussis* is not known to play a role in disease, but smooth LPS may be necessary for virulence. *Bordetella pertussis* LPS has been analyzed and shown to resemble LPS of other gram-negative rods (23,24), although it has several unique features. Both *B. pertussis* LPS (29) and LPS-associated proteins (46) have been shown to be immune adjuvants.

The agglutinogens which will be described in the following section are important surface antigens. Preston maintains that the protective immunity of vaccines is due, at least in part, to agglutinogens 2 and 3 (35). He suggests that 1, 3 strains, but not 1, 2, 3 strains, induce antibody specific for antigen 3. Some of the agglutinogens, including agglutinogen 1, are heat labile.

Bordetella pertussis is amenable to genetic analysis. Plasmids may be transferred into *B. pertussis* by conjugation or transformation (53), and *B. pertussis* can be made into a genetic donor (54). Mutants which have lost hemolysin, or FHA, or AC, or PT have been isolated (56). Mutants deficient in PT, or mutants deficient in both AC and hemolysin showed greatly reduced virulence for infant mice. FHA-deficient mutants were virulent for infant mice in intranasal infections (55).

C. Serology

Workable typing schemes for *B. pertussis* were devised several years ago (1,5). The antigens which induce agglutinating antibody are called agglutinogens, and were designated numerically. Agglutinogens unique to *B. pertussis* are 1, 2, 3, 4, 5, and 6. All *B. pertussis* strains have agglutinogen 1, but the other agglutinogens are variable in their occurrence. Typical serotypes are 1, 2, 4 and 1, 3, 6. However, almost any combination of antigens may occur. Preston has reported that antigen 2 is immunodominant over antigen 3 (35). It also appears that the agglutinogen pattern may vary within a given strain. For example, 1, 2, 4 strains may change into 1, 3, 6 strains (44).

Antigenic variation also occurs in two other ways: phase variation (or degradation) and modulation. Phase variation was first described by Leslie and Gardner in 1931 (25) as a series of antigenically defined serological changes. Most clinical isolates were similar, and were designated phase I, with successively older laboratory-passaged strains designated as phases II, III, and IV. These strains varied in many ways as they changed serologically (45). Unfortunately, a reference antiserum is not available. It is thought that phase I denotes a fully virulent strain, phase II an intermediate strain, phase III a nonvirulent smooth strain, and phase IV a nonvirulent rough strain (18,19).

Many properties vary during strain degradation, including outer-membrane protein (OMP) patterns and the production of various toxins and substances associated with virulence. The changes in the organism may occur en bloc, or singly (45,56). Growth *in vitro,* especially on blood-free medium, selects for degradation (6,33). Phase III or IV cells do not induce protective immunity if used in vaccines.

The genetic approach has been valuable in understanding phase variation (55). Avirulent phase mutants isolated by Tn5 mutagenesis suggested that the Tn5 insertion lay in a regulatory gene which produced an inducer for the virulence-related genes. Studies to date do not suggest a virulence operon but rather an unusual system of coordinate control.

The second type of antigenic variability is termed modulation. Lacey described what he termed X-mode and C-mode forms of *B. pertussis* when he varied sodium and magnesium content of plating media or the temperature of incubation (21). At low magnesium concentrations, or at 35°C, cells were antigenically normal, but when magnesium concentration was elevated or temperature was low, cells lost their phase I antigens. The loss of antigens correlated with changes in cytochromes, toxins, and OMPs, and resembled degradation (see Table I). However, modulation was freely reversible if the ionic conditions or temperature were changed. It was later shown that high levels of nicotinic acid and certain other pyridines also induced modulation (36,41). Two OMPs have been used as markers for modulation (32). These proteins also appear to be markers for degradation to phase III (41). Indeed, the phenotypes of modulated and degraded cells are the same.

Most of the antigens important in pathogenesis are associated with the cell envelope. The major surface antigens of *B. pertussis* are the LPS of the cell wall, the fimbriae, and several OMPs. Agglutinogen 2 is fimbrial in nature (3), and other agglutinogens may be fimbrial. Agglutinogen 1 is not LPS, but its chemical nature is not known. FHA is found on the cell surface, while AC enzymatic activity is extracytoplasmic and PT appears to be associated with the cell envelope. Thus the antigenic mosaic of *B. pertussis* cell surface includes several OMP proteins which are regularly present, fimbrial elements which comprise up to six additional antigens, FHA, PT, AC, and LPS. The latter three substances exert important effects on the human immune system.

III. RESULTS AND DISCUSSION

A. Monoclonal Antibodies to Filamentous Hemagglutinin (FHA)

Monoclonal antibodies to FHA have been isolated in several laboratories for use in pertussis research. The earliest report was from Ashworth *et al.* (3), who showed that FHA-specific monoclonal antibodies did not react with *B. pertussis* fimbriae. Antibody to agglutinogen 2 did, however, react with the fimbriae.

Details of the preparation of these monoclonals were given the following year (16). Mice were immunized with purified FHA, and their spleen cells were fused with the nonsecreting plasmacytoma cell line P3-NS1/1-Ag4-1. An enzyme-linked immunosorbent assay (ELISA) was used to screen for hybrid antibody-secreting cells using the same antigen. Following repeated cloning by limiting dilution, nine stable clones secreting antibody against FHA were isolated and examined in more detail (see Table II).

These antibodies had the following properties: four antibodies reacted with multiple bands when used in immunoblot techniques against purified FHA; all reacted with FHA from *B. pertussis* strains Wellcome 128 and Tohama phase I, and *B. bronchiseptica* strain APM 21; all inhibited FHA-induced hemagglutination. These workers also noted that storage conditions of FHA preparations affected the number of FHA bands detected with some of these antibodies, and suggested that proteolytic breakdown was occurring. They found that a protease inhibitor could prevent both loss of hemagglutination activity and also appearance of new bands upon sodium dodecyl sulfate–polyacrylamide gel electrophoresis (SDS–PAGE).

Three of these monoclonals were later used to assess the role of the FHA antigen in adhesion to Vero cells (12). One monoclonal significantly inhibited adhesion of all *B. pertussis* strains tested to Vero cells, and the other two inhibited some strains under some growth conditions.

Selmer *et al.* (42) prepared monoclonal antibodies to FHA and used the antibody to purify FHA. Mice were immunized with crude preparations enriched

TABLE II

Properties of Monoclonal Antibodies to *Bordetella pertussis*[a]

Number of antibodies	Isotype		Specificity	Immunizing antigen	Positive by immunoblot	Reference
9	5	IgG$_1$	FHA	FHA	4	16
	1	IgG$_{2a}$				
	3	NR				
3	2	IgG$_1$	PT	PTd and PT	3	38
	1	IgG$_{2a}$				
2	1	IgG$_1$	FHA	FHA	2	42
	1	IgG$_2$				
11	10	IgG$_1$	LPS, FHA, PT,	*B. pertussis;* crude	10	7
	1	IgG$_3$	other	PT		
11	5	IgG$_1$	Unknown	*B. pertussis* cells	11	22
	1	IgG$_{2a}$				
	1	IgG$_{2b}$				
	4	Igm				
3	3	IgG$_1$	FHA	FHA	ND	12
4	2	IgG$_1$	PT	PT	ND	12
	1	IgG$_{2a}$				
	1	IgM				
3	3	IgM	AG 1, 2, and 3	Agglutinogens	ND	12
1	1	IgM	OMP7	Detergent extract of outer membrane	ND	12

[a] AG, Agglutinogen; FHA, filamentous hemagglutinin; LPS, lipopolysaccharide; ND, not done; NR, not reported; OMP, outer-membrane protein; PT, pertussis toxin; PTd, detoxified pertussis toxin.

in FHA from *B. pertussis* 18334. Spleen cells from immunized mice were fused with P3x63 Ag 8. 653 myeloma cells, and culture fluids were screened against immobilized whole bacteria by an ELISA test. Two clones which produced highly reactive supernatant fluids were chosen for further study. In immunoblots, each monoclonal reacted with several high molecular weight polypeptides in a pattern consistent with FHA. Authentic FHA was purified from a high ionic strength extract of *B. pertussis* by immunoaffinity chromatography using either of the antibodies. Elution of bound FHA from the columns was optimal with O. 1 *M* phosphate buffer (pH 11.5) containing 1.0 *M* KSCN. Monoclonal F10 inhibited hemagglutination, while F6 did not.

Frank and Parker also described a hybrid cell line, P12H3, which produced anti-FHA (7). The myeloma cell line used for fusion was P3x63 Ag 8. 653. These workers showed that FHA is exposed on the bacterial surface by fluorescent-antibody staining of *B. pertussis*, using the monoclonal as primary antibody. This monoclonal was prepared by immunizing mice with a crude preparation of PT. Antibody-producing hybrids were identified with ELISA tests against a panel of antigens, including concentrated *B. pertussis* culture supernatant fluids, whole-cell lysates, and LPS.

B. Monoclonal Antibodies to Pertussis Toxin (PT)

Frank and Parker isolated hybrid cell lines after immunizing with a fraction enriched for PT (7). Two monoclonals which reacted with PT were studied in detail (8). These monoclonals were identified following fusion of cell line P3x63 Ag 8. 653 with spleen cells of mice immunized with crude PT. One antibody reacted with subunit 2 (S2) of PT in immunoblots, while the other was not reactive in immunoblots.

Both monoclonals were able to purify PT when used in immunoaffinity chromatography columns. Immunoaffinity purifications yielded twice as much PT as conventional purifications, even though the elution buffer for the immunoaffinity column consisted of 4 M sodium thiocyanate–2 M urea. PT is stable and soluble in the chaotropic eluant, although the antibodies are stable for only a limited time.

Attempts to purify PT by immunoprecipitation were less satisfactory. In a high-salt buffer (0.5 M NaCl in 25 mM Tris), monoclonal P11B10 immunoprecipitated S2, although the controls gave a high background, and SDS–PAGE analysis showed that the precipitate was not pure. Monoclonal P7B10, which was negative in immunoblots, was unreactive in immunoprecipitation studies.

Neither of these monoclonals neutralized the toxicity of PT, as examined by ability to block sensitization of mice to histamine lethality.

Hybrid cell lines which produce monoclonal antibodies to PT which neutralize toxicity have been reported (38). Immunization was started with PT toxoid, and completed 3 months later with PT. Fusion was with myeloma cell line SP2/0-Ag14. More than 60 clones secreting antibody to PT were isolated, but only 3 were characterized in detail. Two clones, 1B7 and 3F10, secreted antibody to S1 of PT, and one clone (1H2) produced antibody specific for S4. All three antibodies prevented PT-induced hemagglutination. One monoclonal to S1 (1B7) neutralized the toxicity of PT for mice, and passively protected mice against aerosol and intranasal challenge.

Antibody 1B7 neutralized toxicity and protected mice as well as a polyclonal reference antiserum, and could reverse PT-induced lymphocytosis when given 1 day after the toxin (38). This finding suggests that monoclonal antibodies could be useful in therapy of severe whooping cough. A more immediate use for the monoclonals may be in the assay of the PT content of vaccines, or in diagnostic techniques.

Four monoclonal antibodies to PT were reported to be somewhat effective in preventing adhesion of *B. pertussis* to Vero cells (12). The level of inhibition of adhesion was dependent on the strain and on the growth conditions. These studies are in agreement with findings that PT is associated with the cell envelope, but is not always found on the surface. The finding that some anti-S1 antibodies neutralize toxicity serves to confirm the biochemical findings regarding toxin structure (50).

C. Monoclonal Antibodies to Other *Bordetella pertussis* Antigens

Larsen *et al.* (22) isolated 11 hybrid cell lines which secreted monoclonal antibodies to unidentified components after immunizing with *B. pertussis* cells. Techniques for isolation of hybrid cell lines were the same as described above, for Selmer *et al.* (42). Five of these antibodies were shown to be useful in purifying specific components from *B. pertussis* cell extracts by immunoaffinity chromatography. Two of the antibodies were completely specific for *B. pertussis* when tested in ELISAs for reactivity to *B. parapertussis* and *B. bronchiseptica* and 15 species of other bacteria. The other nine antibodies reacted with other bacteria. Also, these workers demonstrated that proteolytic degradation of some antigens occurred after sample preparation, and that addition of protease inhibitors prevented such degradation.

Frank and Parker (7) described 11 hybrids thay isolated following immunization with whole cells of *B. pertussis* or with crude PT as described above. These include one cell line which produced antibody to FHA and two cell lines producing antibody to PT. Five cell lines produced antibody to LPS, one produced antibody to a 91-kDa OMP of *B. pertussis* (2a), and two produced antibody which reacted with unidentified cell components.

These monoclonals were reacted against a degraded strain of *B. pertussis*, *B. parapertussis*, *B. bronchiseptica*, *Haemophilus influenzae*, *Escherichia coli*, and *Salmonella typhimurium* in ELISA tests. The monoclonal antibodies to LPS reacted with other *Bordetella* species, but not with non-*Bordetella* species. One antibody to LPS, P6H3, reacted quite strongly with all *Bordetella* species examined, while two others reacted only to *B. pertussis* and *B. bronchiseptica*. Only the anti-LPS antibodies reacted with a degraded (phase III) mutant of *B. pertussis*, indicating that virulence associated-antigens PT and FHA were missing. Monoclonal antibodies directed against proteins showed no cross-reactivity outside genus *Bordetella*.

Fluorescence microscopy of intact bacterial cells with the latter 11 antibodies serving as primary antibody showed that antibodies specific for LPS gave strongly positive reactions with *B. pertussis;* anti-FHA and anti-91-kDa protein gave weaker positive reactions; and the remaining antibodies did not appear to react with intact bacteria. The monoclonals to LPS and to FHA seem good candidates for use in the standard fluorescent-antibody technique to diagnose whooping cough. More extensive testing may show that *Bordetella* LPS cross-reacts with other bacterial antigens. However, FHA, PT, and AC are found only in members of this genus.

Gorringe *et al.* (12) reported isolation of a monoclonal antibody to a *B. pertussis* OMP, as well as monoclonals to agglutinogens 1, 2, and 3. These monoclonals were examined for their effects on *B. pertussis* adhesion to Vero cells, together with monoclonals specific for FHA and PT, as described above. The monoclonals to agglutinogen antigens did not agglutinate *B. pertussis* under conditions of the assay. The antibodies did, however, inhibit adherence of such cells to Vero cells. The antiagglutinogen antibodies were the most effective inhibitors, with anti-FHA, anti-PT, and anti-OMP7 showing successively less inhibition. However, each of these antibodies was capable of inhibiting adhesion in some instances. Their data also demonstrate that these antigens are on the bacterial cell surface.

Montaraz and co-workers (28) described cell lines which secrete monoclonal antibodies to an OMP of *B. bronchiseptica* and *B. pertussis*. These workers used whole-cell *B. bronchiseptica* vaccine to immunize mice, fused their spleen cells with P3-NS1/1-Ag4-1) myeloma cells, and screened for antibody against a cell surface fraction of *B. bronchiseptica*. Two clones were characterized which secreted antibody reactive with a 68-kDa protein found both in *B. bronchiseptica* and in *B. pertussis*. The antibodies also reacted with a 71-kDa protein of*B. parapertussis*. One monoclonal passively protected mice from death and nasal pathology which follow aerosol challenge with *B. bronchiseptica*. The protective monoclonal was used to purify the 68-kDa protein by immunoaffinity chromatography. Bound antigen was eluted from the column with 3 *M* NaSCN in these studies. Affinity-purified 68-kDa protein was effective in inducing active immunity to *B. bronchiseptica* challenge.

IV. CONCLUSIONS

Monoclonal antibodies to several *B. pertussis* components have been produced in recent years. Standard procedures of immunization and fusion with myeloma cells are reported by laboratories isolating hybrid cell lines. Hybrid cell lines studied to date yield predominantly IgG_1 antibodies, but other antibody classes are also found. Hybrid cell lines producing antibody of defined specificities are not yet numerous. However, no obstacle to definition of all major *B. pertussis* antigens with monoclonal antibodies is apparent.

The value of monoclonal antibody techniques in the pertussis field was demonstrated by the first report of monoclonal antibody to *B. pertussis* components (3). The fimbriae seen on *B. pertussis* cells by electron microscopy had been assumed to be FHA, since FHA spontaneously forms filaments when it is purified. However, monoclonals to FHA did not bind to the fimbriae. Additional study showed that the agglutinogen 2 antisera reacted with the fimbriae. These findings disproved a widely held assumption about the form and location of FHA. The power and specificity of monoclonal antibodies to identify specific cell components makes them particularly valuable when pure antigens are usually unavailable, as is the case for *B. pertussis*.

The isolation of a monoclonal antibody which neutralizes PT (38) is a major advance. The neutralizing monoclonal reacts with S1, the enzymatically active subunit of the toxin. This antibody protects mice from intoxication with pure PT, and also prevents death from intranasal or intracerebral challenge with live bacteria.

Using monoclonal antibodies, Selmer *et al.* purified FHA (42), Frank and Parker purified PT (7,8), and Montaraz *et al.* purified a protective outer-membrane component of *B. bronchiseptica* (28). Their findings suggest that these and other components of *B. pertussis* may be amenable to purification using monoclonals. FHA and PT are the two components in the new Japanese vaccine, and are purified by biochemical and biophysical means (40). Immunoaffinity purification of FHA and PT might prove useful to vaccine manufacturers. In any event, monoclonals should be useful in assessing the content of relevant antigens in vaccines.

Adhesion of *B. pertussis* cells to cultured eukaryotic cells does not involve binding to cilia, and thus may not be completely analogous to the pathophysiology of disease. However, Gorringe and co-workers (12) have used Vero cell cultures and several monoclonal antibodies to investigate the role of certain antigens on adhesion. The elegance of this study lies in the use of monoclonal antibodies reacting with several defined antigens. The multifactorial nature of *B. pertussis* virulence is supported by this study, and the monoclonality of the antisera used allows interpretation of the data. Polyclonal sera would be unconvincing and nondiscriminating in this study, if such sera were available.

Monoclonal antibody experiments have demonstrated the following:

1. Agglutinogen antigen 2 of *B. pertussis* is located on a fimbrial structure.
2. FHA antigen is not fimbrial but is located on the bacterial surface.
3. FHA, PT, and other components can be purified by immunoaffinity chromatography.
4. The OMP7 protein and the 91-kDa protein of the outer membrane are located on the bacterial surface.
5. Monoclonal neutralizing antibody to PT is against the enzymatically active subunit, S1.

6. Antibodies to several surface antigens, including agglutinogens 1, 2, and 3, FHA, PT, and OMP7, are able to inhibit *B. pertussis* adhesion to Vero cells.

V. PROSPECTS FOR THE FUTURE

Monoclonal antibodies should play an increasingly important role in basic research on *B. pertussis,* and several applications appear likely. These antibodies will find use in structure–function studies of important *B. pertussis* proteins, such as PT and AC. Monoclonals will be used for epitope mapping of several proteins and identification of the epitopes which may be important in vaccines. Monoclonals may also be used to purify selected cell components, to identify recombinant clones which produce certain antigens, and for electron microscopic localization of structural proteins.

Applications of monoclonal antibody technology include vaccine production, production of purified cell components such as PT and AC for research use, and diagnosis of disease. Identification and quantitation of specific bacterial components in vaccines or in purified pertussis products can be reliably performed with monoclonal antibodies. One purified component, PT, is used to study receptor-mediated regulatory processes of eukaryotic cells, adjuvant effects, etc. The AC and FHA proteins may also be of commercial interest, along with LPS and LPS-associated proteins of the outer membrane, and monoclonals could be used in purification or to assay purity.

Antibodies to LPS or to specific phase I antigens could be used for diagnosis of whooping cough by identification of antigen in respiratory secretions. Such an antigen detection method, or an antibody detection method, or both could replace current direct microscopy and culture methods.

VI. SUMMARY

Bordetella pertussis, the causative agent of whooping cough, is known for its frequent antigenic variation. The major antigens for identifying and serotyping *B. pertussis* are six agglutinogens, so called because they induce agglutinating antibody. *Bordetella pertussis* also produces a variety of noxious substances involved in pathogenesis of the disease. Major virulence antigens include pertussis toxin (PT), adenylate cyclase, and filamentous hemagglutinin (FHA).

Several monoclonal antibodies have been induced to *B. pertussis* and its products, such as FHA, PT, outer membrane proteins, lipopolysaccharide, and unidentified antigens. Antibodies to FHA showed that FHA is not fimbrial in nature but lies on the cell surface. Antibodies to PT have shown reactions with specific subunits of the toxin, neutralizing toxicity only if they react with subunit

1. Monoclonal antibodies have been used in immunoaffinity chromatography to purify both FHA and PT from culture fluids. Monoclonal antibodies are likely to play an important role in defining the antigens of *B. pertussis*, in providing diagnostic reagents, and in purifying cell components.

REFERENCES

1. Andersen, E. K. (1953). Serological studies on *H. pertussis*, *H. parapertussis*, and *H. bronchisepticus*. *Acta Pathol Microbiol. Scand.* **33**, 202–224.
2. Arai, H., and Sato, Y. (1976). Separation and characterization of two distinct hemagglutinins contained in purified leukocytosis-promoting factor from *Bordetella pertussis*. *Biochim. Biophys. Acta* **444**, 765–782.
2a. Armstrong, S. K., and Parker, C. D. (1986). Heat-modifiable envelope proteins of *Bordetella pertussis*. *Infect. Immun.* **54** (in press).
3. Ashworth, L. A. E., Irons, L. I., and Dowsett, A. B. (1982). Antigenic relationship between serotype-specific agglutinogen and fimbriae of *Bordetella pertussis*. *Infect. Immun.* **37**, 1278–1281.
4. Confer, D. W., and Eaton, J. W. (1982). Phagocyte impotence caused by an invasive bacterial adenylate cyclase. *Science* **217**, 948–950.
5. Eldering, E. K., Eveland, W. C., and Kendrick, P. L. (1962). Fluorescent antibody reactions in *Bordetella pertussis* cultures. *J. Bacteriol.* **83**, 745–749.
6. Field, L. H., and Parker, C. D. (1979). Differences observed between fresh isolates of *Bordetella pertussis* and their laboratory passaged derivatives. *In* "International Symposium on Pertussis" (C. Manclark and J. Hill, eds.), pp. 124–132. DHEW Publ. No. (NIH) 79-1830, U. S. Dep. Health, Educ. Welfare, Bethesda, Maryland.
7. Frank, D. W., and Parker, C. D. (1984). Isolation and characterization of monoclonal antibodies to *Bordetella pertussis*. *J. Biol. Stand.* **12**, 353–365.
8. Frank, D. W., and Parker, C. D. (1984). Interaction of monoclonal antibodies with pertussis toxin and its subunits. *Infect. Immun.* **46**, 195–201.
9. Gabay, J., and Schwartz, M. (1982). Monoclonal antibody as a probe for structure and function of an *Escherichia coli* outer membrane protein. *J. Biol. Chem.* **257**, 6627–6630.
10. Gill, D. M. (1978). Seven toxic peptides that cross cell membranes. *In* "Bacterial Toxins and Cell Membranes" (J. Jeljaszewicz and T. Wadstrom, eds.), pp. 291–332. Academic Press, New York.
11. Goldman, W. E., Klapper, D. G., and Baseman, J. B. (1982). Detection, isolation and analysis of a released *Bordetella pertussis* product toxic to cultured tracheal cells. *Infect. Immun.* **36**, 782–794.
12. Gorringe, A. R., Ashworth, L. A. E., Irons, L. I., and Robinson, A. (1985). Effect of monoclonal antibodies on the adherence of *Bordetella pertussis* on Vero cells. *FEMS Microbiol. Lett.* **26**, 5–9.
13. Hall, G. W., Dobrogroz, W. J., Ezzell, J. W., Kloos, W. E., and Manclark, C. (1982). Repression of adenylate cyclase in the genus *Bordetella*. *Microbios* **33**, 45–52.
14. Hewlett, E., and Wolff, J. (1976). Soluble adenylate cyclase from the culture medium of *Bordetella pertussis:* Purification and characterization. *J. Bacteriol.* **127**, 890–898.
15. Imaizumi, A., Suzuki, Y., Ono, S., Sato, H., and Sato, Y. (1983). Heptakis (2, 6-*o*-dimethyl) beta cyclodextrin: A novel growth stimulant for *Bordetella pertussis* phase I. *J. Clin. Microbiol.* **17**, 781–786.
16. Irons, L. I., Ashworth, L. A., and Wilton-Smith, P. (1983). Heterogeneity of the filamentous

hemagglutinin of *Bordetella pertussis* studied with monoclonal antibodies. *J. Gen. Microbiol.* **129,** 2769–2778.

17. Jebb, W. H. H., and Tomlinson, A. H. (1955). The nutritional requirements of *Haemophilus pertussis. J. Gen. Microbiol.* **13,** 1–8.

18. Kasuga, T., Nakase, Y., Ukishima, K., and Takatsu, K. (1953). Studies on *Haemophilus pertussis.* Part I: Antigen structure of *H. pertussis* and its phases. *Kitasato Arch. Exp. Med.* **26,** 121–134.

19. Kasuga, T., Nakase, Y., Ukishima, K., and Takatsu, K. (1954). Studies on *Haemophilus pertussis.* Part III: Some properties of each phase. *Kitasato Arch. Exp. Med.* **27,** 37–48.

20. Katada, T., and Ui, M. (1982). Direct modification of the membrane adenylate cyclase system by islet-activating protein dud to ADP-ribosylation of a membrane protein. *Proc. Natl. Acad. Sci. U.S.A.* **79,** 3129–3133.

20a. Kume, K., Nakai, T., Samejima, Y., and Sugimoto, C. (1986). Properties of dermonecrotic toxin prepared from sonic extracts of *Bordetella bronchiseptica. Infect. Immun.* **52,** 370–377.

21. Lacey, B. W. (1960). Antigenic modulation of *Bordetella pertussis. J. Hyg.* **58,** 57–93.

22. Larsen, F. S., Selmer, J. C., and Hertz, J. B. (1984). Purification of *Bordetella pertussis* antigens using monoclonal antibody. *Acta Pathol. Microbiol. Immunol. Scand., Sect. C* **92,** 271–277.

23. LeDur, A., Caroff, M., Chaby, R., and Szabo, L. (1978). A novel type of endotoxin structure present in *Bordetella pertussis. Eur. J. Biochem.* **84,** 579–589.

24. LeDur, A., Chaby, R., and Szabo, L. (1980). Isolation of two pure and protein-free lipopolysaccharides from *Bordetella pertussis* phenol-extracted endotoxin. *J. Bacteriol.* **143,** 78–88.

25. Leslie, P. H., and Gardner, A. D. (1931). The phases of *Haemophilus pertussis. J. Hyg.* **31,** 423–434.

26. Livey, I., Parton, R., and Wardlaw, A. C. (1978). Loss of heat-labile toxin from *Bordetella pertussis* grown in modified Hornibrook medium. *FEMS Microbiol. Lett.* **3,** 203–205.

27. McPheat, W. L., Wardlaw, A. C., and Novotny, P. (1983). Modulation of *Bordetella pertussis* by nicotinic acid. *Infect. Immun.* **41,** 516–522.

28. Montaraz, J. A., Novotny, P., and Ivanyi, J. (1985). Identification of a 68-kilodalton protective protein antigen from *Bordetella bronchiseptica. Infect. Immun.* **47,** 744–751.

29. Munoz, J. J., and Bergman, R. K. (1977). ''*Bordetella pertussis:* Immunological and Other Biological Activities.'' Dekker, New York.

30. Parker, C. (1976). Role of the genetics and physiology of *Bordetella pertussis* in the production of vaccine and the study of host–parasite relationships in pertussis. *Adv. Appl. Microbiol.* **20,** 27–42.

31. Parton, R., and Durham, J. P. (1978). Loss of adenylate cyclase activity in variants of *Bordetella pertussis. FEMS Microbiol. Lett.* **4,** 287–289.

32. Parton, R., and Wardlaw, A. C. (1975). Cell-envelope proteins of *Bordetella pertussis. J. Med. Microbiol.* **8,** 47–57.

33. Peppler, M. S. (1982). Isolation and characterization of isogenic pairs of domed hemolytic and flat nonhemolytic colony types of *Bordetella pertussis. Infect. Immun.* **35,** 840–851.

34. Pittman, M. (1979). Pertussis toxin: The cause of harmful effects and prolonged immunity of whooping cough. A hypothesis. *Rev. Infect. Dis.* **1,** 401–412.

35. Preston, N. W. (1975). Vaccine composition in relation to antigenic variation of the microbe: Is pertussis unique? *Prog. Drug Res.* **18,** 347–355.

36. Pusztai, S., and Joo, I. (1967). Influence of nicotinic acid on the antigenic structure of *Bordetella pertussis. Ann. Immunol. Hung.* **10,** 63–67.

37. Rowatt, E. (1957). The growth of *Bordetella pertussis:* A review. *J. Gen. Microbiol.* **17,** 297–326.

38. Sato, H., Ito, A., Chiba, J., and Sato, Y. (1984). Monoclonal antibody against pertussis toxin: Effect on toxin activity and pertussis infections. *Infect. Immun.* **46,** 422–428.

39. Sato, Y., Izumiya, K., Sato, H., Cowell, J. L., and Manclark, C. R. (1981). Role of antibody to leukocytosis-promoting factor hemagglutinin and to filamentous hemagglutinin in immunity to pertussis. *Infect. Immun.* **31,** 1223–1231.
40. Sato, Y., Kimura, M., and Fukumi, H. (1984). Development of a pertussis component vaccine in Japan. *Lancet* **1,** 122–126.
41. Schneider, D. R., and Parker, C. D. (1982). Effect of pyrimidines on phenotypic properties of *Bordetella pertussis. Infect. Immun.* **38,** 548–553.
42. Selmer, J. C., Larsen, F. S., Hertz, J. B., and Parton, R. (1984). Purification and partial characterization of filamentous hemagglutinins from *Bordetella pertussis* using monoclonal antibodies. *Acta Pathol Microbiol. Immununol. Scand., Sect. C* **92,** 279–284.
43. Stainer, D. W., and Scholte, M. J. (1971). A simple, chemically defined medium for the production of phase I *Bordetella pertussis. J. Gen. Microbiol.* **83,** 211–220.
44. Stanbridge, T. N., and Preston, N. W. (1974). Variation of serotype in strains of *Bordetella pertussis. J. Hyg.* **73,** 305–310.
45. Standfast, A. F. B. (1951). The phase I of *Haemophilus pertussis. J. Gen. Microbiol.* **5,** 531–545.
46. Sultzer, B., Craig, J. P., and Castagna, R. (1985). The adjuvant effect of pertussis endotoxin protein in modulating the immune response to cholera toxoid in mice. *In* ''Developments in Biological Standardization. Volume 61. Proceedings of the Fourth International Symposium on Pertussis'' (C. M. Manclark and W. Hennessen, eds.), pp. 225–232. S. Karger, New York.
47. Tamura, M., Nogimori, K., Murai, S., Yajima, M., Ito, K., Katada, T., Ui, M., and Ishii, S. (1982). Subunit structure of islet-activating protein pertussis toxin in conformity with the A-B model. *Biochemistry* **21,** 5516–5522.
48. Tamura, M., Nogimori, K., Yajima, M., Ase, K., and Ui, M. (1983). A role of the B-oligomer of islet-activating protein, pertussis toxin, in development of the biological effects on intact cells. *J. Biol. Chem.* **258,** 6756–6761.
49. Tuomanen, E., and Weiss, A. (1985). Characterization of two adhesins of *Bordetella pertussis* for human ciliated respiratory–epithelial cells. *J. Infect. Dis.* **152,** 118–125.
50. Ui, M., Katada, T., Murayama, T., and Nakamura, T. (1984). Islet-activating protein, pertussis toxin, as a probe for receptor-mediated signal transduction. *In* ''Calcium Regulation in Biological Systems'' (S. Ebashi, M. Endo, K. Imahori, S. Kakiuchi, and Y. Nishizuka, eds.), pp. 157–169. Academic Press, Tokyo.
51. Wardlaw, A. C., and Parton, R. (1983). *Bordetella pertussis* toxins. *Pharmacol Ther.* **19,** 1–53.
52. Wardlaw, A. C., Parton, R., and Hooker, M. J. (1976). Loss of protective antigen, histamine-sensitizing factor and envelope polypeptides in cultural variants of *Bordetella pertussis. J. Med. Microbiol.* **9,** 89–100.
53. Weiss, A. A., and Falkow, S. (1982). Plasmid transfer to *Bordetella pertussis:* Conjugation and transformation. *J. Bacteriol.* **152,** 549–552.
54. Weiss, A. A., and Falkow, S. (1983). Transposon insertion and subsequent donor formation promoted by Tn501 in *Bordetella pertussis. J. Bacteriol.* **153,** 304–309.
55. Weiss, A. A., and Falkow, S. (1984). Genetic analysis of phase change in *Bordetella pertussis. Infect. Immun.* **43,** 263–269.
56. Weiss, A. A., Hewlett, E. L., Myers, G. A., and Falkow, S. (1983). Tn5-induced mutations affecting virulence factors of *Bordetella pertussis. Infect. Immun.* **42,** 33–41.
57. Weiss, A. A., Hewlett, E. L., Myers, G. A., and Falkow, S. (1984). Pertussis toxin and extracytoplasmic adenylate cyclase as virulence factors of *Bordetella pertussis. J. Infect. Dis.* **150,** 219–222.
58. Wolff, J. G., Cook, G. H., Goldhammer, A. R., and Berkowitz, S. A. (1980). Calmodulin activates prokaryotic adenylate cyclase. *Proc. Natl. Acad. Sci. U.S.A.* **77,** 3841–3844.

8

Molecular Structures of Bacteria Elucidated by Monoclonal Antibodies with Special Reference to Antigenic Determinants of the Methanogens' Envelopes

**EVERLY CONWAY DE MACARIO
AND ALBERTO J. L. MACARIO**
*Wadsworth Center for Laboratories and Research
New York State Department of Health
Albany, New York*

I. INTRODUCTION

A general introduction to the advantages of antibody probes, monoclonal in particular, to study methanogens was presented in Volume I of this treatise (27). The significance of immunologic studies of methanogens for public health, most

MONOCLONAL ANTIBODIES
AGAINST BACTERIA
Volume III

of all for environmental (sanitary) engineering, and for biotechnology were pointed out.

Characterization of monoclonal antibodies for generating probes of considerable precision and resolving power was discussed in Volume II (28). A comparison of poly- and monoclonal antibody probes was presented to show their differences and their potential as complementary reagents to study and manipulate methanogens. Specific properties of monoclonal antibody probes such as specificity spectrum and fine (molecular) specificity pattern were described, as well as methods for using them, for example, inhibition-blocking procedures designed to learn the structure of the antigenic determinants found in the mosaics of methanogens. Various panels of monoclonal antibody probes made against several reference methanogens were also described.

This chapter contains information on the antibody panels and data obtained with them in analyzing the antigenic mosaics of methanogens. It also contains an overview of materials and methods useful for the molecular analyses of methanogens or any other bacteria, with extensive cross referencing to other chapters of this treatise.

II. BACKGROUND

A. Immunogens and Antigens

A variety of materials have been used as immunogens to prepare lymphocytes for fusion with myeloma cells to construct hybridomas that will produce antibacterial antibodies (Table I). One or more doses of a single immunogen are used as

TABLE I

Immunogens and Antigens

Immunogens:	Whole bacterial cells (fixed or not)
(one)	Envelope, cell wall, S layer, sheath, and fractions thereof
	Purified antigen (not necessary)
	Analogs
Antigens:	Whole bacterial cells (fixed or not)
(more than	Envelope, cell wall, S layer, sheath, and fractions thereof
one)	Purified antigen (necessary in special cases)
	Compounds of known composition
	Compounds of known structure (analogs)
	Modified antigen
	Denatured (heat, other)
	Enzyme treated
	Other
	Cross-reactive antigen(s)
	Related molecule(s)

a rule for immunization of the lymphocyte donor. However, in screening hybri-domas for detecting antibody producers, it is convenient to use more than one antigen, that is, the immunogen and some other bacteria or bacterial product cross-reacting with the former. These cross-reactive antigens should be identified using polyclonal antibody probes before the start of the hybridizations. The latter probes help in choosing a panel of antigens for preparing a set of monoclonal antibodies whose specificity spectra will be varied, and will encompass a wider range of antigenic structures than a panel of antibodies with identical or very similar specificities. Sets of monoclonal antibody probes differing in specificity spectra are very useful for resolving antigenic mosaics into their components, elucidating the structure of the latter (determinants), understanding antigenic relationships at the molecular level, gaining insights into the biologic and func-tional roles of bacterial components, and screening samples from a variety of ecologic niches in the search for methanogens or their "footprints."

B. Uses of Monoclonal Antibodies against Bacteria

Monoclonal antibodies are useful for a variety of purposes in bacterial immu-nology (Table II), which can be summarized as follows: diagnosis and control of infection, identification and classification, and biotechnologic manipulations (26).

Bacterial structures that can be targeted for analysis with monoclonal anti-bodies are also varied (Table III). It is possible to undertake the purification and characterization of the molecule that carries the antigenic determinants recog-nized by the antibodies in the panel, and then proceed to the identification of the determinants themselves, and to the elucidation of the bacterial structure of which the antigen molecule is a part. In performing these studies, the categories of information obtained are very diverse (Table IV).

C. Methods

Methodologic tactics for bacterial analyses with monoclonal antibodies, in-cluding the characterizarion of the binding properties of the antibody themselves, are listed in Table V.

Antibody–antigen inhibition-blocking experients complement direct-binding assays and are useful for determining the fine (molecular) specificity of the antibodies (6). This topic was discussed in detail in Volume II (28). Suffice it to say here that the same kind of experiments provide information on the structure and/or composition of the determinants, and thus are the starting point in the elucidation of the structure of the antigen molecule (6,14,18,28).

Antibody–antibody inhibition tests are useful for establishing whether or not two antibodies recognize the same determinant (12,15,16,19,24,34,44). If it is known that the two antibodies do recognize different determinants, antibody–

TABLE II

Uses of Monoclonal Antibodies against Bacteria

Identification of new isolates
Elucidation of complex microbial communities
Taxonomy
Chemotaxonomy
Ecology
Laboratory diagnosis and monitoring infections and response to therapy
    Bacterial cells
    Bacterial antigens: shed, secreted
Epidemiologic surveys
    Individuals (humans, animals)
    Environment (water, soil)
In vivo diagnosis (localization)
Detection of bacterial toxins in food
Serotherapy
    Toxic syndromes
    Infections (local, general)
Vectoring molecules to poison bacteria (*in vivo*)
Study of pathogenetic mechanisms (adhesion, toxins)
Modulation of immune response (adjuvants, T- and B-cell stimulants)
Molecular immunochemistry
    Composition
    Structure
    Domains
    Topography
    Structure–function
Genetic engineering
    Vaccines
    Other
Bacterial manipulation
    Selection (positive, negative)
    Retention
    Other
Industry: Biotechnology
Search for molecular "signatures" of bacteria in
    Ecologic niches
    Organisms
    Other

antibody inhibition tests are instrumental for mapping the determinants on the antigen molecule.

Figure 1 illustrates possible outcomes of antibody–antibody inhibition assays. The antigen (bacteria or molecule) is assumed to bear one copy each of several determinants $(1, 2, 3, \ldots n)$ (5,28). Their corresponding monoclonal antibodies are a1, a2, a3, and an. They are reacted with the antigen in pairs, usually one

TABLE III

Bacterial Structures That Can Be Studied Immunochemically with Monoclonal Antibodies

Molecule
    Simple (one chain)
    Complex (multimer)
Determinant
Supramolecular structure
    Polymer
    Bacterial envelope
    Cell wall
    S Layer
    Pili
    Flagella
    Toxins
    Membrane proteins
    Other

TABLE IV

Categories of Information Obtained by Immunochemical Analyses with Monoclonal Antibodies

Composition
Structure
    Chains
    Domains
Structural domains + function
Mapping of determinants
Determinant
Location, topography
    Cell
    Cell structure
    Tissue
    Organ
    Other
Biologic role
    Protective immunity (vaccine)
    Adjuvant
    Toxin
    Pathogenicity
    Other

TABLE V

Methods

Indirect: Antibody–antigen inhibition blocking
Antibody–antibody inhibition
Antibody–ligand inhibition
Antibody–antigen–antibody tandem
Adsorptions
Comparative survey of antigens
Reaction with modified antigen
Direct: Purify antigen (and/or determinant; biochemically or by genetic engineering)
Chemical composition
Structure
Direct-binding assays
Visualization of antibody–antigen
EM
Biophysical methods
Immunoblotting
Bacterial genetics combined with immunochemistry
Other

---

after the other. The effect of the binding of the antibody reacted first on the one added in the second step is observed. If the second antibody does not bind, or binds only partially (some antibody molecules remain unbound), it is concluded that the two determinants are close to each other, or that an allosteric effect has been brought about by the binding of the first antibody.

When the two determinants being recognized by the two antibodies used in the inhibition assay are close to one another, steric hindrance may be the cause of lack, or impaired binding of the second antibody. The same effect on the binding of the second antibody can be due to allosteric changes in the antigen molecule induced by the first antibody. These allosteric changes may alter the determinant for the second antibody to a point at which it becomes unrecognizable, or at which it is recognized and bound but with considerably less affinity. Likewise, binding of the first antibody may originate allosteric changes that cause an increase in the affinity of the second antibody for its corresponding determinant.

Steric hindrance, allosteric changes, and other molecular mechanisms may be involved in the generation of the results obtained by antibody–antibody inhibition tests. Although understanding these molecular mechanisms is sometimes difficult, antibody–antibody inhibition assays are extremely useful for the structural analyses of bacterial components and for elucidating structure–function relationships (e.g., in studying membrane transport and the action of toxins). In the latter studies, antibody–ligand inhibition assays are instrumental (Fig. 2). For these assays, the tactics and types of information obtained are similar to those of antibody–antibody inhibition.

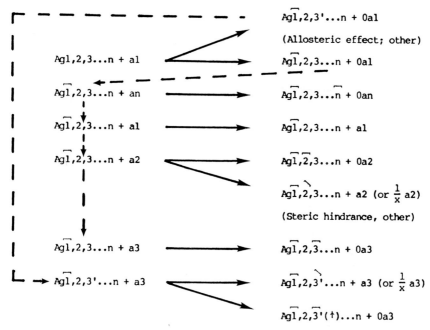

Fig. 1. Antibody–antibody inhibition. $Ag1,2,3, \ldots n$ represents a bacterial antigen (whole cell or molecule) bearing determinants 1, 2, and so on, whose corresponding monoclonal antibodies are a1, a2, and so on. A prime symbol by a determinant (e.g., $3'$) indicates that the latter has been modified in its capacity to interact with its corresponding antibody (a3) due to the binding of another determinant (e.g., 1) to its antibody (i.e., a1). A horizontal bracket capping a determinant means that the latter is bound to (covered by) antibody; a slanted bracket indicates that antibody cannot bind, or that it binds with lower affinity than in the absence of another antibody being bound to its corresponding determinant. A zero (0) indicates absence of free antibody after a reaction (e.g., 0a1 means no free a1 left after reacting $Ag1,2,3, \ldots n$ with a 1), while $1/x$ indicates that a fraction of antibody remains free. A vertical arrow pointing upwards within parentheses shows determinant bound to antibody with higher affinity than in the absence of another determinant–antibody reaction occurring somewhere else in the antigen molecule. A plus symbol indicates a reaction mixture (e.g., $Ag1,2,3, \ldots n$ + a1 means that the antigen and a1 have been mixed), while the horizontal or slanted arrows pointing to the right show the outcome of the reaction. Dashed lines show experimental sequences.

A number of antigen–ligand systems have been studied by means of monoclonal antibodies involving viruses, toxins, C-reactive protein, enzymes, bacterial adherence structures, and their specific binding sites on cell surfaces or molecules (1,2,10–12,20,35,36,38,42,44,47).

Similar to antibody–antibody inhibition, antiserum–antibody inhibitions are performed but for a different purpose (10,14,19,25).

Antiserum–antibody inhibition assays are most useful for elucidating the antibody composition of an immune serum (Fig. 3). A panel of monoclonal anti-

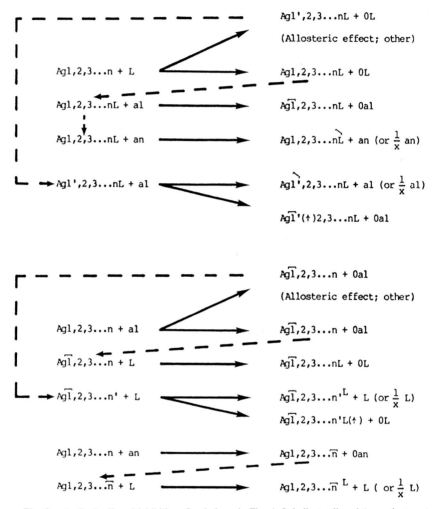

Fig. 2. Antibody–ligand inhibition. Symbols as in Fig. 1; L indicates ligand (e.g., the target molecule of a toxin or the substrate of an enzyme).

bodies of predefined specificities against the antigen for which antibodies must be identified in the immune serum is necessary. The antigen is incubated first with the immune serum and then with a monoclonal antibody. If the latter does not bind, it is concluded that antibodies recognizing the same determinant as that recognized by the monoclonal antibody are present in the serum. The same experiment is repeated with the other monoclonal antibodies in the panel, until a more complete picture of the antibody populations in the serum is obtained. Interpretation of results is subjected to the same rules followed in antibody–antibody and antibody–ligand inhibition assays.

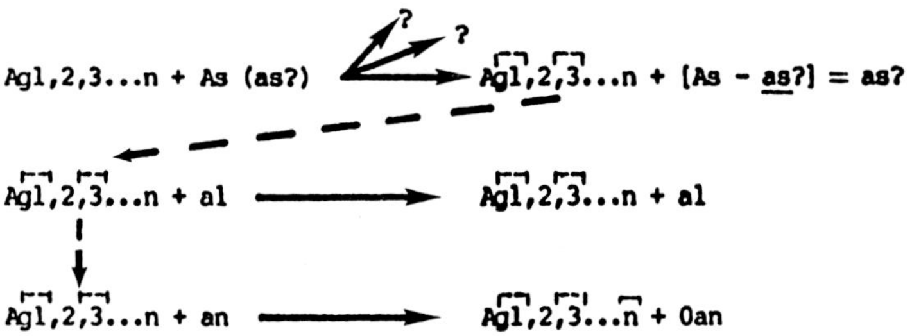

Fig. 3. Antiserum–antibody inhibition. Symbols as in Fig. 1; As, antiserum; as, antibody populations with different specificities in the antiserum; question marks show uncertainties as to which antibody populations are present in the antiserum, or which are bound and which remain free after reacting the antiserum with antigen; [As − *as*?] indicates that after reacting the antiserum (As) with antigen, some antibody populations (*as*?) have been subtracted from the antiserum, leaving behind, free, others (i.e., as?). Dashed brackets capping the determinants indicate that their binding to serum antibodies cannot be ascertained directly.

Information obtained by means of antiserum–antibody inhibition assays is relevant to the monitoring of serum antibody levels in relation with disease status, progression or regression of infection, response to treatment with antibiotics, and other functional or pathologic parameters. In this way it is possible to establish a precise correlation between a given antibody population from among the many present in the serum after a bacterial infection (or immunization) and protective immunity, for example. These types of correlative studies are, in turn, of paramount importance for the identification of the antigenic determinant most relevant to the elicitation of protective immunity, and therefore to the preparation of a vaccine.

Antibody–antigen–antibody tandem involves the use of two monoclonal antibodies recognizing different determinants on the same antigen, or just one antibody if the determinant expresses many copies on the antigen molecule (37). Tandem assays are useful for detecting antigen in fluid samples (biologic and environmental).

Other experimental tactics used to elucidate antigenic mosaics and learn the structure of determinants involve binding assays in which antigen bound to a solid phase, or in solution, is reacted with antibody (see Table V). Antigen may be used in its native state, or denatured, or treated chemically or enzymatically to modify the determinant in a more or less controlled manner, and thus infer which structures are crucial for antibody binding (9,21–23,38–43,45,47). A combination of bacterial genetics with immunochemistry using monoclonal antibodies can accomplish similar objectives in analyzing, for example, mutants in contrast with a wild-type molecule (10,12,46).

A panel of different antigens (e.g., cross-reactive materials) may be used to obtain a series of data that might help establish the structure of a functional molecule as opposed to a nonfunctional mutant. These binding assays and other

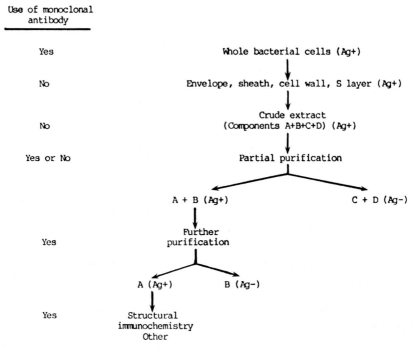

Fig. 4. Schematic representation of the sequential steps involved in the purification and identification of a bacterial antigen using a monoclonal antibody recognizing a determinant on this antigen. Ag+ (or Ag−), antigen detectable (or not detectable) with the monoclonal antibody. Reproduced, simplified, with permission from Garberi, Macario, and Conway de Macario, *J. Bacteriol.*, 1985 (13).

direct methods are efficient complement to the indirect ones mentioned in the foregoing paragraphs (see Table V).

The most powerful method of analysis is direct examination of purified antigen (12,19). This can be accomplished in many cases by virtue of the purity and monospecificity of monoclonal antibodies through a series of steps (Fig. 4). Bacterial genetics and genetic engineering (10,12,17,33,35,46) can help further in producing workable amounts of pure antigen for quantitative analysis and for other practical uses, such as preparation of diagnostic kits or vaccines (26).

III. RESULTS AND DISCUSSION

A. Antigenic Mosaics of Methanogens

Several panels of well-characterized monoclonal antibody probes have been prepared against these reference methanogens: *Methanobacterium thermoauto-*

trophicum strain ΔH (6,7), *Methanobrevibacter smithii* strain PS (8), *Methanobrevibacter arboriphilus* strain DH1 (6), *Methanococcus vannielii* strain SB (4), *Methanogenium cariaci* strain JR1c (3,31,32), *Methanospirillum hungatei* strain JF1 (3,6), *Methanosarcina barkeri* strain 227 (13), and *Methanothrix soehngenii* strain Opfikon (30).

Various antigenic determinants have been identified in the mosaics of the methanogens listed above with the monoclonal antibodies as follows: six in ΔH, PS, and SB, three in 227, two in JR1c, and one in DH1 and JF1. Studies with *Mt. soehngenii* are currently under way, and the results suggest a plurality of determinants in this methanogen, too.

These determinants of methanogens are expressed on the surface of whole bacterial cells regardless of whether these cells are fresh (unfixed) or fixed by formalin, heat, or drying. They have been demonstrated with monoclonal antibodies by slide immunoenzymatic assay (SIA) (6), indirect immunofluorescence (IIF) (6), and immunoelectron microscopy (4), and each of them has been identified by a combination of methods (see Table V). In all cases the determinants are expressed on the surface of the immunogen (i.e., the methanogen used to generate the monoclonal antibodies) with the following two exceptions: one for ΔH and one for 227. In these two cases, the determinant was found to be hidden (not accessible to antibody) in whole bacterial cells of the immunogen, but superficially expressed in a cross-reactive strain (i.e., GC1 for ΔH, and R1M3 for 227).

Each determinant thus far identified is recognized by one monoclonal antibody exclusively. Therefore, each antibody is a specific reagent for its corresponding determinant. Using these antibodies, studies have been performed to elucidate the structure of the determinants and the distribution in nature of these structures.

B. Immunochemistry of Antigenic Determinants

Structural information on five of six determinants in *Mb. thermautotrophicum* ΔH is available (Fig. 5) (6,7). Residues involved are *N*-acetyl-D-glucosamine, *N*-acetyl-D-galactosamine, and L-talosaminuronic acid (a typical component of pseudomurein, not present in eubacteria's murein), each in one determinant, and γ-glutamylalanine in two determinants. These structural data were obtained chiefly by inhibition-blocking assays with compounds of known composition (28).

The compositions of the six determinants described thus far in *Mbr. smithii* strain PS have not been elucidated yet, although it has been established that Orn, Glu and Lys are involved in one of them [Orn being characteristic of PS's pseudomurein (8)]. These determinants were distinguished from one another by a comparative survey of antigens (see Table V), which consisted of extensive testing of 46 *Mbr. smithii* isolates, and thus determining their distinctive distributions (Table VI) (8). Although determinants 6b and 6f show the same distribu-

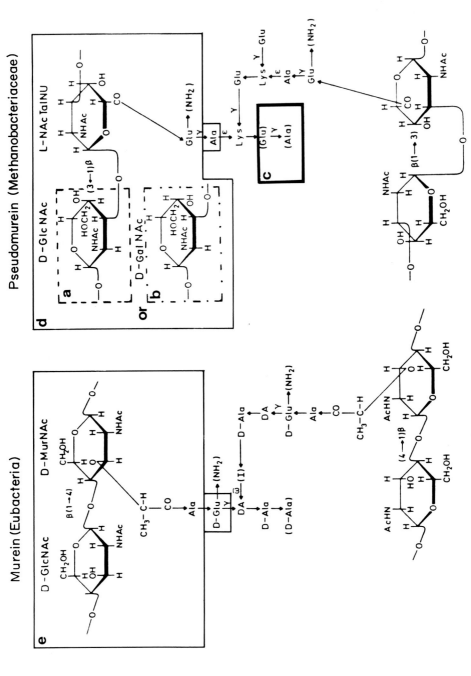

Fig. 5.

TABLE VI

Distinctive Distribution of the Antigenic Determinants of *Methanobrevibacter smithii* among Bacterial Isolates Shown by Monoclonal Antibodies[a]

Bacterial isolate number	Reaction with monoclonal antibody[b]					
	6C	6E	6D	6A	6B	6F
1–5	5p	5p	5p	5p	5p	5p
6–12	7n	7p	6p; 1n	6p; 1n	7p	7p
13–21	9n	9n	9p	8p; 1n	9p	9p
22–24	3n	3n	3n	3p	2p; 1n	2p; 1n
25–30	6n	6n	6n	6n	6p	6p
	(5p; 25n)	(12p; 18n)	(20p; 10n)	(22p; 8n)	(29p; 1n)	(29p; 1n)

[a] Reproduced, modified, with permission from Conway de Macario, Macario, and Pastini, *Arch. Microbiol.*, 1985 (8).

[b] p, Positive; n, negative. Determined by direct-binding assay using SIA and IIF. Examples: determinant 6c (recognized by antibody 6C) is present in isolates 1–5 only; determinant 6e (recognized by antibody 6E) is present in isolates 1–5 and also in isolates 6–12, but it is absent in the rest of the isolates; and so forth. Present or absent means detectable (or undetectable) by antibody on the surface of whole bacterial cells.

tion, they are different structures inasmuch as they express distinctive binding properties.

The determinant that has been identified in *Mbr. arboriphilus* DH1 contains γ-Glu-Ala as shown by inhibition-blocking and direct-binding assays (see Table V) (6).

The determinants that have been found in *Msp. hungatei* JF1 and *Mc. vannielii* SB are proteins. These have been resolved by electrophoresis of the JF1 strain's sheath (Fig. 6) and SB strain's S layer (Fig. 7), respectively (3,4,6). Lys, Phe, and Thr are involved in one of the six determinants found in strain SB; Ser, Try, and Tyr are in another, and Arg, Lys, and Phe are in a third. The superficial location of strain SB's determinants was shown by immunoelectron microscopy with monoclonal antibodies (4). The distribution and frequency of the determinants along the S layer could be visualized.

One of the three determinants that have been described in *Ms. barkeri* 227 was purified through a series of steps (see Fig. 4) in which the pertinent monoclonal antibody was instrumental in following the determinant-bearing molecule

Fig. 5. Primary structure of murein (left) and pseudomurein (right), showing, in boxes, the structures found to be involved in the determinants of *Methanobacterium thermoautotrophicum* strain ΔH that is, GlcNAc, GalNAc, γ-Glu-Ala, and L-NAc-TalNU. Reproduced from Conway de Macario, Macario, Magarinos, König, and Kandler, *Proc. Natl. Acad. Sci, U.S.A.* **80,** 6346–6350, 1983 (7).

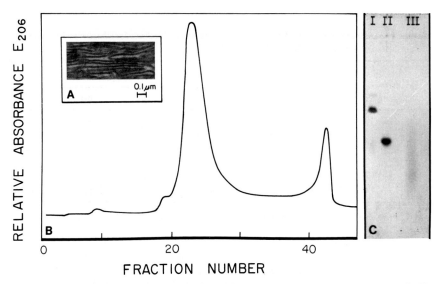

Fig. 6. Location of a antigenic determinant distinctive of *Methanospirillum hungatei* strain JF1 in a fraction of this strain's protein sheath (A). A sheath preparation was separated in a TSK column (B). Fractions 20–30 were pooled and examined by sodium dodecyl sulfate–polyacrylamide gel electrophoresis (SDS–PAGE) (C, lane III); lanes I and II, molecular weight standards, trypsin inhibitor (21.5 kDa) and cytochrome c (12.5 kDa), respectively. Reproduced with permission from Conway de Macario, König, and Macario, *Arch. Microbiol.,* 1986 (3).

throughout the procedure and, finally, to isolate it (13). This determinant contains glucose, predominantly (Table VII).

The two determinants that have been found in *Mg. cariaci* JR1c are proteins of its S layer as shown by monoclonal antibody testing of electrophoretically resolved components (Fig. 8) (3,32). One of these determinants contains Ala, Gly, Ser, and Glu.

These two determinants of JR1c, as well as that of *Msp. hungatei* JF1, are present on the surface of the immunogens, exclusively. These determinants are absent on the surface of all other reference methanogens assayed (30 in all, encompassing the entire range of families and genera) (3,32).

Fig. 7. Location of the antigenic determinants of *Methanococcus vannielii* strain SB in protein components of the S layer resolved by SDS–PAGE (A). Lanes: II, crude S layer; III, S layer; and IV, solubilized S layer. Lanes I and V are molecular weight standards: (a) albumin, 67K; (b) catalase, 60K; (c) lactate dehydrogenase, 36K; and (d) ferritin subunit, 18.5K. (B), densitometric scan of lane II showing the major protein components (scan:gel ratio = 2.39:1). Reproduced with permission from Conway de Macario, König, Macario, and Kandler, *J. Immunol.* **132**, 883–887, 1984 (4).

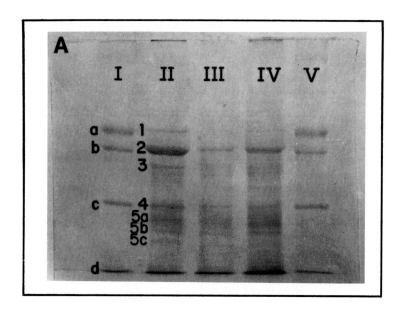

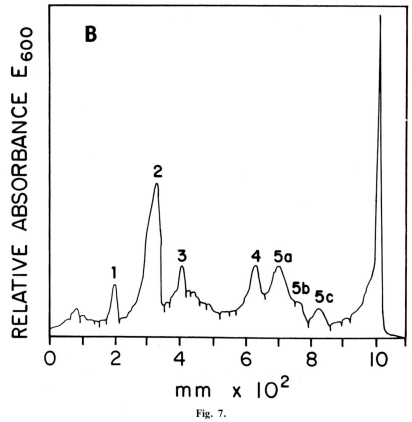

Fig. 7.

TABLE VII

Carbohydrate Composition of an Antigen Purified from
Methanosarcina barkeri Strain 227 Using Its Specific
Monoclonal Antibody[a]

Carbohydrate	Methanol extract[b]		Purified antigen (%)
	%[c]	M_r[d]	
Rhamnose	9.6	0.3	ND[e]
Mannose	56.1	1.7	ND
Glucose	34.0	1.0	100
Glucosamine	0.3	<0.1	ND

    [a] Reproduced with permission from Garberi, Macario, and Conway de Macario, *J. Bacteriol.*, 1985 (13).

    [b] Starting material obtained from strain 227.

    [c] Moles of each carbohydrate (e.g., rhamnose)/moles of total carbohydrates × 100.

    [d] Molar ratio to glucose: moles of each carbohydrate (e.g., rhamnose)/moles of glucose.

    [e] Not detectable.

IV. CONCLUSIONS

Elucidation of the architectural features of bacterial envelopes is progressing thanks to sophisticated immunochemical methods based on the use of monoclonal antibodies.

Various determinants have been identified in the antigenic mosaics of seven reference methanogens. The structures of several of these determinants have been partially elucidated. For this purpose, a combination of complementary procedures proved useful. Direct binding and indirect (adsorption, inhibition-blocking) assays provided data, in some cases confirmed by purification of antigen or chemical analyses of cell walls, S layers, and sheaths. The data indicate considerable antigenic diversity among methanogens, and suggest a number of potential uses of monoclonal antibodies in taxonomy, ecology, bio-

---

Fig. 8. Location of the antigenic determinants of *Methanogenium cariaci* strain JR1c in protein components of the S layer resolved by SDS–PAGE (A). Lane I, crude S-layer preparation; lane II same as lane I but 10 times less concentrated; lane III, molecular weight standards: (a) albumin, 67 kDa; (b) catalase, 60 kDa; (c) lactate dehydrogenase, 36 kDa; (d) ferritin subunit, 18.5 kDa. (B) Densitometric scan of lane I showing the major protein components tested for antigenicity with antibodies. Reproduced with permission from Conway de Macario, König, and Macario, *Arch. Microbiol.*, 1986 (3).

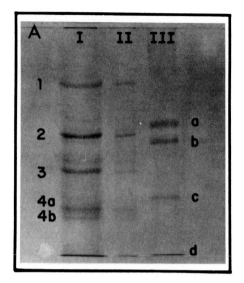

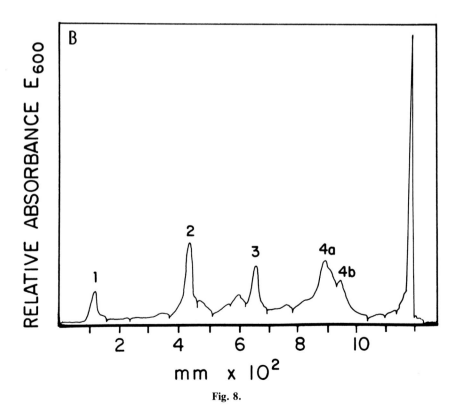

Fig. 8.

chemistry, and biotechnology. Several panels of these antibodies are now available, whose specific complementary determinants on the bacterial envelope are known. Surveys of practically all reference methanogens are revealing the specificity spectra of the antibodies and are providing insights into the distribution in nature of the structures they so specifically recognize. Examples have been found of structures restricted to the immunogen, that is, absent in the surface of all other methanogens. These unique structures can be considered a marker of the methanogen used to generate the antibodies, and the antibodies recognizing them, as extremely useful probes. These probes have a great potential for detecting the particular strain they recognize in a variety of samples, for isolating it, and for any other purpose requiring specific interaction between the antibody and one strain, with the exclusion of everything else in a mixture, for example.

Immunoelectron microscopy has shown the precise location of determinants in the bacterial envelope. Images provided by monoclonal antibodies have been discrete and have shown the spaced distribution of multiple copies of a single determinant in contrast to images obtained with polyclonal antisera. The latter reveal a plurality of determinants, making it impossible to establish the distribution and frequency of each of them.

V. PROSPECTS FOR THE FUTURE

One interesting topic for investigation in the immediate future will be the distribution of determinants in the mosaics of methanogens among these bacteria, other archaebacteria, and other organisms. This will provide insights on the usefulness of antigenic determinants as markers of taxa or of strains of interest. Survey of methanogens with the monoclonal antibodies in the panels already available will also establish which ones are specific probes for a given strain or for a given structure. Such probes will then be utilized for detecting and measuring the strain (or the structure) in unknowns. Molecular signatures (chemical footprints) left by methanogens in sediments, fossils, wastes, other organisms, and so forth, will be traceable with these monoclonal antibodies. Research underway has already demonstrated that antibody probes specifically and quantitatively measures methanogens and molecules released by them in complex microbial communities (29).

Another promising area of research is the elucidation of the architectural features that characterize methanogens. A portrait of supramolecular structures of taxonomic, evolutionary, or functional significance is likely to be obtained aided by monoclonal antibodies. This, along with structural studies such as the ones described in this chapter, will contribute to understanding the full extent of the antigenic diversity of methanogens. Questions that might be answerable in the not too distant future are the following: How many antigenic determinants are there on the surface of a bacterial cell? What is the variability of this number of determinants in different strains, or species, or at various stages of bacterial growth? How are the number and variability influenced by nutritional factors, antibiotics, host reactions, and other environmental parameters?

Last, a multitude of applications may be envisaged for monoclonal antibodies in methanogenic biotechnology. These have been discussed elsewhere (29). Briefly, monoclonal antibodies are potentially useful instruments for monitoring wastes and bioreactors and for developing optimal process controls.

VI. SUMMARY

This is a continuation of two preceding chapters in Volumes I and II of this treatise. The three chapters form a unit in which we have attempted to describe the "birth" and very early stages of a novel area of research concerned with the immunology of methanogens. The core of this chapter is a summary of data on antigenic mosaics of methanogens and on their components (determinants) obtained with monoclonal antibodies. In Section II a general discussion, with cross references to other chapters in this treatise, was included of scientific strategies and methodologic tactics that have proved useful for immunochemical analyses of bacteria, and molecules thereof, utilizing antibody probes (particularly monoclonal). The field is so new that far-reaching generalizations cannot yet be made from the data available. For methanogens, as for other bacterial groups, research with monoclonal antibodies is at a stage of development which involves mostly preparation and characterization of probes and exploratory surveys of reference strains or of molecules characterized by biochemical means. The biologic or practical significance of the findings is only beginning to be understood. Six determinants have been identified in *Methanobacterium thermoautotrophicum* strain ΔH, six in *Methanobrevibacter smithii* strain PS, six in *Methanococcus vannielii* strain SB, three in *Methanosarcina barkeri* strain 227, two in *Methanogenium cariaci* strain JR1c, one in *Methanospirillum hungatei* strain JF1, and one in *Methanobrevibacter arboriphilus* strain DH1. Studies on *Methanothrix soehngenii* strain Opfikon have just begun. Structures that are immunodominant epitopes have been identified for several of the determinants. Emphasis has been given to studying determinants that are accessible to antibody on the surface of whole bacterial cells, whether the immunogen or a cross-reactive methanogen. Extensive surveys of reference methanogens with the antibodies are ongoing. Three determinants have already been found only in the immunogen (they are absent in all other methanogens tested spanning all families and genera). Overall the results are encouraging inasmuch as they demonstrate the excellent resolution power of monoclonal antibodies, the antigenic diversity of methanogens, and their relationships, and suggest various uses of these antibodies in science and biotechnology.

ACKNOWLEDGMENTS

Work done by the authors referred to in this chapter was supported in part by grant DE-FG02-84ER 13197 from the U.S. Department of Energy, and grant 261.82 from the North Atlantic Treaty Organization (NATO).

REFERENCES

1. Carrasco, N., Viitanen, P., Herzlinger, D., and Kaback, H. R. (1984). Monoclonal antibodies against the *lac* carrier protein from *Escherichia coli*. 1. Functional studies. *Biochemistry* **23**, 3681–3687.
2. Chung, H. K., Park, S. C., and Rhee S. G. (1984). Conformation-specific monoclonal antibodies to glutamine synthetase in *Escherichia coli*. *J. Biol. Chem.* **259**, 11756–11762.
3. Conway de Macario, E., König, H., and Macario, A. J. L. (1986). Antigenic determinants distinctive of *Methanospirillum hungatei* and *Methanogenium cariaci* identified by monoclonal antibodies. *Arch. Microbiol.* **144**, 20–24.
4. Conway de Macario, E., König, H., Macario, A. J. L., and Kandler, O. (1984). Six antigenic determinants in the surface layer of the archaebacterium *Methanococcus vannielii* revealed by monoclonal antibodies. *J. Immunol.* **132**, 883–887.
5. Conway de Macario, E., and Macario, A. J. L. (1983). Monoclonal antibodies for bacterial identification and taxonomy. *ASM News* **49**, 1–7.
6. Conway de Macario, E., Macario, A. J. L., and Kandler, O. (1982). Monoclonal antibodies for immunochemical analysis of methanogenic bacteria. *J. Immunol.* **129**, 1670–1674.
7. Conway de Macario, E., Macario, A. J. L., Magarinos, M. C., König, H., and Kandler, O. (1983). Dissecting the antigenic mosaic of the archaebacterium *Methanobacterium thermoautotrophicum* by monoclonal antibodies of defined molecular specificity. *Proc. Natl. Acad. Sci. U.S.A.* **80**, 6346–6350.
8. Conway de Macario, E., Macario, A. J. L., and Pastini, A. (1985). The superficial antigenic mosaic of *Methanobrevibacter smithii:* Identification of determinants and isolates by monoclonal antibodies. *Arch. Microbiol.* **142**, 311–316.
9. Dale, J. B., Hasty, D. L., and Beachey, E. H. (1985). Structure–function analysis of Group A streptococcal M proteins with hybridoma antibodies. This treatise, vol. II, pp. 1–21.
10. DiRienzo, J. M. (1986). Application of monoclonal antibodies to the study of oral bacteria and their virulence factors. This volume, pp. 249–293.
11. Fernandez-Pol, J. A. (1985). Epidermal growth factor receptor of A431 cells. Characterization of a monoclonal anti-receptor antibody noncompetitive agonist of epidermal growth factor action. *J. Biol. Chem.* **260**, 5003–5011.
12. Gabay, J., Schenkman, S., Desaymard, C., and Schwartz, M. (1985). Monoclonal antibodies and the structure of bacterial membrane proteins. This treatise, vol. II, pp. 249–282.
13. Garberi, J. C., Macario, A. J. L., and Conway de Macario, E. (1985). Antigenic mosaic of methanosarcinae: Partial characterization of *Methanosarcina barkeri* 227 surface antigens by monoclonal antibodies. *J. Bacteriol.* **164**, 1–6.

14. Gmür, R., and Wyss, C. (1985). Monoclonal antibodies to characterize the antigenic heterogeneity of *Bacteroides intermedius*. This treatise, vol. I, pp. 91–119.

15. Heckels, J. E., and Virji, M. (1985). Monoclonal antibodies against gonococcal pili: Uses in the analysis of gonococcal immunochemistry and virulence. This treatise, vol. I, pp. 1–35.

16. Herion, P., Siberdt, D., Francotte, M., Urbain, J., and Bollen, A. (1984). Monoclonal antibodies against plasma protease inhibitors: II. Production and characterization of 25 monoclonal antibodies against human α_1-trypsin. Correlation between antigenic structure and functional sites. *Biosci. Rep.* **4,** 139–147.

17. Holmans, P. L., Loftus, T. A., and Hansen, E. J. (1985). Cloning and surface expression in *Escherichia coli* of a structural gene encoding a surface protein of *Haemophilus influenzae* Type b. *Infect. Immun.* **50,** 236–242.

18. Holme, T., and Gustafsson, B. (1985). Monoclonal antibodies against group- and type-specific antigens of *Vibrio cholerae* O:1. This treatise, vol. I, pp. 167–189.

19. Ivanyi, J., Morris, J. A., and Keen, M. (1985). Studies with monoclonal antibodies to mycobacteria. This treatise, vol. I, pp. 59–90.

20. Kilpatrick, J. M., Kearney, J. F., and Volanakis, J. E. (1982). Demonstration of calcium-induced conformational change(s) in C-reactive protein by using monoclonal antibodies. *Mol. Immunol.* **19,** 1159–1165.

21. Kosunen, T. U., and Hurme, M. (1986). Monoclonal antibodies against *Campylobacter* strains. This volume, pp. 99–117.

22. Lam, J. S., Mutharia, L. M., and Hancock, R. E. W. (1985). Application of monoclonal antibodies to the study of the surface antigens in *Pseudomonas aeruginosa*. This treatise, vol. II, pp. 143–157.

23. Li, X.-M, and Krakow, J. S. (1985). Characterization of nine monoclonal antibodies against the *Escherichia coli* cyclic AMP receptor protein. *J. Biol. Chem.* **260,** 4378–4383.

24. Lillehoj, H.-S., Choe, B.-K., and Rose, N. R. (1982). Monoclonal antibodies to human prostatic acid phosphatase: Probes for antigenic study. *Proc. Natl. Acad. Sci. U.S.A.* **79,** 5061–5065.

25. Lim, P. L. (1986). Diagnostic uses of monoclonal antibodies to *Salmonella*. This volume, pp. 29–75.

26. Macario, A. J. L., and Conway de Macario, E. (1984). Antibacterial monoclonal antibodies and the dawn of a new era in the control of infection. *Surv. Synth. Pathol. Res.* **3,** 119–130.

27. Macario, A. J. L., and Conway de Macario, E. (1985). A preview of the uses of monoclonal antibodies against methanogens in fermentation biotechnology: Significance for public health. This treatise, vol. I, pp. 269–286.

28. Macario, A. J. L., and Conway de Macario, E. (1985). Monoclonal antibodies of predefined molecular specificity for identification and classification of methanogens and for probing their ecologic niches. This treatise, vol. II, pp. 213–247.

29. Macario, A. J. L., and Conway de Macario, E. (1985). Antibodies for methanogenic biotechnology. *Trends Biotechnol.* **3,** 204–208.

30. Macario, A. J. L., and Conway de Macario, E. (1986). Immunologic probes for *Methanothrix soehngenii*. *ASM Abstr. Annu. Meet., 86th,* p. 186.

31. Macario, A. J. L., Dugan, C. B., and Conway de Macario, E. (1984). Monoclonal antibody analysis of immuno- and antigenicity of a saltwater archaebacterium. *Fed. Proc., Fed. Am. Soc. Exp. Biol.* **43,** 1773.

32. Macario, A. J. L., Dugan, C. B., and Conway de Macario, E. (1986). *Methanogenium cariaci:* Expression of two private antigenic determinants in strain JR1c. In preparation.

33. Matson, S. W., and Wood, E. R. (1985). Production of antibodies directed against *Escherichia coli* helicase III and the molecular cloning of the helicase III gene. *J. Biol. Chem.* **260,** 11811–11816.

34. Millan, J. L., and Stigbrand, T. (1983). Antigenic determinants of human placental and testicular placental-like alkaline phosphatases as mapped by monoclonal antibodies. *Eur. J. Biochem.* **136,** 1–7.

35. Nunberg, J. H., Rodgers, G., Gilbert, J. H., and Snead, R. M. (1984). Method to map antigenic determinants recognized by monoclonal antibodies: Localization of a determinant of virus neutralization on the feline leukemia virus envelope protein gp70. *Proc. Natl. Acad. Sci. U.S.A.* **81,** 3675–3679.

36. Oguma, K., Syuto, B., Kubo, S., and Iida, H. (1985). Analysis of antigenic structure of *Clostridium botulinum* type C_1 and D toxins by monoclonal antibodies. This treatise, vol. II, pp. 159–163.

37. Praputpittaya, K., and Ivanyi J. (1985). Detection of an antigen (MY4) common to *M. tuberculosis* and *M. leprae* by "tandem" immunoassay. *J. Immunol. Methods* **79,** 149–157.

38. Sato, H. (1986). Monoclonal antibodies against *Clostridium perfringens* O toxin (perfringolysin O). This volume, pp. 203–228.

39. Sethi, K. K. (1985). Monoclonal antibodies against *Legionella pneumophila* serogroup 1 antigens: Characterization and their potential applications. This treatise, vol. I, pp. 121–136.

40. Söderström, T. (1985). *Escherichia coli* capsules and pili: Serological, functional, protective, and immunoregulatory studies with monoclonal antibodies. This treatise, vol. II, pp. 185–212.

41. Sugasawara, R. J. (1985). The use of the monoclonal antibodies for detecting and serotyping *Neisseria meningitidis*. This treatise, vol. II, pp. 61–79.

42. Svennerholm, A.-M., Wikström, M., Lindholm, L., and Holmgren, J. (1986). Monoclonal antibodies and immunodetection methods for *Vibrio cholerae* and *Escherichia coli* enterotoxins. This volume, pp. 77–97.

43. Thompson, N. E., Bergdoll, M. S., Meyer, R. F., Bennett, R. W., Miller, L., and MacMillan, J. D. (1985). Monoclonal antibodies to the enterotoxins and to the toxic shock syndrome toxin produced by *Staphylococcus aureus*. This treatise, vol. II, pp. 23–59.

44. Tzartos, S. J., Rand, D. E., Einarson, B. L., and Lindstrom, J. M. (1981). Mapping of surface structures of electrophorus acetylcholine receptor using monoclonal antibodies. *J. Biol. Chem.* **256,** 8635–8645.

45. Viljanen, M. K., Linko, L., Arstila, P., Lehtonen, O.-P., and Weintraub, A. (1986). Monoclonal antibodies to the lipopolysaccharide and capsular polysaccharide of *Bacteroides fragilis*. This volume, pp. 119–142.

46. Yoshimori, T., and Uchida, T. (1986). Monoclonal antibodies against diphtheria toxin: Their use in analysis of the function and structure of the toxin and their application to cell biology. This volume, pp. 229–248.

47. Yurchenco, P. D., Speicher, D. W., Morrow, J. S., Knowles, W. J., and Marchesi, V. T. (1982). Monoclonal antibodies as probes of domain structure of the Spectrin α subunit. *J. Biol. Chem.* **257,** 9102–9107.

9

Monoclonal Antibodies against *Clostridium perfringens* θ toxin (Perfringolysin O)

HIROKO SATO

Department of Applied Immunology
National Institute of Health
Tokyo, Japan

I. INTRODUCTION

Clostridium perfringens is the best known pathogen of the histotoxic clostridia. It causes severe infection of muscle, gas gangrene (myonecrosis), either

MONOCLONAL ANTIBODIES
AGAINST BACTERIA
Volume III

alone or in combination with a number of different clostridia such as *C. oedema-tiens (C. novyi), C. septicum, C. bifermentans, C. sordellii, C. histolyticum, C. sporogenes,* and *C. fallax* (41,66,71,72). In spite of the time that has elapsed since gas gangrene and its associated pathogens were discovered, the pathogenesis of this disease is little understood. None of these histotoxic clostridia is a highly invasive pathogen, but all release a variety of extracellular toxins and enzymes (mostly designated by Greek letters in order of importance or discovery for each species). For example, *C. perfringens* produces at least 12 distinct toxins such as α toxin (phospholipase C), κ toxin (collagenase), or μ toxin (hyaluronidase), some of which share common biological and immunological properties with that produced by the other clostridia (34,41,43).

The pathogenesis of gas gangrene has been complicated by the fact that the development of the disease does not depend solely on the mixed infection with different bacteria, but on the complexities of their numerous products. Purification of most of these products has not yet progressed to a point where their *in vivo* effects can be analyzed, not even to the limited extent possible with products from *C. perfringens.* Nevertheless, a great part of the identification or classification of the pathogenic clostridia depends on their toxins and enzymes. In fact, *C. perfringens* toxins are used to group the species into five toxigenic types: A, B, C. D, and E. Cell-associated antigens are not so useful for grouping or typing these pathogens (66,71,72).

The importance of clostridial toxins is not limited to the medical field. In fact, many clostridial toxins are utilized in biological, immunological, and biochemical fields for their unique enzymatic or biological properties. Thus, purified toxins or specific antibodies are potentially useful for studies of pathogenesis and other interesting biological problems.

θ Toxin, or perfringolysin O (PLO), is one of the important toxins of *C. perfringens,* and is well known as a member of the group of thiol-activated cytolytic toxins (called oxygen-labile hemolysin in the past) produced by taxonomically related gram-positive bacteria (8). These toxins have common biological properties: (a) they are cytolytic not only to erythrocytes but also to various mammalian cells; (b) they are cardiotoxic and lethal; (c) their biological activities are inhibited by masking of the thiol group(s) by oxidation, and are reactivated by reduction; (d) their biological activities are inhibited by cholesterol; and (e) their activities are neutralized by antibodies against not only homologous but also heterologous toxins.

At least 16 toxins have been described in this group (Table I) (1,2,7,8,67). Some toxins, for example, streptolysin O (SLO) (2,5), pneumolysin (35), cereolysin (9,17), alveolysin (22), thuringiolysin (8), lysteriolysin (8), tetanolysin (6,47), and PLO (43,45,73), have been purified to an extent which has allowed the characterization of some physicochemical and biological properties (1,8,67). The other eight cytolytic toxins have been disregarded for almost 30 years since

TABLE I

Thiol-Activated Cytolytic Toxins[a]

Organism		Toxin
Streptococcus	*pyogenes*	Streptolysin O
Streptococcus	*pneumoniae*	Pneumolysin
Bacillus	*cereus*	Cereolysin
Bacillus	*thuringiensis*	Thuringiolysin O
Bacillus	*alvei*	Alveolysin
Bacillus	*laterosporus*	Laterosporolysin
Listeria	*monocytogenes*	Listeriolysin
Clostridium	*perfringens*	Perfringolysin O (θ-toxin)
Clostridium	*tetani*	Tetanolysin
Clostridium	*oedematiens*	Oedematolysin O (δ-toxin)
Clostridium	*bifermentans*	Bifermentolysin
Clostridium	*sordellii*	Sordelliolysin[b]
Clostridium	*septicum*	Septicolysin O (δ-toxin)
Clostridium	*chauvoei*	Chauveolysin (δ-toxin)
Clostridium	*histolyticum*	Histolyticolysin (ϵ-toxin)
Clostridium	*botulinum*	Botulinolysin

[a] See the following reviews written in the past decade on the thiol-activated cytolytic toxins (1,2,8,43,67).

[b] Sordelliolysin is the name used in this chapter (Section III,B).

they were discovered (27–29,53,58), and, surprisingly, almost all of them are produced by histotoxic clostridia. The common properties of the thiol-activated cytolytic toxins cited above have been confirmed for most of the purified toxins (1,2,6,8,15,16–18,22,36,47,48,67).

Since it is assumed that the mechanism of action of these toxins is very likely identical or at least closely similar, knowledge obtained from any one of the toxins can be applied to all the other toxins in this group.

Despite this assumed functional similarity, dissimilarities among cytolytic toxins have been reported. The amino acid compositions of PLO, cereolysin, listeriolysin, alveolysin, SLO, and pneumolysin show differences (2,67). In addition, their half-cystine content, which must be important for their function, is also different: one in PLO (73), two in both cereolysin (17) and pneumolysin (3,24), and four in alveolysin (22,24). The fact that PLO has only one thiol group in the toxin molecule and that alveolysin has one essential half-cystine of four thiol groups for its membrane-disrupting activity (24) may be important in evaluating the role of the thiol group in the biological activities of the toxins.

Recently, studies on gene cloning of SLO and cereolysin were reported showing that the genetic determinants of the toxins might be expected to share a considerable degree of DNA sequence homology, but no homology occurred between cloned SLO DNA sequences and DNA isolated from bacteria expressing cereolysin, pneumolysin, listeriolysin, PLO, histolyticolysin, or oedematolysin (39,40), nor between cloned cereolysin determinant and DNA isolated from SLO- and listeriolysin-producing bacteria (30). These genetic studies suggested that if homology exists between the DNA sequence encoding SLO or cereolysin and the determinants of other cytolytic toxins examined, it is less than that which can be easily detected by Southern blot hybridization experiments (40).

In spite of these structural differences, similarities in the biological activities among the cytolytic toxins and their immunologic relatedness suggest the existence of common primary, and/or three-dimensional structures which may be located in a restricted region.

Antibodies are useful tools for the detection of the microheterogeneity and microhomogeneity of the toxins. However, the usefulness of immunological assays has been complicated by the heterogeneity of all antisera obtained by conventional methods. The polyclonality of antisera results in multiple antibodies against different parts of each antigen. Even if the same antigen preparation is used, each antiserum contains a different proportion of antibodies. It is impossible to generate repeatedly antisera that have the same proportion of antibodies. Development of hybridoma technology made it possible to generate monoclonal antibodies routinely and increased the usefulness of antibodies as research tools. Monoclonal antibodies have many advantages over polyclonal antibodies; for example, once a useful hybridoma has been generated, the exact same antibody can be used by many different groups. Structure–function relationships of toxins can be studied using PLO, since it is available in highly purified form and possesses a large number of common biological functions, as can SLO, which is considered the prototype of the cytolytic toxins.

In this chapter, monoclonal antibodies against PLO will be described as a useful tool for studies on thiol-activated cytolytic toxins.

II. BACKGROUND

Several reviews have been published in the past on thiol-activated cytolytic toxins (1,2,7,8,34,43,67). Therefore, in this section, the focus will be on PLO as it relates to the results in Section III.

A. Chemical Aspects

PLO is produced in culture media with various toxins and enzymes by every type of *C. perfringens* (41,43), and it is responsible for the clear hemolytic zones surrounding colonies on a blood agar plate. Toxin production is greatly influenced by the composition of the nutrient media. PLO can be produced in chemically defined media in the quantity as in complex media (50,51,68); 5–10 μg/ml of PLO (i.e., <1% of total extracellular protein) are produced during the logarithmic growth phase in either medium. SLO is also produced in chemically defined media, but the yield is much lower than that in complex media. In the latter, 5 μg/ml of SLO at most (1000 hemolytic units/ml) are produced (2). According to studies on PLO production in chemically defined media, high-potency extracellular proteases are produced, especially in media with Ca^{2+}, which destroy PLO as well as other toxins (64,69). These proteases and other cell products cause inactivation of the toxin during purification, which results in low yields. As the same problems have been hindering many investigators who have attempted to purify other cytolytic toxins, improvement in purification methods for the toxins can be expected (2,3,22,38). Even the purification of SLO, which is considered a prototype of these cytolytic toxins, still poses a serious problem, and its reported amino acid composition is still regarded as tentative (2). Many publications have described isolation protocols for the toxin since its discovery (31,32), but a consensus regarding such basic parameters as molecular weight, isoelectric point, and hemolytic capacity of the toxin has not yet been achieved.

Purified PLO showed a single band on sodium dodecyl sulfate–polyacrylamide gel electrophoresis (SDS–PAGE) with a molecular weight in the 51,000–62,000 range (43). Furthermore, PLOs and SLOs having different molecular weights and isoelectric points, but the same biological activity, have been reported (10,45).

The amino acid composition of purified PLO has been reported by two groups (45,73), and their results differ. Mitsui *et al.* (45) did not find cysteine in their preparation, but Yamakawa *et al.* (73) found one cysteine residue using performic acid-oxidized protein. The former investigators, however, suggested in a later paper (46) that the active form of the toxin has free thiol groups in its active site. It has been believed that thiol-activated cytolytic toxin could be oxidized easily by oxygen as indicated by the expression "oxygen-labile hemolysin" used in the past in referring to PLO. However, purified PLO is not so labile against aeration. Purified-reduced SLO is also not oxidized readily on storage in air or even under a current of pure oxygen, although crudely reduced or partially purified SLO material undergoes reversible oxidation on storage or during the purification process (2). The findings that purified toxins are rather stable to oxidation by air and that PLO produced in chemically defined media contained much less of the oxidized form than that produced in complex media (68) suggest that various chemical substances in the culture media take part in the generation of the oxidized form (73).

The biological activity of PLO is inhibited by many thiol-blocking agents, such as *p*-chloromercuribenzoate (PCMB), 5,5-dithiobis(2-nitrobenzoic acid)

(DTNB), or N-[p-(2-benzimidazolyl)phenyl]maleimide (BIPM), which can be reversed by adding thiols (34,43,46). These reversible chemical modifications are well known in other cytolytic toxins too (1,2,8).

B. Biological Aspects

Although PLO is cytolytic for erythrocytes and for other mammalian cells (43), hemolysis has been examined most frequently using erythrocytes of various animal species. Since the hemolytic activity of PLO is very high, it is not difficult to detect less than 1 ng of the toxin (1,67). Quantitative determination of the toxin in crude or purified material is usually based on the estimation of hemolytic activity of the toxin expressed as hemolytic doses (HD) or hemolytic units (HU). The HD is usually expressed in terms of the reciprocal of the highest dilution showing complete hemolysis (HD_{100}) or 50% hemolysis (HD_{50}). Since the assay system of the toxin is different from laboratory to laboratory, or from experiment to experiment, and no common reference toxin or antitoxin is used, severalfold differences in the hemolytic activity found in different laboratories or experiments probably reflect only these technical differences (2,67). It should thus be emphasized that a supply of standardized toxins and/or antitoxins is important for the progress of studies on toxins. Utilization of monoclonal antibodies could help in this regard.

It has been known from early studies with pneumolysin, SLO, and PLO that the lytic process of erythrocytes involves two sequential steps (1,54,56,67). The first step consists of toxin binding on the surface of the cytoplasmic membrane. Toxin binding was found to be temperature independent and could be inhibited by cholesterol.

The second step involves membrane damage as evidenced by the release of hemoglobin. It is relatively slow and is temperature dependent; it does not take place at 0°C.

It is also well known that cholesterol and related sterols prevent not only hemolysis but also other biological activities of the cytolytic toxins. Many detailed studies on the structural requirements and on the mechanism of sterol inhibition of toxin activity have been performed (1,2,4,8,16,20,30a,54,67). However, studies on the stoichiometry of cholesterol binding are hampered by the limited solubility of this compound and its tendency to form micelles (1,67). Recently, the binding of cholesterol by pneumolysin, alveolysin, and SLO has been demonstrated. Properties of the cytolytic toxin–cholesterol interaction paralleled those of cytolytic toxin–erythrocyte interaction in that the reaction is rapid and temperature independent. However, oxidized or p-hydroxymercuribenzoate-treated toxin showed no decrease in cholesterol-binding activity, whereas the ability of the toxin to bind to erythrocytes was modified by such treatment (36).

When erythrocytes or erythrocyte ghosts were treated with PLO, rings and arc-shaped structures with diameters of around 30 nm were observed on the cell membrane by electron microscopy (48). This was also true on treatment with SLO, tetanolysin, and cereolysin. These rings and arc-shaped structures have been considered to be toxin–cholesterol complexes. However, at high concentration of toxin, such structures have also been reported in the absence of cholesterol (18,48). Additionally, these structures have been considered as sites of pore formation (1). Relationships between these structures and membrane damage by the cytolytic toxins have been reported using PLO (48), cereolysin (18), SLO (7), or tetanolysin (6). When erythrocytes treated with PLO or cereolysin were examined by freeze–fracture electron microscopy, these structures did not appear to form holes through the membrane (18,48). Recently, it was reported for SLO that these structures isolated from the membrane do not contain cholesterol but only a toxin oligomer, and that these toxin oligomers most probably form very large transmembrane pores in the target bilayer (10,11). On the other hand, it was reported that tetanolysin seems to act by causing lipid perturbations (12). The possibility that mechanisms of toxin–membrane interaction and membrane damage are not identical for all cytolytic toxins has not been excluded (13,19). In any case, more information is needed for the elucidation of the mechanism of membrane damage.

It is considered that the almost instantaneous lethal effects of the cytolytic toxins on laboratory animals are largely due to the direct cardiotoxicity of the toxin. The cardiotoxicity of SLO, tetanolysin, pneumolysin, and listeriolysin has been investigated (2,8), but direct evidence for the cardiotoxicity of PLO has not been reported.

C. Immunological Aspects

Cross-neutralization of hemolytic activity of thiol-activated cytolytic toxins by heterologous antisera has been demonstrated in the past by many investigators (8). This immunological relatedness among PLO, pneumolysin, SLO, and tetanolysin was found early in the 1900s. Since neutralization of hemolytic activity with antisera could be observed so easily with crude antigens and serum antibodies—even in the case of clostridial toxins for which purification had not yet been attempted—their cross-neutralization was recognized very early. Inhibition of the hemolytic activity of cultures of *C. sordellii, C. bifermentans, C. histolyticum,* and *C. botulinum* with antisera to either PLO, tetanolysin, histolyticolysin, or sordelliolysin was described at almost the same time these toxins were discovered (27–29). Septicolysin O and chauveolysin were also reported to be cross-neutralized by mutual antisera, neutralized by anti-SLO serum, and by the normal sera of humans and animals such as rabbits, guinea pigs, oxen, and horses (49). These antigenic relationships were always evident when hyperimmunized horse sera were used. Since nonspecific neutralization of hemolytic activity of the toxins by normal serum is always observed, one should take into account this fact in studying the neutralization of antisera.

The cross-reactivity of 10 anti-SLO human sera containing monoclonal-hypergammaglobulinemia was also studied using pneumolysin, tetanolysin, PLO, and SLO (42). With one exception, there was no cross-neutralization in the 30 possible combinations involving the first three antigens. This exception was remarkable because the serum sample neutralized pneumolysin and SLO equally well.

The antigenic relatedness among cytolytic toxins has also been demonstrated by immunoprecipitation. Cereolysin, SLO, and PLO formed cross-immunoprecipitates when they reacted with heterologous horse antisera against tetanolysin, SLO, and PLO. These findings indicated that thiol-activated cytolytic toxins share several (not just one) common antigenic structure (15,65). It is still unclear whether the common antigenic sites are localized in the region related to the biological activity of the toxin.

Two types of anti-SLO antibodies have been reported (2,56): some neutralizing anti-SLO antibodies from horse sera and from human myeloma sera prevented toxin fixation on the cell surface but did not prevent cell lysis after toxin binding (antifixation antibodies). However, other neutralizing antibodies prevented subsequent hemolysis after reduced SLO had become fixed to them at 0°C (antilytic antibodies). On the basis of these findings a speculative model of SLO molecule interaction with erythrocyte membrane was proposed (1). In this regard, cross-neutralization of SLO, alveolysin, botulinolysin, listeriolysin, PLO, pneumolysin, and tetanolysin was investigated using three horse anti-SLO sera which contained different proportions of two types of neutralizing antibodies (antifixation and antilytic antibodies), and the immunological relatedness of these seven toxins was considered with respect to the fixation and lytic regions of SLO (23).

Exploration of antigenic relatedness of the cytolytic toxins using heterogeneous horse antitoxins provides only indirect evidence of antigenic similarities. Monoclonal antibodies are potentially much better tools for this purpose.

III. RESULTS AND DISCUSSION

A. Production and Properties of Monoclonal Antibodies against PLO

Table II is a list of anti-PLO monoclonal antibodies discussed in this section which were used for studying thiol-activated cytolytic toxins as well as PLO. The monoclonal antibodies were prepared as described by Oi and Herzenberg (55).

TABLE II

Binding and Antihemolytic Activities of Monoclonal Antibodies to PLO[a]

| | | | Activities[d] | |
| | | Protein[c] | Binding (ELISA) | Antihemolytic |
Group[b]	Antibody	(μg/ml)	(U/ml)	(μg/ml)
I	1C3	760	2.49	>380
	1B9	670	2.73	>335
	2D4	1036	9.50	>518
	3F11	1228	8.48	>614
II	4D8	100	0.58	14
	2C5	564	4.28	17
	3H10	1280	10.96	1
	PAb	343	1.00	3

[a] Adapted from Sato *et al.* (59), with permission.

[b] Monoclonal antibodies were divided into two groups (I, nonneutralizing, and II, neutralizing) on the basis of their effect on PLO.

[c] Monoclonal antibodies were purified from ascites fluids by protein A–Sepharose column chromatography. The reference polyclonal antibody (PAb) was purified by PLO–Sepharose affinity chromatography (see text) from pooled sera of mice immunized with purified PLO toxoid. The protein concentration of the antibodies was estimated using the value of the extinction coefficient ($E\vert_{cm}^{\%} = 14$) at 280 nm.

[d] Binding activity was measured by ELISA using polystyrene microtiter plates coated with purified PLO (1 μg), and expressed in ELISA (U/ml) as a value relative to the reference polyclonal anti-PLO antibody (PAb). For estimation of antihemolytic activity, equal volumes (50 μl) of PLO (10 ng/ml) and antibody diluted serially twofold were mixed at room temperature. After 30 min, 1% sheep red blood cells (100 μl) were added and incubation was continued at 37°C for 30 min. After centrifugation at 4°C, the absorbance of the supernatant at 405 nm was measured. The antihemolytic activity is expressed as the protein antibody concentration (μg/ml) at 50% hemolysis calculated from the absorbance values.

Since purified PLO shows high lethality (6000 LD_{50}/mg) to mice by intravenous injection, the toxin was detoxified before the immunization of mice. PLO (400 μg/ml) purified from a culture supernatant of *C. perfringens* strain PB6K, as described previously (73), was detoxified by dialysis for 1 day against 1/60 *M* phosphate-buffered saline (PBS), pH 7.0, containing 0.3% formalin and 0.05 *M* L-lysine. Hemolytic activity as well as the lethality of the formalinized toxin (PLO toxoid) were also reduced by this mild treatment, but the antigenicity estimated by agar gel immunodiffusion remained unchanged. A BALB/c mouse was primed with an intraperitoneal injection of the alum-precipitated PLO toxoid (100 μg protein per mouse) supplemented with 12.5 μg of pertussis toxoid prepared as reported previously (62). Seven weeks later, the mouse was boosted with 80 μg of the PLO toxoid without adjuvant by intravenous injection. Three days after the booster injection, the spleen cells of the immune mouse were fused to SP2/0-Ag14 myeloma cells by polyethylene glycol (55). Initial screening of the hybridoma producing specific antibodies was carried out by PLO-ELISA using polystyrene microtiter plates coated with purified PLO (1 μg/ml) (70), and by antihemolytic activity to PLO. More than 80% of the hybrid cell cultures were positive to PLO-ELISA, and about half of them showed antihemolytic activity. Seven distinct clones of hybridoma producing monoclonal antibody against PLO were selected by repeated cloning by limiting dilution. Three antibodies were neutralizing to PLO and four were not. All antibodies were IgG_1 as determined by double immunodiffusion (59).

High antibody titer can be obtained in ascites fluid of BALB/c mice injected with the hybridomas. Monoclonal antibodies obtained from the culture medium or from ascites fluid should have the identical characteristics, but all ascites fluids of mice injected with any hybridoma showed antihemolytic activity, not only with PLO but also with other toxins such as SLO or tetanolysin. To avoid this nonspecific inhibition to the toxins by ascites fluid, the neutralizing activity of every monoclonal antibody has to be analyzed using either immunoglobulin purified from the ascites fluid, or culture supernatants.

Purification of the monoclonal antibodies was carried out by affinity chromatography with PLO–Sepharose (a conjugate of purified PLO and CNBr-activated Sepharose 4B), protein A–Sepharose (from Pharmacia Fine Chemicals), or a DEAE Affi-gel blue (Bio-Rad Laboratories) column (14,21). Since it was expected that PLO–Sepharose affinity chromatography had to be the best way to obtain a highly specific antibody to PLO, a polyclonal anti-PLO mouse antibody preparation was applied on the PLO–Sepharose column. After washing the column with PBS, antibody bound to PLO–Sepharose was eluted with 0.17 M glycine HCl containing 0.5 M NaCl, pH 3. A 2.5-ml portion of the eluate was collected in a tube having 0.4 ml of 0.5 M Tris-HCl, pH 8.0, to neutralize the pH of the eluate at once. Antibody fractions were dialyzed against PBS to serve as the reference antibody.

The activity of monoclonal antibodies in ELISA (ELISA U/ml) was expressed as values relative to this affinity-purified polyclonal antibody (PAb) by the parallel-line assay method as reported previously (60). When monoclonal antibodies 1C3 and 1B9 were applied to the PLO–Sepharose column, the activity of the antibodies was recovered chiefly in the wash fractions although the other monoclonal antibodies were eluted at pH 3, the same as PAb. In spite of the low affinity of 1C3 and 1B9 for PLO–Sepharose, both monoclonal antibodies showed a good dose response in PLO-ELISA, and their regression lines on log-log graph paper showed identical slopes as compared with the other monoclonal antibodies or with PAb.

Protein A–Sepharose column chromatography worked successfully for purification of every monoclonal antibody. Antibodies bound to the protein A–Sepharose column at pH 8.0 and were eluted with citrate buffer at pH 6.0 (21). DEAE Affi-gel blue column chromatography (14) also gave good results for purification of 3H10 and 2C5. Antibodies purified by either method showed no nonspecific antihemolytic activity to the toxins (59).

Binding activity of three monoclonal antibodies (1C3, 2D4, and 3H10) to PLO modified chemically in its thiol group with DTNB or BIPM was examined (59). All these antibodies could bind to the modified PLO but a difference in binding capacity was observed between 1C3 and 2D4. This result may suggest that these three antibodies recognize different antigenic sites not masked with DTNB or BIPM.

The passive hemagglutination reaction using formalinized sheep red blood cells (SRBC) sensitized with PLO was also carried out. Antibodies 1C3, 1B9, 2D4, and 3F11 agglutinated the SRBC, although these antibodies did not form a precipitin line with PLO with the double-immunodiffusion test as reported for SLO (57). Synergistic effects of the monoclonal antibodies on binding and neutralizing activities were also examined but none was observed (59).

B. Cross-Reactivity

Six types of specificity spectra of anti-PLO monoclonal antibodies can be expected considering their possible cross-reactivities with other toxins (Table III). In our previous paper (59), only SLO was examined as a heterologous toxin, but to investigate immunological relatedness among all the cytolytic toxins, an attempt was made to reactivate clostridial toxins that had been dormant for a long

TABLE III

Expected Types of Specificity Spectra of Antitoxin Monoclonal Antibodies[a]

Toxin group	Type	Homologous[b]		Heterologous[c]	
		B[d]	N[e]	B	N
I	1	+	−	−	−
	2	+	−	+	−
	3	+	−	+	+
II	4	+	+	−	−
	5	+	+	+	−
	6	+	+	+	+

[a] Adapted from Sato *et al.* (59), with permission.
[b] Toxin used for immunization of mice to generate hybridomas producing monoclonal antibodies. (PLO is the homologous toxin in this review.)
[c] The other thiol-activated cytolytic toxins.
[d] Binding ability to the toxin (+, binding; −, not binding).
[e] Neutralizing ability to toxin activities (+, neutralizing; −, not neutralizing).

time (28,29,53,58). *Clostridium bifermentans* SJ2 and *C. sordellii* 1620 (52), kindly donated by Nakamura, were chosen for two main reasons:

1. Since they produce phospholipase C, which is neutralized by antibody against α toxin (phospholipase C) of *C. perfringens* (44,71,72), a closer relation of their cytolytic toxins to PLO might be expected.

2. Since the organisms are distinct but very similar to one another, it was interesting to study if differences between their toxins existed.

The hemolysin produced by *C. sordellii* has not been given any proper name; we refer to it as sordelliolysin in this chapter. Oedematolysin, the δ toxin of *C. oedematiens*, was also examined because the organism, as well as that of *C. perfringens*, has been known as one of the important pathogens of gas gangrene, but it produces phospholipase C that is immunologically distinct from the *C. perfringens* α toxin (71,72). Tetanolysin was also reinvestigated, although it was not included in our previous work (59), for its nonreactivity with monoclonal antibodies. These four toxins were purified by affinity chromatography with 2C5– or 3H10–Sepharose, which was a conjugate of purified 2C5 or 3H10 and CNBr-activated Sepharose 4B (detailed in Section III,D,1), and were used for all the experiments discussed in this chapter.

Table IV shows the cross-reactivity of the seven monoclonal antibodies with the five other toxins. None of the four nonneutralizing antibodies (1C3, 1B9, 2D4, and 3F11) reacted with any of the heterologous toxins, namely, all of them were type 1 antibodies for the five toxins as described in Table III. Antibody 4D8 was type 4 for all heterologous toxins except sordelliolysin, to which 4D8 showed a weak binding activity. Thus it was not clear whether 4D8 was type 4 or type 5 for sordelliolysin. Antibodies 2C5 and 3H10 showed antihemolytic activity to SLO, bifermentolysin, and sordelliolysin (type 6), but showed no activity to tetanolysin and oedematolysin (type 5). We failed to detect hybridoma producing tetanolysin-ELISA-positive antibody in previous work (59) in which insufficiently purified tetanolysin was used. A culture supernatant of *C. tetani*, strain A47, was concentrated, fractionated with ammonium sulfate between 20 and 40% saturation, and applied to a column of DE 52 as described in an earlier paper (61). The fractions passed through were pooled and concentrated as partially purified tetanolysin. When tetanolysin, purified from this partially purified toxin preparation with 3H10–Sepharose, was used for coating the microtiter plate, both 2C5 and 3H10 showed positive reaction with ELISA. This unexpected result made us aware that we should be more cautious in the determination of binding activity of the antibodies to the toxins.

The binding of antibodies to the toxins was also examined by Western blotting analysis. Each toxin treated with 1% SDS at 50°C for 30 min was applied to a 1% SDS–10% polyacrylamide slab gel. After electrophoresis, the toxins in the gel were transblotted by electrophoresis on a nitrocellulose membrane, and the binding of the monoclonal antibodies to each toxin was determined using the ELISA

TABLE IV

Specificity Spectra of Seven Anti-PLO Monoclonal Antibodies with Five Other Thiol-Activated Cytolytic Toxins

Antibody (IgG$_1$)	Toxin[a]											
	PLO		SLO		BL		SL		TL		OL	
	B[b]	N[c]	B	N	B	N	B	N	B	N	B	N
1C3	+	−	−	−	−	−	−	−	−	−	−	−
1B9	+	−	−	−	−	−	−	−	−	−	−	−
2D4	+	−	−	−	−	−	−	−	−	−	−	−
3F11	+	−	−	−	−	−	−	−	−	−	−	−
4D8	+	+	−	−	−	−	∓	−	−	−	−	−
2C5	+	+	+	+	+	+	+	+	+	−	±	−
3H10	+	+	+	+	+	+	+	+	+	−	±	−
PAb[d]	+	+	+	+	+	+	+	+	+	+	+	+

[a] SLO was purified from a culture supernatant of *Streptococcus pyogenes* strain D58 as reported previously (5,59). Bifermentolysin (BL) was purified by 2C5–Sepharose column chromatography from a concentrated culture supernatant of *Clostridium bifermentans* SJ2 as shown in Table VI. Sordelliolysin (SL) was purified by 2C5–Sepharose column chromatography from a concentrated culture supernatant of *Clostridium sordellii* 1620 as shown in Table VI. Tetanolysin (TL) was purified by 3H10-Sepharose column chromatography from the partially purified preparation used in Sato *et al.* (59) as shown in Table VI. Oedematolysin (OL) was purified by 3H10–Sepharose column chromatography from a concentrated culture supernatant of *C. oedematiens* strain 140 as shown in Table VI.

[b] Binding activity by ELISA using polystyrene microplates coated with each toxin.

[c] Neutralizing activity determined by antihemolytic activity.

[d] Reference polyclonal antibody (see text).

system (Bio-Rad Laboratories). In spite of the positive binding activity of 2C5 and 3H10 antibodies to tetanolysin, they did not show antihemolytic activity to the toxin. This result suggests weakness of affinity of the monoclonal antibodies for tetanolysin in solution or for the target cells. This speculation should be confirmed by estimating the affinity constants of the monoclonal antibodies for each toxin, since the strength of the binding force and the toxin-neutralizing activity of the antibody are closely related. Oedematolysin also showed tetanolysinlike reactivity to 2C5 and 3H10 antibodies.

Figure 1 shows dose–response curves of antihemolytic activity of 2C5, 3H10, 4D8, and PAb to different toxins. The regression lines of the linear portion of these curves are represented by the equation $Y = a + b \log X$, where Y represents percentage hemolysis and X the concentration of antibody.

Antibody 2C5 showed almost the same slope ($b = -78$) for the toxins except for tetanolysin and oedematolysin, but 3H10 showed a steeper slope for SLO ($b = -163$), bifermentolysin ($b = -150$), and sordelliolysin ($b = -150$). For

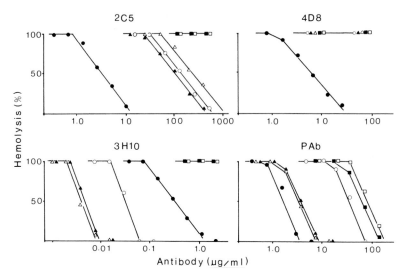

Fig. 1. Dose–response curves of antihemolytic activity of monoclonal antibodies. Antibodies were diluted serially twofold in a microtiter plate (V-bottom) and equal volumes (50 μl) of test toxin were added. The mixture was incubated at room temperature for 30 min. 0.3% SRBC (100 μl) were then added. After incubation at 37°C for 30 min, the plates were centrifuged at 4°C, and the supernatants (150 μl) were transferred to another plate (flat-bottom) to measure the absorbance at 405 nm with an autoreader (MR 580, Dynatech). Hemolysis was expressed as the percentage of the maximum absorbance by the test toxin. Test dose of each toxin was 2 HD_{100}, which corresponded to 5 ng/ml of PLO. Symbols: PLO (●), SLO (○), BL (△), SL (▲), TL (□), OL (■).

PLO, antibodies 3H10, 2C5, and 4D8 showed similar slopes. PAb also showed rather steep slopes ($b = -108$ to -150) for each toxin.

Steeper slopes can be taken to represent stronger affinities of the monoclonal antibodies for the toxins. Although other explanations are possible, this is the simplest and seems to be consistent with the results.

Based on their binding properties, antibodies (2C5 and 3H10) were used for the purification of the toxins by affinity chromatography (see Section III,D,1).

The results shown in Fig. 1 suggest that there is a structure near the active site(s) which is common to the toxins, but the results also indicate that there is microheterogeneity at the level of the common structure. These findings suggest that monoclonal antibodies would be a useful tool in the investigation of structure–function relationships along with the alkylating agents tosyl phenylalanine chloromethyl ketone (TPCK) and tosyl lysine chloromethyl ketone (TLCK) (3).

Neutralizing activities of monoclonal antibodies other than their antihemolytic activity were also investigated; for example, cardiotoxicity of PLO, SLO, and tetanolysin for cultured mouse myocardial cells.

The anticardiotoxic activity of antibodies 1C3, 2D4, 2C5, and 3H10 was investigated by the method reported by Goshima *et al.* (26) and Honda *et al.* (33). The myocardial cells were isolated from 16-day-old BALB/c mouse fetuses according to the method of Goshima (25). The heart cell suspension was distributed in a microtiter plate (1×10^4 cells per 0.1 ml per well). After cultivation in a 5% CO_2 incubator at 37°C overnight, a 10-μl portion of the toxin diluted with Eagle minimum essential medium was added to each well in which active beating of the myocardial cells was observed. By addition of the toxin (2 ng of PLO per well), the beating of the cells was accelerated immediately and then stopped. With high concentrations of the toxin (≥ 10 ng of PLO per well), the mouse myocardial cells abruptly stopped beating and degenerated. Three toxins tested—PLO, SLO, and tetanolysin—showed the same pattern of cardiotoxicity to the cultured cells; they stopped beating of the cells and destroyed cells depending on the concentration of each toxin. Quantification of the cardiotoxic activity of the toxin was so difficult that several doses of each toxin were tested for testing the anticardiotoxicity of the monoclonal antibodies. An appropriate dose of test toxin was mixed with an equal volume of the antibody diluted serially twofold, and was allowed to react for 30 min at room temperature. The mixture (20 μl) was added to the cultured beating heart cells (100 μl) under a phase-contrast microscope. Two antibodies showing antihemolytic activity (2C5 and 3H10) neutralized the cardiotoxic activity of PLO and SLO, but the other two (1C3 and 2D4), did not. None of the four antibodies neutralized tetanolysin at any test dose of the toxin. This result suggests that the epitope(s) involved in hemolysis is also involved in cardiotoxicity.

C. Binding Site of the Monoclonal Antibodies on the Cytolytic Toxins

The existence of two active fixing (f) and lytic (l) sites in the cytolytic toxins has been a matter of interest since the speculative model for SLO was proposed (1), but there has been little direct evidence favoring the model for other toxins (56) (Section II,C). This model's validity was investigated using four toxins (PLO, SLO, bifermentolysin, and sordelliolysin) to discover whether three neutralizing monoclonal antibodies (4D8, 2C5, and 3H10) were anti-f antibody or anti-l antibody. 1C3 was used as the negative control for antihemolysis. As shown in Table V, every antibody having antihemolytic activity in system I inhibited the hemolysis even after the toxin was fixed to the erythrocyte at 0°C (system II), although cholesterol could not inhibit the hemolysis under such conditions. Similarly, toxin–SRBC complexes washed with and resuspended in PBS at 0°C were saved from subsequent hemolysis with the antibodies, but this effect was not observed with cholesterol. From these results, all of these antibodies were considered to react with the region related to the lytic site, namely, they are anti-l antibodies. To my disappointment, there were no anti-f antibodies

TABLE V

Antihemolytic Activity of the Monoclonal Antibodies against Toxin–SRBC Complex[a]

Inhibitor[b]	Conc. (μg/ml)	PLO		SLO		BL		SL	
		I	II	I	II	I	II	I	II
1C3	150	96	107	108	100	ND[c]		ND	
4D8	20	3	0	100	103	ND		ND	
2C5	200	3	0	12	16	ND		ND	
3H10	5	0	3	0	0	0	1	0	0
PAb	30[d]	1	17	0	1	ND		ND	
Cholesterol	25	3	94	0	91	0	83	0	101
PBS	—	100	100	100	100	100	100	100	100

[a] The following two assay systems, I and II, were employed. System I: Each toxin, $2HD_{100}$ (50 μl), was reacted with an equal volume of the inhibitor at 0°C for 30 min, then 0.3% SRBC (100 μl) were added and the mixture was incubated at 0°C for 30 min and at 37°C for 30 min. System II: Each toxin (50 μl) was reacted with 0.3% SRBC (100 μl), first at 0°C for 30 min to form toxin–SRBC complexes. Then each inhibitor was allowed to react with the complexes for 30 min at 0°C and at 37°C for 30 min. Reaction mixtures in both systems were centrifuged at 4°C. Percentage hemolysis was estimated from the absorbance of the supernatant as described in the legend to Fig. 1.

[b] IC3, 4D8, 2C5, and 3H10 are monoclonal antibodies; PAb: polyclonal antibody control; PBS: phosphate-buffered saline (see text for details).

[c] Not done.

[d] For SLO, 150 μ/ml of PAb was used.

in the panel of three tested. If both types of antibodies were obtained in the future, the understanding of the lytic process of erythrocytes with the cytolytic toxins would certainly progress.

D. Application of the Monoclonal Antibodies

1. Purification of Toxin by Affinity Chromatography by Sepharose Coupled with Monoclonal Antibody

By taking advantage of the cross-reactivity of the monoclonal antibodies with the heterologous cytolytic toxins, purification of several different toxins by affinity chromatography with 2C5– or 3H10–Sepharose columns was attempted. Purified toxins were obtained by one-step chromatography using concentrated culture supernatant on the columns. By using the monoclonal antibody having weak affinity for each toxin, the latter could be eluted under mild conditions and was obtained in good yield. Table VI shows the conditions of buffer elution used for the purification of six different toxins using 2C5– or 3H10–Sepharose columns. This purification method was especially useful for bifermentolysin, sor-

TABLE VI

**Elution Conditions of Six Distinct Cytolytic Toxins
from 2C5– and 3H10–Sepharose Columns**

Affinity absorbent	Elution condition	Toxin					
		PLO	SLO	BL	SL	TL	OL
2C5–Sepharose[a]	Pass through	−[b]	−	−	−	ND[c]	±
	Wash buffer	−	−	−	−	ND	+
	1.5 *M* NaSCN	+	+	+	+	ND	−
	3.0 *M* NaSCN	−	−	−	−	ND	−
3H10–Sepharose	Pass through	−	ND	−	−	—	±
	Wash buffer	−	ND	−	−	+	+
	1.5 *M* NaSCN	+	ND	−	−	−	−
	3.0 *M* NaSCN	−	ND	+	+	−	−

[a] 2C5– or 3H10–Sepharose columns were used (except for TL and OL) as follows: Columns were washed successively with at least 10 column volumes of 0.1 *M* borate buffer containing 1.0 *M* NaCl, pH 8.0, and PBS containing 1 m*M* EDTA, pH 6.8. After washing the column, the toxin was eluted with 1.5 *M* NaSCN in PBS and 3.0 *M* NaSCN in PBS, successively. The eluate was collected in PBS containing 10% glycerol, 1 m*M* EDTA, and 1 m*M* DTT to lower the concentration of NaSCN to 0.5 *M* and to keep the toxin in a stable active state. TL and OL were applied on the column and washed with PBS containing 1 m*M* EDTA, pH 6.8. The treatment following with NaSCN solution was the same as for the other toxins.

[b] −, Toxin absent; +, toxin present.

[c] Not done.

delliolysin, or oedematolysin, for which purification had not yet been accomplished and for the partially purified toxin tetanolysin. The slopes of antihemolytic activity of the monoclonal antibodies against each toxin delineated in Fig. 1 reflect the binding strength between toxin and antibody shown in Table VI. From the 2C5–Sepharose column, four toxins, PLO, SLO, bifermentolysin, and sordelliolysin, were eluted with 1.5 *M* NaSCN, and from the 3H10–Sepharose column, PLO was eluted with 1.5 *M* NaSCN, but the latter two were with 3 *M* NaSCN. SLO was not applied to the 3H10–Sepharose column. Tetanolysin and oedematolysin were eluted in the wash fractions from both columns, using PBS containing 1 m*M* EDTA without NaSCN because of their very weak affinity for the 3H10– or 2C5–Sepharose column. Contaminant proteins of the partially purified tetanolysin were eliminated very effectively.

The elution profiles of tetanolysin were reproducible, and the purified toxin showed high specific activity and one major band on SDS–PAGE, although four major bands and several minor ones were observed in the partially purified tetanolysin. All purified toxins analyzed by SDS–PAGE and Western blot showed a molecular size very similar to PLO.

Similarly, affinity chromatography may be utilized for the isolation of a certain protein fragment containing an epitope related to the biological activity of the toxin, if the monoclonal antibodies still recognize the fragment of which the native conformation is presumably changed or lost. Such fragments will be obtained as products of protein chemistry or gene-cloning technology.

2. Toxin Estimations by ELISA

Figure 2 shows dose–response curves of PLO using the ELISA system with microtiter plates coated with monoclonal antibody 3H10 or SRBC membrane. With the 3H10-ELISA methods, less than 100 pg/ml (5 pg per well) of PLO could be measured. This sensitivity is higher and the linear range of the dose response is longer than that obtained by hemolysis with SRBC. A combination of both assay methods should be convenient for the analyses of toxins or toxin fragments activated or inactivated by various treatments. 2C5, 4D8, and 2D4-ELISA also gave similar results.

ELISA can be utilized for studies of competition between monoclonal antibodies using enzyme-conjugated monoclonal antibody. The other toxins were also measured by the 3H10-ELISA, but the sensitivity was rather low. Anti-PLO rabbit IgG was used here, which might not contain sufficient amounts of common antibodies that react with sites of the toxin not occupied by 3H10. If such

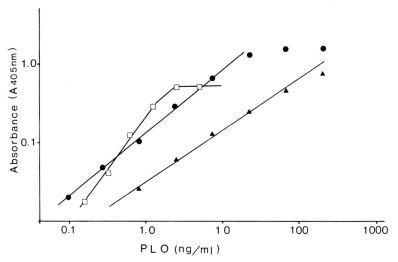

Fig. 2.   Measurement of PLO by 3H10-ELISA (●), SRBCmembranes-ELISA (▲) and hemolysis (□) systems. PLO (50 µl) diluted serially was allowed to react with 3H10 (2 µg/ml), or SRBC membrane (20 µg/ml), anti-PLO rabbit immunoglobulin (50 µl), alkaline phosphatase–anti-rabbit IgG conjugate (50 µl), and p-nitrophenyl phosphate (200 µl) in microtiter plates as reported previously (60,63). After 20 min at room temperature, the absorbance at 405 nm was measured by the autoreader (MR 580, Dynatech). Hemolysis was measured as described in the legend for Fig. 1.

antibody to each toxin were available, even if it were not monospecific, the 3H10-ELISA could become useful for the toxins or their fragments. Since this specific method can be used with impure toxins, it can be expected to be useful for differential assays of toxin preparations containing different hemolytic toxins.

IV. CONCLUSIONS

In this chapter, an attempt has been made to describe the various applications of monoclonal antibodies to the investigation of structure–activity relationships in thiol-activated cytolytic toxins based only on our own published data (59) and on our unpublished results that are still in the initial stages of investigation.

The immunological relatedness of six thiol-activated cytolytic toxins, PLO, tetanolysin, bifermentolysin, sordelliolysin, oedematolysin, and SLO, was investigated using seven monoclonal antibodies against PLO. Three antibodies, 4D8, 2C5, and 3H10, were neutralizing to PLO (group II in Table II) and the other four, 1C3, 1B9, 2D4, and 3F11, were not (group I in Table II). All the toxins seem to share common structure around the biologically active site because they reacted only with antibodies in group II. Thus, antibodies of group I were type 1 for the five heterologous toxins. This observation is not inconsistent with the data reported in the past, and does not exclude the possibility that some structures apart from the active center are common among the toxins. The experiments presented here do not provide evidence in favor of an immunological distinctiveness for all clostridial toxins with regard to SLO, or that histotoxic clostridia share more common epitopes than the others. However, the data indicate that each toxin has microheterogeneity in the region common to the six toxins.

Behavior of tetanolysin and oedematolysin toward the monoclonal antibodies was very similar. They showed very weak affinity to 2C5– and 3H10–Sepharose, and their hemolytic effect was not inhibited by the antibodies.

Toxin typing with monoclonal antibodies (Table III) showed that 2C5 and 3H10 belong to type 5 for tetanolysin and oedematolysin, and to type 6 for SLO, bifermentolysin, and sordelliolysin. Possible identification of bifermentolysin and sordelliolysin is still inconclusive because of the weak reactivity of sordelliolysin with 4D8 that was observed with 4D8– and SRBCmembrane-ELISA as well as with sordelliolysin-ELISA.

It may be possible that the cytolytic toxins are separated into several subgroups. Only SLO was used as a nonclostridial toxin in this paper, and further investigations are necessary to elucidate fully the immunological relatedness among the cytolytic toxins in this group.

The anticardiotoxic activity of the monoclonal antibodies against PLO, SLO, and tetanolysin was estimated with an *in vitro* assay system using mouse myocardial cells, and it was consistent with their antihemolytic activity, although one must bear in mind that the measurements are still only semiquantitative.

A two-site model for the hemolysis with SLO was also confirmed with PLO, bifermentolysin, and sordelliolysin, using the neutralizing antibodies and cholesterol (all neutralizing monoclonal antibodies used here were antilytic antibodies).

Three clostridial cytolytic toxins, bifermentolysin, sordelliolysin, and oedematolysin, were purified from the culture supernatants for the first time by affinity chromatography using 2C5– and 3H10–Sepharose. The molecular size of these purified toxins was almost identical to that of PLO by SDS–PAGE and Western blotting analysis. Purification by affinity chromatography should be applied to other toxins, and this strategy will become instrumental for further developments in studies on cytolytic toxins.

V. PROSPECTS FOR THE FUTURE

A. Prospects as Chemical Reagents

Structure–activity relationships are one of the most important and attractive subjects for the investigation of toxins. Monoclonal antibodies are promising reagents as specific inhibitors or affinity-labeling reagents to restricted site(s) of the toxin (Section III,B). An antibody fragment, Fab, might also be useful to diminish the problem of steric hindrance. Several clues from protein chemical, biochemical, or immunochemical studies indicate that monoclonal antibodies might play an important role in studies on clostridia toxins. Separation of the two steps by the interaction of anti-f and anti-l monoclonal antibodies with binding or lytic site of the toxin in a course of hemolysis must be achieved to enhance our understanding of the hemolytic process. This strategy should be effective for the investigation of relationships between the formation of ring- or arc-shaped structure on the erythrocytes with the toxin and the subsequent hemolysis resulting from the toxin fixation. Also, antiidiotype antibodies against these monoclonal antibodies may also become necessary probes for the study of structure–activity relationships.

There is no doubt that monoclonal antibodies are superior to polyclonal antibodies for analytical comparison of various epitopes among thiol-activated cytolytic toxins. Small differences between the toxins can be more easily detected by monoclonal antibodies because antibodies to many more determinants, even to minor determinants, can be obtained by hybridoma technology. For determination of the immunological relatedness, systematic studies with more monoclonal antibodies are necessary. However, to obtain the hybridoma-producing antibodies against various epitopes which are common or uncommon to other toxins, many different toxins and assay systems must be used from the outset. It may be possible to prepare a variety of monoclonal antibodies, but this will still depend on chance. Collaborated efforts of different researchers should speed progress in this area. Also, a combination of hybridoma and gene-cloning technologies as reported for several cytolytic toxins (30,37,40) should also help in the investigation of the relationships between a common structure and the biological activity of the cytolytic toxins produced by many different but closely related gram-positive bacteria.

B. Prospects as Immunoadsorbents

As described in Section III,D,1, it is expected that affinity chromatography will be useful in the purification of every cytolytic toxin using the proper monoclonal antibody. A monoclonal antibody offers several advantages over a polyclonal antibody as immunoadsorbent for purification of the toxin. A pure monospecific antibody helps to obtain highly purified toxin. By choosing the antibody with proper affinity for the toxin, the latter can be eluted under mild conditions, and severe damage to the toxin can be avoided. Isolation of common or uncommon fragments of the cytolytic toxins should also be made easier by affinity chromatography with the antibodies.

Qualitative and quantitative assays for the toxins will be improved in specificity and sensitivity by using an adequate monoclonal antibody as immunoadsorbent, as described in Section III,D,2.

C. Prospects for Investigation of Clostridial Toxins and Pathogenesis of *Clostridia*

Thiol-activated cytolytic toxins are not considered as important as a virulence factor for each pathogen, so that the role of the toxin in the development of the clostridial infection has been little studied. For investigation of the biological action of an individual toxin *in vivo*, purification of the toxin is necessary. Most clostridial toxins have not been purified in spite of their importance in various biological aspects, as described in Section I. Existence of several other immunologically related clostridial toxins, such as phospholipase C, have been well known for a long time. Since hybridoma technology made it possible to generate pure antibodies from impure antigens, a similar development, as demonstrated here, can be expected for the various clostridial toxins using monoclonal antibodies. Purification of toxins by affinity chromatography using the monoclonal antibodies obtained from impure (or pure) toxin will be feasible. Once purified toxin is obtained, many approaches from various directions or on various levels will become possible. We are now attempting continuous or simultaneous purification of PLO and phospholipase C using monoclonal antibodies against each toxin. Since monoclonal antibodies also show distinct reactivity with phospholipase C, they are expected to become useful tools for studies on the pathogenesis and on the biological interactions between enzymes and their targets (molecule or cell surface, for example).

Toxigenicity of the pathogen is an important factor in the identification or classification of clostridia. Monospecific antitoxins against various toxins are therefore desirable. Monoclonal antibodies will be the best candidate as the standard or reference antitoxin for such a purpose. Monoclonal antibodies will become useful reagents with clostridia, and hopefully more attention will be paid to the clostridial toxins.

VI. SUMMARY

Seven monoclonal antibodies—1C3, 1B9, 2D4, 3F11, 4D8, 2C5, and 3H10, against perfringolysin O (θ toxin), a thiol-activated cytolytic toxin of *Clostridium perfringens*—were generated from hybridomas of BALB/c mouse spleen cells and SP2/0-Ag14 myeloma cells. Three antibodies (4D8, 2C5, and 3H10) showed antihemolytic activity to perfringolysin O, and they were all antilytic antibodies which prevented hemolysis after binding of the toxin to the erythrocytes at 0°C. Only two antibodies, 2C5 and 3H10, showed cross-reactivity with bifermentolysin, sordelliolysin, oedematolysin, tetanolysin, and streptolysin O, but they did not neutralize hemolysis with oedematolysin and tetanolysin. Also, 2C5 and 3H10 antibodies showed anticardiotoxic effect on perfringolysin O and streptolysin O in an *in vitro* assay system using mouse myocardial cells, but did not on tetanalysin. These results suggest that the structural environment on the antibody–binding site of the toxin is different from toxin to toxin. The thiol-activated cytolytic toxins may be separable into several subgroups by their structural relatedness.

By taking advantage of the cross-reactivity of 2C5 and 3H10 antibodies with bifermentolysin, sordelliolysin, and oedematolysin, these three toxins were purified for the first time by affinity chromatography using Sepharose coupled with 2C5 or 3H10. The molecular size that was observed by sodium dodecyl sulfate–polyacrylamide gel electrophoresis and Western blotting analysis of these three toxins was almost identical to that of perfringolysin O.

ACKNOWLEDGMENTS

I am grateful to Y. Sato, Department of Bacteriology, National Institute of Health, Japan, for his help in carrying out the research described in this chapter. This investigation was supported in part by a grant-in-aid for Fundamental Scientific Research from the Ministry of Education, Japan.

REFERENCES

1. Alouf, J. E. (1976). Cell membranes and cytolytic bacterial toxins. *In* "Specificity and Action of Animal, Bacterial and Plant Toxins" (P. Cuatrecasas, ed.), pp. 221–270. Chapman & Hall, London.
2. Alouf, J. E. (1980). Streptococcal toxins (streptolysin O, streptolysin S, erythrogenic toxin). *Pharmacol. Ther.* **11,** 661–717.
3. Alouf, J. E., and Geoffroy, C. (1984). Structure–activity relationships in sulfhydryl-activated toxins. *In* "Bacterial Protein Toxins" (J. E. Alouf, F. J. Fehrenbach, J. H. Freer, and J. Jeljaszewicz, eds.), pp. 165–171. Academic Press, London.
4. Alouf, J. E., Geoffroy, C., Pattus, F., and Verger, R. (1984). Surface properties of bacterial sulfhydryl-activated cytolytic toxins: Interaction with monomolecular films of phosphatidylcholine and various sterols. *Eur. J. Biochem.* **141,** 205–210.
5. Alouf, J. E., and Raynaud, M. (1973). Purification and some properties of streptolysin O. *Biochimie* **55,** 1187–1193.
6. Alving, C. R., Habig, W. H., Urban, K. A., and Hardegree, M. C. (1979). Cholesterol-dependent tetanolysin damage to liposomes. *Biochim. Biophys. Acta* **551,** 224–228.
7. Bernheimer, A. W. (1974). Interactions between membranes and cytolytic bacterial toxins. *Biochim. Biophys. Acta* **344,** 27–50.
8. Bernheimer, A. W. (1976). Sulfhydryl activated toxins. *In* "Mechanisms in Bacterial Toxinology" (A. W. Bernheimer, ed.), pp. 85–97. Wiley, New York.
9. Bernheimer, A. W., and Grushoff, P. (1967). Cereolysin: Production, purification and partial characterization. *J. Gen. Microbiol.* **46,** 143–150.
10. Bhakdi, S., Roth, M., Sziegoleit, A., and Tranum-Jensen, J. (1984). Isolation and identification of two hemolytic forms of streptolysin O. *Infect. Immun.* **46,** 394–400.
11. Bhakdi, S., Tranum-Jensen, J., and Sziegoleit, A. (1985). Mechanism of membrane damage by streptolysin-O. *Infect. Immun.* **47,** 52–60.
12. Blumenthal, R., and Habig, W. H. (1984). Mechanism of tetanolysin-induced membrane damage: Studies with black lipid membranes. *J. Bacteriol.* **157,** 321–323.
13. Bremm, K. D., Brom, H. J., Alouf, J. E., Konig, W., Spur, B., Crea, A., and Peters, W. (1984). Generation of leukotrienes from human granulocytes by alveolysin from *Bacillus alvei*. *Infect. Immun.* **44,** 188–193.
14. Bruck, C., Portelle, D., Gleneur, C., and Bollen, A. (1982). One-step purification of mouse monoclonal antibodies from ascitic fluid by DEAE Affi-gel blue chromatography. *J. Immunol. Methods* **53,** 313–319.
15. Cowell, J. L., and Bernheimer, A. W. (1977). Antigenic relationships among thiol-activated cytolysins. *Infect. Immun.* **16,** 397–399.
16. Cowell, J. L., and Bernheimer, A. W. (1978). Role of cholesterol in the action of cereolysin on membranes. *Arch. Biochem. Biophys.* **190,** 603–610.
17. Cowell, J. L., Grushoff-Kosyk, P., and Bernheimer, A. W. (1976). Purification of cereolysin and the electrophoretic separation of the active (reduced) and inactive (oxidized) forms of the purified toxin. *Infect. Immun.* **14,** 144–154.
18. Cowell, J. L., Kim, K., and Bernheimer, A. W. (1978). Alteration by cereolysin of the structure of cholesterol-containing membranes. *Biochim. Biophys. Acta* **507,** 230–241.
19. Duncan, J. L. (1974). Characteristics of streptolysin O hemolysis: Kinetics of hemoglobin and [86]rubidium release. *Infect. Immun.* **9,** 1022–1027.
20. Duncan, J. L., and Buckingham, L. (1980). Resistance to streptolysin O in mammalian cells treated with oxygenated derivatives of cholesterol: Cholesterol content of resistant cells and recovery of streptolysin O sensitivity. *Biochim. Biophys. Acta* **603,** 278–287.

21. Ey, P. L., Prowse, S. J., and Jenkin, C. R. (1978). Isolation of pure IgG1, IgG2a and IgG2b immunoglobulins from mouse serum using protein A-Sepharose. *Immunochemistry* **15**, 429–436.

22. Geoffroy, C., and Alouf, J. E. (1983). Selective purification by thiol-disulfide interchange chromatography of alveolysin, a sulfhydryl-activated toxin of *Bacillus alvei*: Toxin properties and interaction with cholesterol and liposomes. *J. Biol. Chem.* **258**, 9968–9972.

23. Geoffroy, C., and Alouf, J. E. (1984). Antigenic relationship between sulfhydryl-activated toxins. *In* "Bacterial Protein Toxins" (J. E. Alouf, F. J. Fehrenhach, J. H. Freer, and J. Jeljaszewicz, eds.), pp. 241–243. Academic Press, London.

24. Geoffroy, C., Gilles, A.-M., and Alouf, J. E. (1981). The sulfhydryl groups of the thiol-dependent cytolytic toxin from *Bacillus alvei*: Evidence for one essential sulfhydryl group. *Biochem. Biophys. Res. Commun.* **99**, 781–788.

25. Goshima, K. (1969). Synchronized beating of and electrotonic transmission between myocardial cells mediated by heterotypic strain cells in monolayer culture. *Exp. Cell Res.* **58**, 420–426.

26. Goshima, K., Honda, T., Hirata, M., Kikuchi, K., Takeda, Y., and Miwatani, T. (1977). Stopping of the spontaneous beating of mouse and rat myocardial cells *in vitro* by a toxin from *Vibrio parahemolyticus*. *J. Mol. Cell. Cardiol.* **9**, 191–213.

27. Guillaumie, M. (1950). Hémolysines bactériennes et anti-hémolysines. *Ann. Inst. Pasteur, Paris* **79**, 661–671.

28. Guillaumie, M., Fagonde, A. P., and Kréguer, A. (1950). Hémolysine oxydable de *Cl. bifermentans*. *Ann. Inst. Pasteur, Paris,* **79**, 20–32.

29. Guillaumie, M., and Kréguer, A. (1950). Nouvelles recherches sur les hémolysines oxydables. *Ann. Inst. Pasteur, Paris* **78**, 467–480.

30. Hartlein, M., Hughes, C., Muller, D., Kreft, J., and Goebel, W. (1984). Haemolysin genes from gram-negative and gram-positive bacteria. *In* "Bacterial Protein Toxins" (J. F. Alouf, F. J. Fehrenbach, J. H. Freer, and J. Jeljasxewicz, eds.), pp. 39–46. Academic Press, London.

30a. Hase, J., Mitsui, K., and Shonaka, E. (1976). *Clostridium perfringens* exotoxins. IV. Inhibition of θ-toxin induced hemolysis by steroids and related compounds. *Jpn. J. Exp. Med.* **46**, 45–50.

31. Herbert, D. (1941). A simple colorimetric method for the estimation of haemolysis and its application to the study of streptolysin. *Biochem. J.* **35**, 1116–1123.

32. Herbert, D., and Todd, E. W. (1941). Purification and properties of a haemolysin produced by group a haemolytic streptococci (streptolysin O). *Biochem. J.* **35**, 1124–1139.

33. Honda, T., Goshima, K., Takeda, Y., Sugino, Y., and Miwatani, T. (1976). Demonstration of the cardiotoxicity of the thermostable direct hemolysin (lethal toxin) produced by *Vibrio parahemolyticus*. *Infect. Immun.* **13**, 163–171.

34. Ispolatovskaya, M. V. (1971). Type A *Clostridium perfringens* toxin. *In* "Microbial Toxins. Vol. IIA: Bacterial Protein Toxins" (S. Kadis, T. C. Montie, and S. J. Ajl, eds.), pp. 109–158. Academic Press, New York.

35. Johnson, M. K. (1972). Properties of purified pneumococcal hemolysin. *Infect. Immun.* **6**, 755–760.

36. Johnson, M. K., Geoffroy, C., and Alouf, J. E. (1980). Binding of cholesterol by sulfhydryl-activated cytolysins. *Infect. Immun.* **27**, 97–101.

37. Johnson, M. K., Johnson, E. J., Geoffroy, C., and Alouf, J. E. (1984). Physiologic and genetic regulation of the synthesis of sulfhydryl-activated cytolytic toxins. *In* "Bacterial Protein Toxins" (J. E. Alouf, F. J. Fehrenbach, J. H. Freer, and J. Jeljaszewicz, eds.), pp. 55–63. Academic Press, London.

38. Johnson, M. K., Knight, R. J., and Drew, G. K. (1982). The hydrophobic character of thiol-activated cytolysins. *Biochem. J.* **207**, 557–560.

39. Kehoe, M., Dougan, G., Foster, T., Kennedy, S., Duncan, J., Timmis, K., Grey, G., and

Fairweather, N. (1984). Genetic analysis of toxins from gram positive cocci. *In* "Bacterial Protein Toxins" (J. E. Alouf, F. J. Fehrenbach, J. H. Freer, and J. Jeljaszewicz, eds.), pp. 47–54. Academic Press, London.

40. Kehoe, M., and Timmis, K. N. (1984). Cloning and expression in *Escherichia coli* of the streptolysin O determinant from *Streptococcus pyogenes:* Characterization of the cloned streptolysin O determinant and demonstration of the absence of substantial homology with determinants of other thiol-activated toxins. *Infect. Immun.* **43**, 804–810.

41. MacLennan, J. D. (1962). The histotoxic clostridial infections of man. *Bacteriol. Rev.* **26**, 177–276.

42. Mansa, B., and Kjems, E. (1970). Further studies on M-components with antistreptolysin O activity. The inactivating effect on different oxygen-labile hemolysins. *Acta Pathol. Microbiol. Scand., Sect. B* **78**, 467–472.

43. McDonel, J. L. (1980). *Clostridium perfringens* toxins (type A, B, C, D, E). *Pharmacol. Ther.* **10**, 617–655.

44. Miles, E. M., and Miles, A. A. (1947). The lecithinase of *Clostridium bifermentans* and its relation to the α-toxin of *Clostridium welchii*. *J. Gen. Microbiol.* **1**, 385–399.

45. Mitsui, K., Mitsui, N., and Hase, J. (1973). *Clostridium perfringens* exotoxins. II. Purification and some properties of θ-toxin. *Jpn. J. Exp. Med.* **43**, 377–391.

46. Mitsui, K., and Hase, J. (1979). *Clostridium perfringens* exotoxins. VI. Reactivity of perfringolysin O with thiol and disulfide compounds. *Jpn. J. Exp. Med.* **49**, 13–18.

47. Mitsui, N., Mitsui, K., and Hase, J. (1980). Purification and some properties of tetanolysin. *Microbiol. Immunol.* **24**, 575–584.

48. Mitsui, K., Sekiya, T., Nozawa, Y., and Hase, J. (1979). Alteration of human erythrocyte plasma membranes by perfringolysin O as revealed by freeze–fracture electron microscopy: Studies on *Clostridium perfringens* exotoxins. V. *Biochim. Biophys. Acta* **554**, 68–75.

49. Moussa, R. S. (1958). Complexity of toxins from *Clostridium septicum* and *Clostridium chauvoei*. *J. Bacteriol.* **76**, 538–545.

50. Murata, R., Soda, S., Yamamoto, A., and Ito, A. (1968). Further investigations on the influence of inorganic cations on growth and toxin production by *Clostridum perfringens* PB6K. *Jpn. J. Med. Sci. Biol.* **21**, 55–70.

51. Murata, R., Soda, S., Yamamoto, A., Sato, H., and Ito, A. (1969). The effect of zinc on the production of various toxins of *Clostridium perfringens*. *Jpn. J. Med. Sci. Biol.* **22**, 133–148.

52. Nakamura, S., Shimamura, T., Hayashi, H., and Nishida, S. (1975). Reinvestigation of the taxonomy of *Clostridium bifermentans* and *Clostridium sordellii*. *J. Med. Microbiol.* **8**, 299–309.

53. Oakley, C. L., Warrack, G. H., and Clarke, P. H. (1947). The toxins of *Clostridium oedematiens (Cl. novyi)*. *J. Gen. Microbiol.* **1**, 91–107.

54. Oberley, T. D., and Duncan, J. L. (1971). Characteristics of streptolysin O action. *Infect. Immun.* **4**, 683–687.

55. Oi, V. T., and Herzenberg, L. A. (1980). Immunoglobulin-producing hybrid cell lines. *In* "Selected Methods in Cellular Immunology" (B. B. Mishell and S. W. Shiigi, eds.), pp. 351–372. Freeman, San Francisco, California.

56. Prigent, D., Alouf, J. E., and Raynaud, M. (1974). Étude de la fixation de la streptolysine O radioiodée sur les érythrocytes. *C. R. Hebd. Seances Acad. Sci., Ser. D* **278**, 651–653.

57. Raynaud, M., Alouf, J. E., Mihaesco, C., and Seligman, M. (1970). Étude quantitative de l'activité anti-streptolysine O d'une proteine myélomateuse IgG humaine. *Ann. Inst. Pasteur, Paris* **118**, 448–458.

58. Rutter, J. M., and Collee, J. G. (1969). Studies on the soluble antigens of *Clostridium oedematiens (Cl. novyi)*. *J. Med. Microbiol.* **2**, 395–421.

59. Sato, H., Ito, A., and Chiba, J. (1984). Cross-reactivity of monoclonal antibodies against *Clostridium perfringens* θ toxin with streptolysin O. *Curr. Microbiol.* **10**, 243–248.
60. Sato, H., Ito, A., Chiba, J., and Sato, Y. (1984). Monoclonal antibody against pertussis toxin: Effect on toxin activity and pertussis infections. *Infect. Immun.* **46**, 422–428.
61. Sato, H., Ito, A., Yamakawa, Y., and Murata, R. (1979). Toxin-neutralizing effect of antibody against subtilisin-digested tetanus toxin. *Infect. Immun.* **24**, 958–961.
62. Sato, H., and Sato, Y. (1984). *Bordetella pertussis* infection in mice: Correlation of specific antibodies against two antigens, pertussis toxin, and filamentous hemagglutinin with mouse protectivity in an intracerebral or aerosol challenge system. *Infect. Immun.* **46**, 415–421.
63. Sato, H., Sato, Y., and Ito, A. (1983). Affinity of pertussis toxin produced by *Bordetella pertussis* for human haptoglobin: Application to the *in vitro* assay of the toxin. *J. Microbiol. Methods* **1**, 99–109.
64. Sato, H., Yamakawa, Y., Ito, A., and Murata, R. (1978). Effect of zinc and calcium ions on the production of alpha-toxin and proteases by *Clostridium perfringens*. *Infect. Immun.* **20**, 325–333.
65. Shany, S., Grushoff, P. S., and Bernheimer, A. W. (1973). Physical separation of streptococcal nicotinamide adenine dinucleotide glycohydrolase from streptolysin O. *Infect. Immun.* **7**, 731–734.
66. Smith, J. W. G., and Smith, G. (1984). Gas gangrene and other clostridial infections of man and animals. *In* "Topley and Wilson's Principles of Bacteriology, Virology, and Immunity. Vol. 3: Bacterial Diseases" (C. R. Smith, ed.), pp. 48–78. Arnold, London.
67. Smyth, C. J., and Duncan, J. L. (1978). Thiol-activated (oxygen-labile) cytolysins. *In* "Bacterial Toxins and Cell Membranes" (J. Jeljaszewicz and T. Wadstrom, eds.), pp. 129–183. Academic Press, New York.
68. Soda, S., Ito, A., and Yamamoto, A. (1976). Production and properties of θ-toxin of *Clostridium perfringens* with special reference to lethal activity. *Jpn. J. Med. Sci. Biol.* **29**, 335–349.
69. Soda, S., Sato, H., and Murata, R. (1969). The effect of calcium on the production of various toxins of *Clostridium perfringens*. *Jpn. J. Med. Sci. Biol.* **22**, 175–179.
70. Voller, A., Bidwell, D., and Bartlett, A. (1980). Enzyme-linked immunosorbent assay. *In* "Manual of Clinical Immunology" (N. R. Rose and H. Friedman, eds.), pp. 359–371. Am. Soc. Microbiol., Washington, D.C.
71. Willis, A. T. (1977). "Anaerobic Bacteriology: Clinical and Laboratory Practice." Butterworth, London.
72. Willis, A. T. (1983). Clostridium: the spore-bearing anaerobes. *In* "Topley and Wilson's Principles of Bacteriology, Virology and Immunity. Vol. 2: Systematic Bacteriology" (M. T. Pasker, ed.), pp. 20–47. Arnold, London.
73. Yamakawa, Y., Ito, A., and Sato, H. (1977). Theta-toxin of *Clostridium perfringens*. I. Purification and some properties. *Biochim. Biophys. Acta* **494**, 301–313.

10

Monoclonal Antibodies against Diphtheria Toxin: Their Use in Analysis of the Function and Structure of the Toxin and Their Application to Cell Biology

T. YOSHIMORI[1] AND T. UCHIDA

Institute for Molecular and Cellular Biology
Osaka University, Osaka, Japan

I. INTRODUCTION

Investigations on diphtheria toxin started about 100 years ago. Since the clinical problems have now been nearly eliminated, the focus of attention has

[1]Present address: Department of Physiology, Kansai Medical University, Osaka 570, Japan.

MONOCLONAL ANTIBODIES
AGAINST BACTERIA
Volume III

turned to the biological activity of the toxin. Recent studies at the molecular level have provided many interesting facts about the toxin, and the main question at present is the structure–function relationship of the toxin molecule; that is, what function is involved in the action of the toxin and which domain (or site) in the toxin molecule is related to each function, and, especially, the entry of the toxin into sensitive cells. Employing antibodies against the toxin should be one way of analyzing the structure–function relationship. Already, polyclonal antisera against the toxin have been used for the analysis of the structure of the toxin, but although some results have been obtained in this way, the value of this approach is limited by the heterogeneity of polyclonal antisera. With the recent development of hybridoma technology, it is now possible to obtain monoclonal antibodies directed to a given antigen, and because of their high specificity, these monoclonal antibodies are very useful for further studies on the toxin.

Thus information on the relation between a certain domain and a certain function should be obtainable by comparing the locations of binding sites of monoclonal antibodies with their effects—for example, their inhibition of certain steps in the toxin action. However, there are certain limitations to the use of monoclonal antibodies. For example, a monoclonal antibody may cause a conformational change of a protein antigen that inhibits a certain function, even though the active center for the function is located far from the epitope recognized by the monoclonal antibody. In most cases, however, including that of direct binding of the monoclonal antibody to the active center, inhibition is presumably caused by steric interference. Moreover, it is likely that the nearer the binding site of monoclonal antibody is to the active center, the greater the inhibition (see Fig. 6), although there is no direct evidence for this. While this uncertainty about the mechanism of inhibition is a disadvantage in studies with monoclonal antibodies, significant results may be obtained by assuming simply that the effect of an antibody is nearly epitope-specific.

Studies on the toxin itself have been extended to cell biology and cancer therapy. For example, in the field of cell biology, the functional stability of antibodies introduced into the cytoplasm of living cells was studied with toxin as antigen, using the ability of the antibodies to protect cells from the cytotoxicity of the toxin as an index of their activity (28). In the field of cancer therapy, fragment A is used as the lethal moiety of hybrid toxin to kill malignant cells specifically (5). For such applied studies, as well as for basic studies on the toxin itself, it is very important to understand the structure and function of the toxin completely, and so extensive analyses with monoclonal antibodies are required. Studies with antitoxin monoclonal antibodies should also provide information for developing this cell biological technology.

This article describes the results of recent studies using monoclonal antibodies with emphasis on two problems: the structure–function relationship of toxin and the applicability of antitoxin monoclonal antibodies in the field of cell biology.

II. BACKGROUND

Diphtheria toxin is synthesized and released by *Corynebacterium diphtheriae*. It is a single-chain polypeptide with a molecular weight of 58,348, and its primary amino acid sequence is predicted from the base sequence of the toxin structural gene (9). The intact toxin molecule consists of two functional domains, fragment A and B, which can be separated by trypsin cleavage and reduction: fragment A (M_r 21,167) from the NH_2-terminal region, catalyzes the NAD-dependent ADP-ribosylation of elongation factor 2 (EF-2); and fragment B (M_r 37,199), from the COOH-terminal region, binds to specific receptors on the surface of susceptible eukaryotic cells and is required for the translocation of fragment A into the cells (1,25).

The cytotoxic action of diphtheria toxin is due to a sequence of events: (i) binding of toxin to its receptor, (ii) passage of at least fragment A across the lipid bilayer to the cytoplasm, and (iii) inhibition of cellular protein synthesis as a result of inactivation of EF-2 by fragment A. A single molecule of fragment A in the cytoplasm can kill a cell (27). A number of immunologically cross-reacting materials (CRMs) have been obtained by mutation of the structural gene for the toxin and have contributed to analysis of the functions of different domains within the toxin molecule. (4,18,22).

The action of diphtheria toxin on sensitive cells has attracted attention as a model of receptor-mediated translocation of macromolecules into the cytoplasm across a lipid bylayer. So the mechanism of entry of the toxin into the cell has been investigated extensively and is now partially clarified. The COOH-terminal region of fragment B is essential for binding to the receptor, and a hybrophobic domain in about the middle of fragment B is required for translocation of fragment A (1,24). The toxin (perhaps fragment B) forms ion-permeable channels in artificial membranes at low pH, and it is supposed that fragment A passes through these channels to the cytoplasm (6,14). Toxin is transferred to the cytoplasm *in vivo* also only after exposure to low pH in an endocytotic vesicle (21).

The enzyme reaction catalyzed by fragment A is well understood; fragment A binds a single molecule of NAD^+, then binds to EF-2 and transfers an ADP-ribosyl moiety to "diphthamide," a unique posttranslationally modified histidine residue within EF-2 (26). The COOH-terminal region of fragment A (M_r ~4000) may be required for ADP-ribosyltransferase activity. Recently the NAD-binding site of fragment A of diphtheria toxin was identified as Glu_{148} by photoaffinity labeling (2). It is known that *Pseudomonas aeruginosa* exotoxin A also catalyzes the same enzyme reaction (12).

As mentioned above, the biological action and structure of diphtheria toxin have been more extensively studied than those of other protein toxins, but many questions still remain unanswered, such as the exact process of entry of toxin into cells, the structural features of the toxin and the cellular functions required by the process, and the sites and functions concerned with ADP-ribosyltransferase activity.

For further studies on the toxin, two groups have so far isolated and characterized monoclonal antibodies against diphtheria toxin.

III. RESULTS AND DISCUSSION

A. Location of Monoclonal Antibody-Binding Sites

By immunization with diphtheria toxoid, Hayakawa et al. (10) and Zucker and Murphy (30) independently obtained 14 and 43 monoclonal antibodies, respectively. To locate the positions of the epitopes, they used various CRMs, which are prematurely terminated polypeptide chains lacking some of the COOH-terminal region (see Table I). Figure 1 summarizes the location of binding sites of the monoclonal antibodies obtained by the two groups. Hayakawa et al. (10) tested the binding of their antibodies to the toxin, fragment A, CRM 30, and CRM 45 by radioimmunoprecipitation. They found that two antibodies reacted only with fragment A, one antibody reacted only with toxin, and the remainder reacted with both the toxin and CRM 45 but did not react with CRM 30. Thus they divided the toxin into three epitope regions as shown in Fig. 1. Zucker and

TABLE I

Diptheria Toxin and Immunologically Related Proteins

	MW		Cytotoxicity (%)	Activity of fragment A (%)	Binding activity to receptor (%)
Toxin	58,348		100	100	100
Fragment A	21,167		0	100	0
Fragment B	37,199		0	0	100
CRM 1	~17,000	x^a	0	0	—
CRM 2	~23,000	x	0	100	—
CRM 3	~31,000	x	0	100	—
CRM 30	~27,000	x	0	100	0
CRM 45	41,984	x	0	100	0
CRM 111	~44,000	x	—	—	—
CRM 176	~58,348	x ?x	0.5	10	100
CRM 197	58,329	x	0	0	100
CRM 228	58,395	x x x x x	0	0	20

^{a} x, Mutation sites.

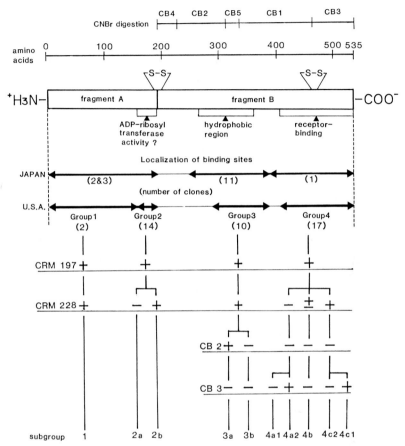

Fig. 1. Locations of epitopes recognized by antitoxin monoclonal antibodies and their subdivision based on antibody reactivity with various CRMs and CNBr peptides of fragment B. Modified with permission from Zucker, D. R., and Murphy, J. R., Monoclonal antibody analysis of diphtheria toxin, I. Localization of epitopes and neutralization of cytotoxicity. *Mol. Immunol.* **21**, 785–793. Copyright 1984 Pergamon Press.

Murphy (30) also tested the reactivities of their monoclonal antibodies with various CRMs by Western blot analysis, and from the results they classified their antibodies into four groups (Fig. 1). Group 1 antibodies bound to fragment A and CRM 1, group 2 bound to fragment A only, and groups 3 and 4 were anti-fragment B, the former reacting with CRM 45 but not CRM 3, and the latter reacting with the toxin but not CRMs. Thus, the epitopes recognized by the monoclonal antibodies in the two laboratories were clustered within two similar restricted regions on fragment B.

1. Fragment A

Group 2 antibodies constituted 88% (14 of 16) of the anti-fragment A antibodies obtained in the U.S. laboratory (30). The epitope region of the group 2 antibodies is limited to part of the COOH-terminal of fragment A of about 4000 of 22,000 da. This finding suggests that only this narrow region of fragment A of the toxin molecule has high antigenicity, a possibility that is consistent with an earlier finding that most of the amino acid sequence of fragment A is masked in the toxin molecule. Yoshimori *et al.* (29) obtained several anti-fragment A monoclonal antibodies by immunization with free fragment A and found that none of them bound to whole toxin, and that they bound only weakly to CRM 45. Thus it appears that fragment A in the intact toxin is largely masked by fragment B or differs in conformation from isolated fragment A.

Fragment A of CRMs 197 and 228 have no ADP-ribosyltransferase activity as the result of one and two amino acid substitutions, respectively, due to missense mutations. The complete amino acid sequences of CRMs 197 and 228 were deduced from the sequences of their genes and so the mutation sites were identified (8,13). Group 1 and 2 antibodies both bound to CRM 197, but two antibodies of group 2 failed to bind to CRM 228. Thus group 2 was divided into two subgroups (Fig. 1). Yoshimori *et al.* (29) isolated three monoclonal antibodies against fragment A that caused complete, partial, and no block of the enzymatic activity of fragment A, respectively. They investigated the affinities of these monoclonal antibodies to fragment A of CRMs 197 and 228 by competitive radioimmunoassay. None of the antibodies bound to these mutant A-fragments. Since these three antibodies differ in ability to inhibit ADP-ribosylation of fragment A but have similar affinity constants to wild-type fragment A, they may recognize different epitopes. Thus one and two amino acid substitutions in CRMs 197 and 228, respectively, may bring about changes of the protein conformation that affect its antigenicity.

There is a disulfide bridge within the region recognized by group 2 antibodies, but no antibody of group 2 reacts with a synthetic oligopeptide corresponding to the COOH-terminal region of fragment A spanned by this disulfide bridge.

2. Fragment B

The reactivities of group 3 and 4 anti-fragment B antibodies with CNBr-digested fragments of fragment B were examined by solid-phase ELISA. CB4, which is the NH_2-terminal region of 5000 Da of fragment B, did not react with any antibody, a finding that is consistent with results by CRMs analysis. As seen in Fig. 1, some group 3 and 4 antibodies reacted with CB2 and CB3, respectively. The reactivities of the antibodies with CRMs 197 and 228 were also tested. There is no mutation within fragment B of CRM 197, and all the anti-fragment B antibodies (group 3 and 4) reacted with it. Fragment B of CRM 228 contains three amino acid substitutions and CRM 228 binds less strongly than the normal toxin to the cell surface. The amino acid substitutions in CRM 228 are Gly for Ser_{197}, Ser for Pro_{378}, and Ser for Gly_{431}. The latter two substitutions are perhaps within the regions recognized by group 3 and group 4 antibodies, respectively. All group 3 antibodies bound with CRM 228, but about half those in group 4 did not.

The Japanese group examined the relative distances between the epitopes recognized by monoclonal antibodies on the toxin molecule by measuring the competitions between pairs of antibodies for binding to the toxin. The values obtained were closely related with the effects of these antibodies on the action of the toxin, as described in Section III,B.

B. Effects of Antibodies on Entry of Toxin into Cells

Hayakawa et al. (10) selected four of their anti-fragment B monoclonal antibodies and examined in detail their abilities to inhibit the action of the toxin. Two antibodies, 2 and 7, had quite different effects: antibody 7 seemed to block the binding of the toxin to the cell surface receptor, whereas antibody 2 did not block the binding but inhibited the process of toxin translocation into the cytoplasm after binding. Figures 2–5 show the data supporting this idea.

^{125}I-Labeled toxin (^{125}I-toxin) preincubated with antibody 7 did not bind to cells at 4°C, while when preincubated with antibody 2 or normal mouse IgG, it showed normal binding (Fig. 2).

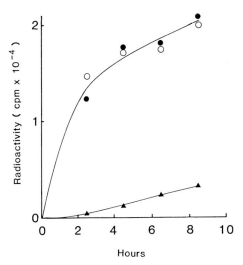

Fig. 2. Effects of antibodies 2 and 7 on the time course of binding of ^{125}I-toxin to cells at 4°C. ^{125}I-Toxin was mixed with antibody, incubated at 37°C for 30 min, and then incubated at 4°C overnight. The mixture was added to Vero cells and incubated at 4°C for the indicated times, and then radioactivity associated with the cells was counted. (○) Antibody 2 and ^{125}I-toxin; (▲) antibody 7 and ^{125}I-toxin; (●) normal mouse IgG and ^{125}I-toxin. Modified from Hayakawa et al. (10).

In a similar experiment with ^{125}I-labeled antibody (^{125}I-antibody) instead of ^{125}I-toxin, ^{125}I-antibody 2 showed binding kinetics in the presence of unlabeled toxin similar to those of ^{125}I-toxin, whereas ^{125}I-antibody 7 did not bind to the cells (Fig. 3). Since ^{125}I-antibody 2 could not bind to the cells without toxin, its association with the cells must be through toxin.

The next step in the action of the toxin after its binding is its internalization into the cytoplasm. Figure 4 shows the effects of the antibodies on toxin translocation into the cytoplasm. ^{125}I-Toxin preincubated with antibody was added to cells and then the cells were incubated at 37°C. It is known that toxin is degraded after its translocation at 37°C. Cell association of ^{125}I-toxin mixed with normal IgG increased for the first hour (translocation) and then decreased (degradation). When toxin prebound to antibody 2 was used, cell association increased, but no decrease was observed. When toxin prebound to antibody 7 was used, no association of toxin with the cells was observed, as expected. From these results it was concluded that antibody 2 inhibited translocation of the toxin into the cytoplasm. Methylamine is known to block toxin translocation but not toxin binding. In the presence of methylamine, toxin accumulates in the cells (perhaps in endocytotic vesicles) as its translocation and degradation are inhibited. The

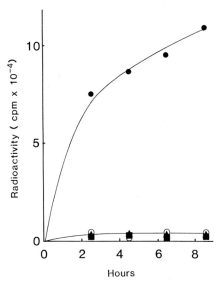

Fig. 3. Binding of ^{125}I-antibody to cells in the presence of toxin. ^{125}I-Antibody was incubated with toxin at 37°C for 30 min and then at 4°C for 14 hr. The mixtures were incubated with Vero cells at 4°C for the indicated times and then the radioactivity associated with cells was counted. (●) ^{125}I-Antibody 2 and toxin; (○) ^{125}I-antibody 7 and toxin; (■) ^{125}I-antibody 2 alone; (▲) ^{125}I-antibody 7 alone. Modified from Hayakawa *et al.* (10).

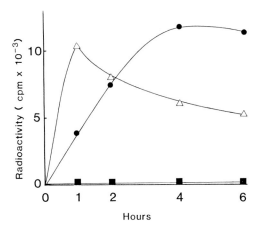

Fig. 4. Effects of monoclonal antibodies 2 and 7 on the association of ^{125}I-toxin with cells at 37°C. ^{125}I-Toxin was incubated with antibody at 37°C for 30 min and then at 4°C for 14 hr. The mixtures were then incubated with Vero cells at 37°C. At indicated times, the radioactivity associated with cells was counted. (●) Antibody 2 and ^{125}I-toxin; (■) antibody 7 and ^{125}I-toxin; (△) normal IgG and ^{125}I-toxin. Modified from Hayakawa *et al.* (10).

time course of the effect of antibody 2 was similar to that of methylamine (Fig. 5).

Preincubation of the toxin with antibody 7 prevented inhibition of protein synthesis by the toxin because it blocked binding of the toxin to the cells. But on preincubation of the cells with toxin at 4°C for 1 hr, removal of unbound toxin, and preincubation of the cells with antibody at 4°C for 2 hr, no neutralization of the toxin by the antibody was observed. Under similar conditions, antibody 2 could block inhibition of protein synthesis by the toxin after preincubation of the cells with toxin, but it could not protect cells when preincubated with the toxin.

Two other monoclonal antibodies, 1 and 5, had effects intermediate between those of 2 and 7. Figure 6 shows the relations between the effects of antibodies on the action of the toxin and their relative binding sites. Relative binding sites were determined by competition between pairs of antibodies for binding to the toxin linked to Sepharose 4B. Since these four antibodies had similar association constants for the toxin of 6 to 9 $\times$ 10^8 M^{-1}, the results indicated the correlation of effects to the relative distances of binding sites.

The reason antibody 2 did not protect cells from the toxin in the toxin–antibody preincubation experiment may be that a very large amount of antibody is required to block translocation of the toxin after its binding. The translocation is presumably very rapid and shows high affinity, and so if there is insufficient antibody some toxin will escape and kill the cells (in the reported experiment the molar toxin:antibody ratio was 1:200). There is also a possibility that binding of

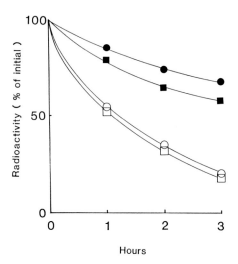

Fig. 5. Effects of monoclonal antibodies 2 and 7 on ^{125}I-toxin bound to cells. ^{125}I-Toxin was incubated with Vero cells at 4°C for 14 hr. The cells were then washed four times, and incubated with antibody or methylamine at 37°C for the indicated times. Then radioactivity associated with the cells was counted. (●) Antibody 2; (○) antibody 7; (□) normal IgG; (■) normal IgG plus methylamine. Modified from Hayakawa *et al.* (10).

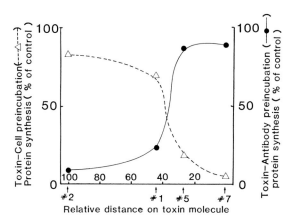

Fig. 6. Relation between the effects of monoclonal antibodies on the action of toxin and their recognition sites on the toxin molecule. The binding of one antibody labeled by ^{125}I to toxin–Sepharose 4B that had been preincubated with an excess of another antibody was taken as a measure of the relative distance between the antibody-binding sites on the toxin. The distance between the sites for antibodies 2 and 7 was taken as 100. Modified from Hayakawa *et al.* (10).

toxin to the receptor at 4°C changes its conformation at 37°C for the entry process and consequently decreases the affinity of antibody 2. If so, more antibody will be required to counteract the decrease in its affinity and inhibit the process of entry of the toxin.

Zucker and Murphy (30) also examined the effects of their monoclonal antibodies on the action of the toxin, though in less detail. They examined 14 antibodies from each epitope group by (i) a test of *in vitro* neutralization of cytotoxicity by preincubation of the toxin with the antibodies; (ii) an *in vivo* rabbit skin test; and (iii) assay of inhibition of toxin binding to cells on preincubation of the toxin with the antibodies. All the antibodies tested neutralized the toxin *in vitro* when present in excess. They reported the molar antibody:toxin ratios of representative antibodies required for neutralization; the values differed for different antibodies (molar ratios of 1:268 in CHO cell assay). In *in vivo* experiments, in most cases even excess antibody (>100-fold excess over toxin) did not cause neutralization. Results of tests on the inhibition of toxin binding to cells were shown as +, ±, or −, and in general correlated with neutralization of cytotoxicity. Since the association constants of the antibodies also varied, more detailed studies are required on the mechanisms of inhibition by these monoclonal antibodies using monoclonal antibodies of high and similar affinity.

Of all the monoclonal anti-diphtheria toxin antibodies obtained, antibodies 2 and A5 are the most interesting. The former appears to block processing of the toxin after its binding to the cells, even when the toxin has already bound to the cells. Little is known about the mechanism of toxin translocation into the cytoplasm, and antibody 2 should provide information on this process. The epitope recognized by antibody 2 is located 30K–45K from the N-terminus of the toxin. This region contains a hydrophobic part that may be important in toxin translocation across the lipid bilayer. Although this monoclonal antibody can bind to the native toxin in which the hydrophobic region is not exposed (1), an interesting possibility is that conformational changes occurring when the toxin binds to the receptor, which are related to expression of the function of the hydrophobic region, are blocked by binding of the antibody near to this region. Antibody A5 is an anti-fragment A antibody obtained by Zucker and Murphy (30). In spite of previous reports that polyclonal anti-fragment A antibody cannot neutralize cytotoxicity (19), we were surprised to find that it did neutralize cytotoxicity and strongly inhibited binding of the toxin to the cells. It also neutralized the ADP-ribosyltransferase activity of fragment A completely, unlike antibody A10, which did not neutralize this activity but inhibited the cytotoxicity and binding. It is noteworthy that none of the anti-fragment A monoclonal antibodies obtained by the Japanese group blocked both binding and cytotoxicity of the toxin. This peculiar effect of antibody A5 suggests that the active site of fragment A is involved in the mechanism of entry of the toxin into the cytoplasm. ATP is known to inhibit toxin binding to cells (16), and Lory and Collier (15) and Proia *et al.* (20) reported that the nucleotide-binding site, named the P-site, is near the C-terminus of fragment B. Moreover, it is suggested that the toxin binds to nucleotides that are involved in the cell surface receptor (E. Mekada, personal communication). These observations and the effect of antibody A5 suggest that the sites of fragment A and B are both involved in the interaction of toxin with the receptor through the nucleotide portion of the receptor. Very recent studies suggest that binding of CRM 197 and of wild-type toxin to target cells differs, because the binding of CRM 197 to cells is not inhibited by ATP and "nicked" CRM 197 shows increased binding ability (15a). This idea, and especially the participation of fragment A, is supported by the facts that in CRM 197, fragment B is not altered but fragment A shows no enzymatic activity, and that hybrid molecules of wild-type fragment A and fragment B of CRM 197 do not bind to cells in the presence of ATP. These findings at least suggest that the functional relation between fragments A and B is more complex than originally thought.

Mouse L cells are more resistant to diphtheria toxin than sensitive monkey Vero cells: the LD_{50} of toxin for L cells is about 10^5 times higher than that for Vero cells. In a toxin–antibody preincubation experiment with L cells, inhibition of cellular protein synthesis by the toxin was blocked by antibody 2 but not antibody 7. This finding supports a previous suggestion that L cells have no binding site for toxin (3,17).

C. Effects of Antibodies on ADP-Ribosyltransferase Activity

There are two papers about the effects of anti-fragment A monoclonal antibodies on ADP-ribosyltransferase activity (29,31), which report similar results. There are three types of monoclonal antibodies for inhibition of ADP-ribosyltransferase activity, namely, those causing complete, partial, and no inhibition. Figure 7 shows results with the monoclonal antibodies obtained by Yoshimori *et al.* (29). Preincubation of fragment A with antibody DA1 neutralized its *in vitro* ADP-ribosylating activity. The inhibition curve indicates that at a molar ratio of about 1.0, DA1 inhibited the enzymatic activity of fragment A. Antibody DA2 also neutralized the activity of fragment A, but less strongly, the molar ratio of DA2 to toxin required for 50% inhibition being 10. Antibody DA3 did not inhibit the activity at all. These antibodies have similar affinity constants to purified fragment A of 4 to $7 \times 10^7 \ M^{-1}$. Zucker *et al.* (31) reported that antibody A5 inhibited fragment A activity at an antibody:fragment A ratio of 0.7, which is similar to that of DA1, while antibodies A1, A3, and A4 inhibited the activity only partially, and antibodies A11 and A13 had no effect.

Interesting results were obtained with antibodies DA1, 2, and 3 and mutant fragment As. CRM 176 has a missense mutation resulting in a single amino acid substitution in fragment A, and reduction of the ADP-ribosylating activity to

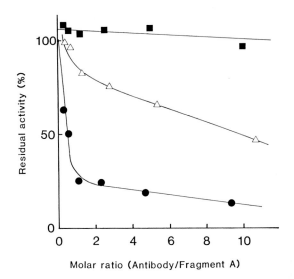

Fig. 7. Effects of antibodies on the ADP-ribosyltransferase activity of wild-type fragment A. Fragment A was incubated with various concentrations of antibody at 37°C for 1 hr and then ADP-ribosylating activity was assayed. (●) Antibody DA1; (△) antibody DA2; (■) antibody DA3. Modified from Yoshimori *et al.* (29).

one-tenth of that of the wild type. As shown in Fig. 8, DA3 did not neutralize the activity of CRM 176 fragment A as in the case of wild-type fragment A, but the inhibition curves of DA1 and DA2 were reversed. DA2, which had only a weak effect on wild-type fragment A, strongly inhibited CRM 176 fragment A at a molar ratio of about 1.0, whereas DA1 inhibited CRM 176 fragment A less than wild-type fragment A. Since these antibodies have association constants similar to fragment A (both that of CRM 176 and that of the wild type), their different effects must reflect differences in their binding sites. Thus the difference between wild-type and CRM 176 fragment A may be not only a single amino acid substitution but also some structural change that is related to reduction of the activity, because the inhibition patterns of the two antibodies DA1 and DA2 are changed. The mechanism by which the structural change occurs in CRM 176 fragment A cannot be deduced from these results only, but this phenomenon is significant in investigations on the structure related with the enzymatic activity of fragment A. Structural changes caused by one and two amino acid substitutions may have occurred in fragment A of both CRM 197 and 228, because none of these antibodies bound to either fragment A (see Section III,A,1).

A difference between the anti-fragment A monoclonal antibodies obtained by the American and the Japanese groups is their ability to bind to whole toxin. The

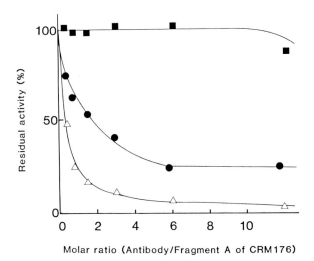

Fig. 8.   Effect of antibody on the ADP-ribosyltransferase activity of mutant fragment A of CRM 176. For experimental conditions, see Fig. 7. Modified from Yoshimori *et al.* (29).

antibodies obtained by the American group were produced by immunization with toxin and so could bind to toxin, whereas the antibodies of the Japanese authors were obtained by immunization with purified fragment A and none of them had any affinity for the toxin, as shown by competitive-binding assays. In addition, the association constants of the latter antibodies with CRM 45, which lacks a C-terminal 17000-Da region of fragment B, were very weak, being 1 to 2×10^6 M^{-1}. Unfortunately the binding sites of these antibodies have not yet been located, and so the relation between the binding sites and inhibition of fragment A activity is not clear.

Although none of the antibodies of the Japanese group affected binding of the toxin or its entry into the cells, antibodies A5 and A10 (group 2b) inhibited toxin binding and cytotoxicity.

Since exotoxin A from *Pseudomonas aeruginosa* catalyzes ADP-ribosylation of EF-2 in a similar way to fragment A of diphtheria toxin, *Pseudomonas* and diphtheria toxin fragments may show homology in the amino acid sequence related to catalytic activity. None of the anti-diphtheria fragment A monoclonal antibodies obtained in either laboratory, however, inhibited the activity of *Pseudomonas* exotoxin A or its purified active fragment.

D. Application of Antibodies in Cell Biology

The cytotoxicity of diphtheria toxin can be employed in other fields of biology or medicine. For instance, anti-fragment A monoclonal antibody and toxin can

be used in a system for selection of cells into which foreign proteins are introduced, as follows: exogenous macromolecules are introduced into living cells by
the red cell ghost fusion method (7), together with anti-fragment A monoclonal
antibody that can neutralize the ADP-ribosyltransferase activity of fragment A.
Then the cells are treated with diphtheria toxin. As a result, the population of
cells that fused with red cell ghosts containing the exogenous macromolecules
and monoclonal antibodies survive, while other cells are killed by the toxin.

To demonstrate the practicality of this system, Vero cells (toxin-sensitive
cells) were fused with red cell ghosts containing monoclonal antibody DA2 with
a fusion efficiency of 40% and were then exposed to various concentrations of
CRM 176. Then their rate of protein synthesis was measured. At a concentration
of CRM 176 that almost completely inhibited protein synthesis of control
cultures, cells fused with red cell ghosts could synthesize protein at about 35% of
the control rate. The value of 35% was almost the same as the fusion efficiency,
indicating that most of the cells into which antibodies were introduced became
resistant to CRM 176. Monoclonal antibody was about 5 times more effective
than conventional anti-fragment A antibody, on a molecular basis for neutralization of CRM 176 fragment A in the cytoplasm of living cells (Fig. 9).

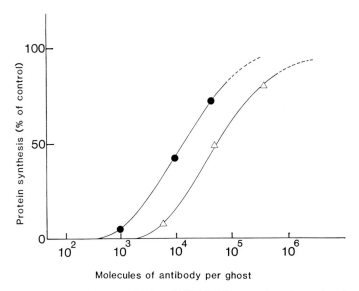

Fig. 9. Dependence of the neutralization of CRM 176 fragment A on the number of molecules
of antibody trapped per ghost. Vero cells were fused with Sendai virus to red cell ghosts containing
various concentrations of antibody. Then the cells were exposed to CRM 176 at 37°C for 6 hr, and
after incubation, their rate of protein synthesis was measured. The rate of protein synthesis of the
control culture (not exposed to CRM 176) × the fusion efficiency was set at 100% on the ordinate.
(●) Monoclonal antibody DA2; (△) polyclonal antifragment A antibody. Modified from Yoshimori
et al. (29).

Wild-type toxin was not suitable in this system because too many antibodies were required for complete neutralization of the wild-type fragment A, even a single molecule of which can kill a cell.

IV. CONCLUSIONS

Studies on diphtheria toxin using monoclonal antibodies are just beginning: there are only four papers on their use from two laboratories. Studies by the American group (30,31) were insufficient for determination of the effects of the antibodies, and those by the Japanese group (10,29) were insufficient for location of the antibody-binding sites. However, these studies resulted in progress that was not possible with conventional antibodies.

The epitopes recognized by the monoclonal antibodies were located in four restricted clusters and were classified into 10 subgroups. Studies on the effects of the monoclonal antibodies showed that one antibody inhibited toxin binding, another inhibited the process of entry of the toxin after its binding, and others had intermediate effects. The effects of monoclonal antibodies on the ADP-ribosyl-transferase activity of fragment A were also examined, and from the results the antibodies were classified into three types: strongly inhibitory, moderately inhibitory, and noninhibitory. The strongly and moderately inhibitory types had the reverse effects on mutant fragment A of CRM 176, and none of the three types reacted with mutant fragment A of CRM 197 or 228. The conclusion from studies with conventional antibodies that most of fragment A is masked in the intact toxin were confirmed by use of monoclonal antibodies.

It is interesting that two clusters of epitopes on fragment B, groups 3 and 4, correspond to the hydrophobic region and receptor-binding domain, respectively. The receptor-binding site of the toxin may be located within a carboxy-terminal region of 15,000 Da of fragment B (23). The finding that antibodies 7, B12, and B19 with epitopes in this region inhibited toxin binding to cells supports this idea. In addition, B12 and B19 did not react with the C-terminal CNBr fragment of fragment B of 8000 Da (CB 3), suggesting that the amino-terminal portion of this region is involved in the receptor-binding site.

As mentioned in Section III,C, antibodies 2 and A5 are very interesting with respect to toxin binding and entry into cells. Antibody 2 inhibited the process of entry of the toxin after its binding, whereas antibody A5 strongly inhibited the enzymatic activity of fragment A and toxin binding to cells. These antibodies will be good probes in further studies on the mechanisms of toxin binding and entry. In addition, antibody 2 will be useful as a tracer in studies on cell binding of the toxin; that is, labeled antibody 2 can be used instead of labeled toxin to measure the amount of cell binding of toxin, since antibody 2 does not interfere with binding of toxin to cells and can bind to the toxin–receptor complex. The merits of its use in this indirect system are that it will result in greater labeling, it is convenient, and its use avoids the complication that the toxin may be inactivated by labeling. The toxin receptor on the cell surface has not yet been purified completely, but antibody 2 can be used as a probe in purification of the receptor and in affinity chromatography.

Monoclonal antibodies against the toxin are available not only for studies on relationships between structure and function of the toxin but also for use in various cell biological techniques. This application opens up new possibilities in studies on the structure and function of the toxin and its monoclonal antibodies and seems an attractive and potentially useful approach.

Diphtheria toxin may be valuable in determining the potentials of use of monoclonal antibodies. Much basic information on the toxin has now been obtained, such as its complete amino acid sequence, but little is known about the regions essential for biological activity and use of monoclonal antibodies to study. This problem should indicate their availability and limitations in molecular investigations on active proteins.

V. PROSPECTS FOR THE FUTURE

For analysis of the structure–function relationships of diphtheria toxin with monoclonal antibodies, more complete, systematic characterization of the monoclonal antibodies must be done. The toxin-binding sites for the monoclonal antibodies must be identified and, for this purpose, experiments with various synthetic peptides corresponding to parts of toxin fragments are now in progress. These synthetic peptides can be used to determine which domain is related to which function by testing their abilities to inhibit the actions of the toxin competitively. Furthermore, the synthetic peptide that is most effective as antigen for neutralizing toxicity should be a very efficient and safe vaccine against diphtheria. Recently, the location of an epitope in feline leukemia virus envelope protein gp70 recognized by a virus-neutralizing monoclonal antibody was determined by use of short DNase 1-generated DNA fragments encoding portions of the virus protein (11). As cDNA of diphtheria toxin has been obtained, this new method will be also useful.

Some investigators consider that the interaction between the toxin molecule and the cell surface receptor involves binding through more than one binding site. Evidence supporting this idea has been obtained from studies on both the toxin and cells. One piece of evidence is the participation of nucleotide. Determination of which antitoxin monoclonal antibodies can inhibit binding between the toxin and nucleotide will clarify the role of nucleotide in the toxin–receptor system. Mutant toxin CRM 228 can bind to nucleotide well but binds to the cell surface only poorly. This CRM 228 toxin amino has an acid substitution in fragment B, and an interesting problem is which part of the toxin–receptor system is obstructed by the mutation. A monoclonal antibody with different effects on wild-type toxin and CRM 228 or different bindings to these toxins is required. Experiments with combinations of various mutant toxins that show altered functions when bound to monoclonal antibodies should be fruitful. Moreover, mutants that can bind to receptor but have no activity for translocation across the lipid bilayer should be available before long and will be very helpful.

Other applications of diphtheria toxin, such as use of hybrid toxins, are now being studied extensively. Thus we are convinced that monoclonal antibodies against diphtheria toxin are useful in cell biological studies as well as in studies on diphtheria toxin itself, and that their use will increase in the future.

VI. SUMMARY

At present the main question on studies of diphtheria toxin is the relationships between structure and function of the toxin molecule. Recently, the use of antitoxin monoclonal antibodies has provided a new means for analyzing the problem and given some information which could not be obtained with polyclonal antibodies. The epitopes recognized by monoclonal antibodies were located in four restricted clusters on the toxin molecule. One antibody inhibited the binding of the toxin to the surface of sensitive cells, while another inhibited the entry of the toxin into the cells after binding. Monoclonal antibodies against fragment A of diphtheria toxin were classified into three types according to the difference of their effect on the ADP-ribosyltransferase activity of fragment A. This effect, or the binding of some of these antibodies changed dramatically when mutant toxins were used. One anti-fragment A antibody inhibited both ADP-ribosyltransferase activity and binding of the toxin to the cells. The conclusion from studies using conventional antibodies that most of fragment A is masked in the intact toxin was confirmed by data obtained with monoclonal antibodies.

Cytotoxicity of diphtheria toxin has been applied in other fields of study, for example, cell biology, where antitoxin monoclonal antibodies should also be useful. A system for selecting cells into which foreign proteins have been introduced was developed by using anti-fragment A monoclonal antibody.

REFERENCES

1. Boquet, P., Silverman, M. S., Pappenheimer, A. M., Jr., and Vernon, W. (1976). Binding of Triton X-100 to diphtheria toxin cross-reacting material 45, and their fragments. *Proc. Natl. Acad. Sci. U.S.A.* **73**, 4449–4453.

2. Carroll, S. F., and Collier, R. J. (1984). NAD binding site of diphtheria toxin: Identification of a residue within the nicotinamide subsite by photochemical modification with NAD. *Proc. Natl. Acad. Sci. U.S.A.* **81,** 3307–3311.
3. Chang, T., and Neville, D. M., Jr. (1987). Demonstration of diphtheria toxin receptors on surface membranes from both toxin-sensitive and toxin-resistant species. *J. Biol. Chem.* **253,** 6866–6871.
4. Collier, R. J. (1975). Diphtheria toxin: Mode of action and structure. *Bacteriol. Rev.* **39,** 54–85.
5. Collier, R. J., and Kaplan, D. A. (1984). Immunotoxins. *Sci. Am.* **251,** 44–52.
6. Donovan, J. J., Simon, M. I., Draper, R. K., and Montal, M. (1981). Diphtheria toxin forms transmembrane chennels in planar lipid bilayers. *Proc. Natl. Acad. Sci. U.S.A.* **78,** 172–176.
7. Furusawa, M., Nishimura, T., Yamaizumi, M., and Okada, Y. (1974). Injection of foreign substances into single cells by cell fusion. *Nature (London)* **249,** 449–450.
8. Giannini, G., Rappuoli, R., and Ratti, G. (1984). The amino-acid sequence of two non-toxic mutants of diphtheria toxin: CRM45 and CRM197. *Nucleic Acid Res.* **12,** 4063–4069.
9. Greenfield, L., Bjorn, M. J., Horn, G., Fong, D., Buck, G. A., Collier, R. J., and Kaplan, D. A. (1983). Nucleotide sequence of the structural gene for diphtheria toxin carried by corynebacteriophage β. *Proc. Natl. Acad. Sci. U.S.A.* **80,** 6853–6857.
10. Hayakawa, S., Uchida, T., Mekada, E., Moynihan, M. R., and Okada, Y. (1983). Monoclonal antibody against diphtheria toxin-effect on toxin binding and entry into cells. *J. Biol. Chem.* **258,** 4311–4317.
11. Hunberg, J. H., Rodgers, G., Gilbert, J. H., and Snead, R. M. (1984). Method to map antigenic determinants recognized by monoclonal antibodies: Localization of a determinant of virus neutralization on the feline leukemia virus envelope protein gp70. *Proc. Natl. Acad. Sci. U.S.A.* **81,** 3675–3679.
12. Iglewski, B. H., Liu, P. U., and Kabat, D. (1977). Mechanism of action of *Pseudomonas aeruginosa* exotoxin A: Adenosine diphosphate-ribosylation of mammalian elongation factor 1 *in vitro* and *in vivo. Infect. Immun.* **15,** 138–144.
13. Kaczorek, M., Delpeyroux, F., Chenciner, N., Streek, R. E., Murphy, J. R., Boquet, P., and Tidlais, P. (1983). Nucleotide sequence and expression of the diphtheria *tox*228 gene in *Escherichia coli. Science* **221,** 855–858.
14. Kagan, B. L., Finkelstein, A., and Columbini, M. (1981). Diphtheria toxin fragment forms large pores in phospholipid bilayer membranes. *Proc. Natl. Acad. Sci. U.S.A.* **78,** 4950–4954.
15. Lory, S., and Collier, J. (1980). Diphtheria toxin: Nucleotide binding and toxin heterogeneity. *Proc. Natl. Acad. Sci. U.S.A.* **77,** 267–271.
15a. Mekada, E., and Uchida, T. (1985). Binding properties of diphtheria toxin to cells are altered by mutation in the fragment A domain. *J. Biol. Chem.* **260,** 12148–12153.
16. Middlebrock, J. L., and Dorland, R. B. (1978). Protection of mammalian cells from diphtheria toxin by exogenous nucleotides. *Can. J. Microbiol.* **25,** 285–290.
17. Middlebrook, J. L., Dorland, R. B., and Leppla, S. H. (1978). Association of diphtheria toxin with Vero cells—demonstration of a receptor. *J. Biol. Chem.* **253,** 7325–7330.
18. Pappenheimer, A. M., Jr. (1977). Diphtheria toxin. *Annu. Rev. Biochem.* **46,** 69–94.
19. Pappenheimar, A. M., Jr., Uchida, T., and Harper, A. A. (1972). Immunological study of the diphtheria toxin molecule. *Immunochemistry* **9,** 891–906.
20. Proia, R. L., Wray, S. K., Hart, D. A., and Eidels, L. (1980). Characterization and affinity labeling of the cationic phosphate-binding (nucleotide-binding) peptide located in the receptor-binding region of the B-fragment of diphtheria toxin. *J. Biol. Chem.* **255,** 12025–12033.
21. Sandvig, K., and Olsnes, S. (1980). Diphtheria toxin entry into cells is facilitated by low pH. *J. Cell Biol.* **87,** 828–832.
22. Uchida, T. (1983). Diphtheria toxin. *Pharmacol. Ther.* **19,** 107–122.

23. Uchida, T., Gill, D. M., and Pappenheimer, A. M., Jr. (1971). Mutation in the structural gene for diphtheria toxin carried by temperature phage beta. *Nature (London), New Biol.* **233**, 8–11.

24. Uchida, T., Mekada, E., and Okada, Y. (1980). Hybrid toxin of the A chain of ricin toxin and s subunit of *Wistaria floribunda* lectin. Possible importance of hydrophobic region for entry of toxin into the cell. *J. Biol. Chem.* **255**, 6687–6693.

25. Uchida, T., Pappenheimer, A. M., Jr., and Harper, A. A. (1972). Reconstitution of diphtheria toxin from two nontoxic cross-reacting mutant toxins. *Science* **175**, 901–903.

26. Van Ness, B. G., Howard, J. B., and Bodley, J. W. (1980). ADP-ribosylation of elongation factor 2 by diphtheria toxin: Isolation and properties. *J. Biol. Chem.* **255**, 10717–10720.

27. Yamaizumi, M., Mekada, E., Uchida, T., and Okada, Y. (1978). One molecule of diphtheria toxin fragment A introduced into a cell can kill the cell. *Cell (Cambridge, Mass.)* **15**, 245–250.

28. Yamaizumi, M., Uchida, T., Mekada, E., and Okada, Y. (1979). Antibodies introduced into living cells by red cell ghosts are functionally stable in the cytoplasm of the cells. *Cell (Cambridge, Mass.)* **18**, 1009–1014.

29. Yoshimori, T., Yamada, M., Sugawa, H., Mekada, E., Uchida, T., and Okada, Y. (1984). Monoclonal antibodies against diphtheria toxin fragment A: Characterization and introduction into living cells. *Exp. Cell Res.* **151**, 344–353.

30. Zucker, D. R., and Murphy, J. R. (1984). Monoclonal antibody analysis of diphtheria toxin, I. Localization of epitopes and neutralization of cytotoxicity. *Mol. Immunol.* **21**, 785–793.

31. Zucker, D. R., Murphy, J. R., and Pappenheimer, A. M., Jr. (1984). Monoclonal antibody analysis of diphtheria toxin, II. Inhibition of ADP-ribosyltransferase activity. *Mol. Immunol.* **21**, 795–800.

11

Application of Monoclonal Antibodies to the Study of Oral Bacteria and Their Virulence Factors

JOSEPH M. DIRIENZO
Department of Microbiology
School of Dental Medicine
University of Pennsylvania
Philadelphia, Pennsylvania

249

I. INTRODUCTION

The number of these Animals in the scurf of a man's Teeth, are so many that I believe they exceed the number of Men in a kingdom.

Antony van Leeuwenhoek (1684). *Philos. Trans. R. Soc. London* **14**, 568.

The beauty of monoclonals is that one does not have to purify a specific antigen. One can use a shotgun approach, using ground-up fly brains to immunize mice and make a collection of hybridomas, each of which produces an antibody to a single molecule of the mixture.

Seymour Benzer (1984). *Science* **223**, 919.

This chapter opens with two quotations which seem to exemplify (i) the monumental task of isolating and identifying human oral bacteria and characterizing virulence factors from the pathogenic strains and (ii) the advantage that monoclonal antibodies provide as an approach to this complex problem. Simply and perhaps naively stated, pathogenic members of the oral microbial flora can be broadly grouped into two major disease categories: those microorganisms that are thought to be associated with the formation and development of dental caries and those microorganisms that are thought to be associated with the initiation and progression of periodontal diseases. The specific bacterial species that can be placed in each disease category, and in some cases in both, are among themselves heterogeneous groups which are often difficult to dissect on the basis of metabolic, genetic, and antigenic criteria. It has been proposed that over 250 species of bacteria can reside in the human oral cavity (78). This figure is probably a conservative estimate because some species may not survive the primary isolation. An example of the complexity of the human oral microbial flora can be ascertained by considering the numerous studies, past and present, that have attempted to define this flora in individuals displaying clinical signs of periodontal disease (76–78,111,112,117,121,129). The results of these investigations have routinely been revised as existing sampling and analytical methods were improved and new methods developed.

The recently developed hybridoma technique is one such method that has the potential to stimulate significant advances in the analysis of the oral microbial flora. The central idea expressed in the opening quotation exemplifies one of the most direct applications of monoclonal antibodies currently in use in the study of oral bacteria. Although fly brains will not be a topic of this chapter, the approach expressed in the quotation is pertinent. Since in many studies of oral bacteria the antigenic composition of the bacterium or identity of a particular virulence factor is unknown, or at least poorly characterized, a ''shotgun'' approach can be used by employing a heterogeneous antigen mixture, such as whole-cell lysates, to immunize mice. A selective screening technique, such as the enzyme-linked immunosorbent assay (ELISA), Western blotting, or dot blotting, can then be used to detect or screen for a specific reactive antigen in the mixture of antigens.

In this chapter a comprehensive review of currently characterized monoclonal antibodies prepared against oral bacteria or potential virulence factors produced by these bacteria will be presented. These monoclonal antibodies have been used for the serological classification of clinical isolates and the identification and characterization of antigens. The antigens that have been studied usually represent cell surface molecules which promote the adherence of the bacterium to hard or soft tissues, cellular antigens which afford protection, in animals, against infection (possible vaccine components), and biological factors (exoenzymes, toxins) which contribute to the overall pathogenicity of the bacterium. Specifically, monoclonal antibodies prepared against *Streptococcus mutans, Actinomyces viscosus, Bacteroides gingivalis, Bacteroides intermedius,* and *Actinobacillus actinomycetemcomitans,* all potential human oral pathogenic bacteria, will be discussed. The particular application (serological, antigen identification or isolation, structural characterization) of each group of monoclonal antibodies will be evaluated and any unusual or interesting approaches used in the production and application of these antibodies will be stressed. Furthermore, the specific application of monoclonal antibodies to the detailed study of a major potential virulence factor, the leukotoxin, of *Actinobacillus actinomycetemcomitans,* the primary suspected etiological agent in juvenile periodontitis, will be presented. An effort has been made to be as current and complete as possible in reporting the existence and details of the characterization of the monoclonal antibodies produced specifically against oral bacteria. In relation to this, various individuals supplied information, prior to publication, which made my effort easier. However, I am responsible if any omissions or misinterpretations of data have occurred.

II. BACKGROUND

A comprehensive review of the literature describing the serology, antigenic profiles, known virulence factors, and the role in oral disease of *S. mutans, Actinomyces viscosus, B. gingivalis, B. intermedius,* and *Actinobacillus actinomycetemcomitans,* prior to the development of monoclonal antibodies, is beyond the scope of this chapter. However, a brief review concerning select aspects of these bacterial species will be presented to orient the reader and to provide background information and rationale for the monoclonal antibody approach. The discussion will be limited to those bacterial species listed above due to the fact that, at the present time, monoclonal antibodies have been produced primarily to these select bacterial species or antigens isolated from them. This is not to imply that these species are the only important microorganisms associated with oral diseases.

A. Role of *Streptococcus mutans* and *Actinomyces viscosus* in Dental Caries

The gram-positive coccus, *S. mutans,* is considered to be a primary contributor to the development of dental caries. Strains of this bacterium exhibit various metabolic activities that, when considered in an additive fashion, impart the destructive properties which lead to the formation of smooth-surface caries. One important property of this bacterium is the biosynthesis of insoluble extracellular polysaccharides (29,57). These extracellular polymers can contribute to the overall adherence of the bacteria to the tooth surface (82,83). In addition, the production of high levels of lactic acid, through the fermentation of carbohydrates, promotes the demineralization of the tooth (100). Both of these properties are closely linked to the efficient metabolism of sucrose by this microorganism. Strains of *S. mutans* contain extracellular glucosyltransferases and fructosyltransferases which catalyze the formation of glucans and fructans from sucrose (29,57). The glucosyltransferases appear to represent a heterogeneous population of enzymes necessary for the synthesis of soluble and insoluble glucans. Some workers have separated two forms of glycosyltransferase, from the same cell, each of which catalyzes the formation of water-soluble and water-insoluble glucans (10,29,82,83). Others have suggested that a single enzyme can alternate forms to catalyze the formation of water-soluble and water-insoluble polymers (75). The glucosyltransferases are therefore considered important virulence factors in *S. mutans*. The inhibition of extracellular glucan synthesis can be envisioned as one mechanism to reduce caries formation by preventing colonization of the teeth by this bacterium.

The oral streptococci contain additional cell surface polymers that have the potential to mediate adherence to teeth. Lipoteichoic acids are major cell surface-exposed polymers found in all serotypes of *S. mutans* (19,67,101). This polymer is composed of alternating residues of glycerol and phosphate and is often substituted with fatty acids and sugars (134). The polyglycerol phosphate backbone is highly conserved and therefore represents a common antigen found within strains of *S. mutans* (54,55). Since lipoteichoic acid is an amphiphile, it has the potential to interact with many types of compounds and is thought to promote binding to the tooth surface (11). In addition, there exists a strong affinity between lipoteichoic acid and glucosyltransferase resulting in the formation of glucan–enzyme–lipoteichoic acid complexes (71). Thus, these polymers, alone and in heterogeneous complexes, contribute to the colonization of the oral cavity by *S. mutans*.

Other characterized cell surface molecules of *S. mutans* include the secreted protein antigens I, II, I/II, and III (94–97). Antigens I and II were found to be associated in a single molecule I/II having a molecular weight of 185,000 (95, 139). When antigen I/II was treated with pronase, a 48,000 MW protein (antigen II) was isolated (95). Antigens I (97) and III (94) are proteins having molecular weights of 150,000 and 44,000, respectively. Although these protein antigens do not appear to play a major role in the adherence of the bacterium, Lehner and co-workers (61) have shown that antigens I and I/II can protect monkeys, when challenged with *S. mutans,* against caries. The implantation of animals with any serotype of *S. mutans* always results in the formation of caries (38,56,72).

There are seven serotypes of *S. mutans,* designated a–g (5,6,89). Serospecific antigens for each of the seven serotypes have been identified and purified. They all represent polysaccharides that are readily extracted in soluble form from whole cells or isolated cell wall preparations. The proposed antigenic determinants for the serotypes a–g are Glc-β(1,6)-Glc (81), α-Gal (80), Glc-α(1,4)-Glc (63,131), Gal-β(1,6)-Glc (64), Glc-β(1,4)-Glc (132), Glc-α(1,6)-Glc (37), and β-Gal (44), respectively. Due to extensive heterogeneity or cross-reactivity, known protein antigens would appear to be of little value in the serotyping of *S. mutans.* For example, in the case of glucosyltransferase, three proteins with different isoelectric points and pH optima were found in a serotype d strain (36), while two glucosyltransferase activities were identified in a serotype a strain (29). Furthermore, similar results have been reported in the case of serotype c (57), b (99), and g (9) strains. The secreted protein antigens I–IV (96) also do not appear to be particularly useful as serospecific markers, since there is a significant degree of cross-reactivity among the various serotypes (94,95,97). These serotypic analyses have been carried out using polyclonal rabbit antisera and, in the case of the carbohydrate determinants, appears to be the most definitive system for the routine typing of *S. mutans.* The data obtained from biotyping (104,105) and genotyping (20) studies resulted in certain discrepancies that could be resolved by the serotypic analyses. The reader is referred to an excellent review of *S. mutans* by Hamada and Slade (39) for a more detailed discussion of the immunochemistry of this microorganism.

The filamentous, gram-positive bacterium *Actinomyces viscosus,* along with other *Actinomyces* species and sometimes *S. mutans,* appear to be the significant microorganisms involved in the formation of root surface caries (123). In experiments employing hamsters, the presence of *A. viscosus* was necessary for the formation of root caries (48), while in gnotobiotic rats *A. viscosus* as well as other gram-positive bacteria were thought to be responsible for the development of the lesion (32,49,120). In the development of root caries the contributing disease mechanisms are not as clearly understood as in the case of smooth-surface caries formation. However, the presence of one of two types of fimbriae on *A. viscosus* virulent strains appears to be responsible for the adherence of these cells to teeth (16,17). The fimbriae represent the major characterized virulence factors of *A. viscosus*. Through the elegant work of Cisar (12) and co-workers, the fimbriae have been classified into two antigenically distinct forms, designated type 1 and type 2. Results suggest that the two types of fimbriae mediate different adherence specificities in the oral cavity, since the type 1 fimbriae appear to bind selectively to saliva-coated teeth (133), while the type 2 fimbriae display lactose-sensitive adherence of *A. viscosus* to oral streptococci (15). Unlike the case of *S. mutans*, genotypic analysis appears to be a more valuable tool for the taxonomic classification of *A. viscosus*. On the basis of numerical taxonomy and serological studies (28), DNA homology (21), and immunofluorescence data (110), *A. viscosus* was divided into four groups, designated typical, atypical, heterogeneous (all human isolates), and animal.

B. *Bacteroides* Species and Chronic (Adult) Periodontitis

Although the gram-negative anaerobic bacteria in general are thought to be the major contributors to the progression of chronic periodontitis, several species within the genus *Bacteroides* (*B. gingivalis* and *B. intermedius*) have recently earned the most attention. This is also evident by the fact that the production of monoclonal antibodies against *Bacteroides* species have, at the time of this review, been limited to these two species (see Table I and Section III,A). The potential virulence factors and antigenic profiles of both *B. gingivalis* and *B. intermedius* have not been well characterized. Members of both species contain lipopolysaccharide and capsules. The lipopolysaccharides have shown only weak endotoxic activity (42); however, the presence of a capsule may be responsible for the ability of these bacteria to resist phagocytosis (88). Strains of *B. gingivalis* are particularly proteolytic, producing a trypsinlike activity (113), collagenase (33,93), fibrinolysin (90), hyaluronidase (119), and heparinase (84).

Gmür and Wyss have thoroughly reviewed the serological aspects of *B. intermedius* in Volume I of this treatise (35). As these authors have discussed, there are apparent discrepancies in the classification of the black-pigmented *Bacteroides* species. Serotypic analyses have shown significant heterogeneity within the subspecies (68,92). Particularly in the case of *B. intermedius*, DNA homology studies indicate extensive genetic heterogeneity (47,130), while classical biochemical schemes cannot distinguish among the genotypes (34).

C. *Actinobacillus actinomycetemcomitans* and Localized Juvenile Periodontitis

Actinobacillus actinomycetemcomitans has probably been the most thoroughly studied periodontal pathogen (65,91,114). There is a strong body of data linking this organism with localized juvenile periodontitis, a rapidly destructive form of periodontal disease affecting children. The role of *A. actinomycetemcomitans* in periodontal disease has been exhaustively treated in a recent review (135). But briefly, almost all patients showing clinical signs of juvenile periodontitis harbor relatively high numbers of *A. actinomycetemcomitans* in diseased sites and usually have significantly elevated antibody titers against this bacterium (62,66). In addition, sera obtained from these patients almost always contain antibodies against a leukotoxin produced by some strains of *A. actinomycetemcomitans* (124). The number of *A. actinomycetemcomitans* in infected lesions has been shown to decrease dramatically following periodontal therapy with a corresponding regression of the disease (116). Concomitantly, the reappearance of *A. actinomycetemcomitans* paralleled disease recurrence. Several possible virulence factors of *A. actinomycetemcomitans* have been identified and their biological activities studied. These include a leukotoxin (2), lymphocyte (103) and fibroblast (102) suppressive factors, epithelial cell proliferation and attachment inhibitory factor (50), collagenase (93), and endotoxin (52, 87). Only the leukotoxin will be considered here. The leukotoxin specifically kills neutrophils and monocytes originating from human and nonhuman primates (124). Greater than 90% of the sera obtained from juvenile periodontitis patients inhibits the killing activity of the leukotoxin (124,127). More recently, it has been shown that sera obtained from cynomolgous monkeys (*Macaca fascicularis*) also neutralized the cytotoxic activity of the leukotoxin (125). Extraction of whole bacteria with the antibiotic polymyxin B, followed by separation of the released material by ion exchange and gel filtration chromatography, revealed a protein of apparent molecular weight of 115,000 (128). Not all strains of *A. actinomycetemcomitans* appear to express the leukotoxin. Strains of this bacterium have been separated into 10 biotypes (115) and 3 serotypes, designated a, b, and c (137), or 4 serotypes (124), depending on the study. Only serotype a and b strains harbor the leukotoxin. The serotype c specific antigen, a mannose-containing cell surface polymer, has also been isolated (138). The other serotype-specific antigens have not yet been identified but appear to represent cell surface components, since they could be detected by immunofluorescent methods employing polyclonal rabbit antisera and whole bacteria (137).

III. RESULTS AND DISCUSSION

A. Monoclonal Antibodies Produced against Oral Bacteria

The use of monoclonal antibodies, produced against bacteria, in oral health-related research is a relatively recent development. Much of the initial work concentrated primarily on *S. mutans,* because this bacterium represented one of the most thoroughly studied oral pathogens at the time. Now, however, monoclonal antibodies against suspected gram-negative periodontal pathogens are

TABLE I

Monoclonal Antibodies against Oral Bacteria

Bacterium	Antigenic specificity	Subclass	Source/ Reference
Streptococcus mutans	I	IgG_1	118
	II	IgG_1	
	I/II	IgG_1, IgG_{2a}	
	III	IgG_1	
	Glucosyltransferase	IgG_1	30
	Lipoteichoic acid	IgG_1, IgG_3, IgM	45
Streptococcus sanguis	Fimbriae	IgG	27
Actinomyces viscosus	Type 2 fimbriae	IgG_1, IgG_{2a}, IgG_{2b}, IgG_3, IgM	13,14
	Type 1 fimbriae	IgG_{2a}	15–17
Bacteroides gingivalis	—	IgG_{2a}, IgG_3	40
	—	IgG_1, IgG_{2b}, IgM	83a,108,108a
Bacteroides intermedius	—	IgG_{2a}	40
B. intermedius[a]	Ag 38, Ag 39, Ag 40	IgG_{2a} IgG_{2a}	34,35
	Ag 37	IgG_{2b}	
Actinobacillus actinomycetemcomitans	Leukotoxin	IgG_1, IgG_2	25
	Surface polysaccharide, lipopolysaccharide	IgG	53,69,70
	—	—	4,18

[a] These monoclonal antibodies prepared against B. intermedius showed extensive cross-reactivity with other Bacteroides species.

being produced. Table I summarizes the available monoclonal antibodies which recognize oral bacteria or their specific components. The list of monoclonal antibodies is surely subject to rapid growth in relation to the diversity of oral bacterial species as well as the number of antigens and biological factors associated with a particular species. The characterization and application of the monoclonal antibodies listed in Table I will be discussed below.

1. Monoclonal Antibodies against Gram-Positive Bacterial Species Associated with Dental Caries

Smith and co-workers (118) constructed hybridomas which produced monoclonal antibodies to the four *S. mutans* serotype c antigens I, II, I/II, III. Pure preparations of these antigens were used to immunize mice for hybridoma production. It was shown in an earlier study that at least two of these antigens, I and I/II, provided protection against dental caries in monkeys (61). Thus, antigens I and I/II may be good components for the production of a caries vaccine. The monoclonal antibodies to antigens I/II and III did not cross-react with either of the other two antigens, while monoclonal antibodies against I and II cross-reacted with antigen I/II. In addition, all monoclonal antibodies cross-reacted to some degree with *S. mutans* serotype f strains. Antibodies to antigens I, II, and III also recognized serotype e strains, while antibodies to antigen I recognized serotype a strains. The binding of the monoclonal antibodies to whole cells and to antigens in ammonium sulfate-precipitated culture supernatants was compared and revealed that specific antigenic determinants in I and I/II were exposed on the cell surface while other determinants in II, I/II, and III were recognized both on the cell surface and in the culture supernatant. Consequently, these monoclonal antibodies may be useful as diagnostic reagents for identifying secreted antigens of *S. mutans* in the oral cavity. Since several of the monoclonal antibodies recognize protective antigens, they may be useful in the production of caries vaccine components. Monoclonal antibodies against another caries-protective antigen from *S. mutans* have also been produced (43). However, the results of this study are of a preliminary nature.

In a separate study, a monoclonal antibody which reacted with a *S. mutans* serotype g glucosyltransferase was isolated and characterized (30). This antibody appeared to inhibit primarily the water-insoluble glucan-synthesizing activity of the enzyme. Although the monoclonal antibody was prepared against purified serotype g glucosyltransferase, strong cross-reactivity was noted with the enzyme from serotype d and minimal activity against serotype a and e enzymes. The production of additional monoclonal antibodies which recognize glucosyltransferase enzymes from other serotypes of *S. mutans* or from various cell fractions which catalyze the formation of either water-soluble or water-insoluble glucans should provide data relevant to the question of glucosyltransferase heterogeneity and its role in the synthesis of different forms of cell surface glucans.

In the study of cell surface interactions of *Actinomyces* species, Cisar and co-workers (13,14) isolated monoclonal antibodies which recognized a lactose-specific lectin on the cell surface of *A. viscosus* T14V. Nine different monoclonal antibodies were recovered following the immunization of mice with whole cells of the bacterium. All of the antibodies reacted with a single type of fimbria (type 2) localized on the bacterial cell surface. These monoclonal antibodies cross-reacted only with strains of *A. viscosus* and *A. naeslundii* that contained the lactose-specific lectin. Since the lectin-containing fimbria appears to be involved in the coaggregation of *A. viscosus* and oral streptococci (12,15), the monoclonal antibodies will be extremely useful as probes for studying bacterial cell surface-mediated interactions. Such intrageneric coaggregation reactions are important considerations in oral microbial ecology. Along these lines, Cisar has used monoclonal antibodies against either type 1 or type 2 fimbriae to isolate fimbria-deficient mutants of *A. viscosus* T14V-J1, a streptomycin-resistant variant of strain T14V (15,17). Spontaneously derived mutants were obtained which lacked type 1 or type 2 fimbriae or both. In order to examine the binding of the monoclonal antibodies to the mutants and parent strain, the antibodies were labeled by reductive methylation with [^{14}C]formaldehyde (15). The antibodies were mixed with [^{14}C]formaldehyde and NaCNBH$_3$, and the reaction was allowed to proceed at room temperature for 2 hr. The ^{14}C-labeled IgG was then purified by chromatography on Sephadex G-50. Specific activities in the range of 1×10^4 cpm/µg of protein were obtained. In a separate study the type 1 and type 1–type 2 fimbriae-deficient mutants adhered poorly to hydroxyapatite, supporting the role of the type 1 fimbriae in the attachment of A. viscosus to teeth. Interestingly, it has been reported that the monoclonal antibodies that recognized type 1 fimbriae failed to inhibit the binding of A. viscosus T14V to saliva-coated hydroxyapatite (16,17).

2. Monoclonal Antibodies against Gram-Negative Bacterial Species Associated with Periodontal Diseases

The anaerobic, gram-negative bacterium B. gingivalis has recently gained attention as a major contributor to chronic or adult periodontitis (35,106). Attempts to clarify the antigenic composition of this species, especially in relation to those of other Bacteroides species, have been made using monoclonal antibodies. In a recent study by Hanazawa et al. (40), 14 hybridomas were recovered which produced antibodies reactive against the immunizing strain of B. gingivalis. Four of these hybridomas were subcloned by limiting dilution and their reactivities with various Bacteroides species examined. All four monoclonal antibodies failed to react with B. melaninogenicus and a nonoral strain of B. asaccharolyticus; however, one of the antibodies (BGF2) also recognized three strains of B. intermedius. Immunoadsorption experiments confirmed the intraspecies cross-reactivity of this monoclonal antibody. This represented an interesting finding, since other investigators have shown that polyclonal antisera made against B. gingivalis did not cross-react with strains of B. intermedius, suggesting that the antigenic compositions of both species were significantly different (58,79,92). In a related study, Gmür and Guggenheim (34) performed the reverse experiment, in which they employed a strain of B. intermedius as the antigen to prepare hybridomas. Among 39 strains of Bacteroides species tested, B. intermedius, B. loescheii, B. melaninogenicus, and B. corporis cross-reacted with one of the monoclonal antibodies (38BI1). This monoclonal antibody demonstrated the antigenic relatedness between B. intermedius and the other former B. melaninogenicus subsp. melaninogenicus strains. None of the monoclonal antibodies produced in this study recognized B. gingivalis. However, it should be noted that only three strains of B. gingivalis were examined. In the latter study mice were initially immunized with whole cells of B. intermedius but were boostered with cell lysate. This may account for the observed cross-reactivity among the various *Bacteroides* species which was not as evident in the former investigation, in which formalin-treated whole cells of *B. gingivalis* were used. The cross-reacting monoclonal antibody could have been produced against a common intracellular enzyme or ribosomal protein, which would be more highly conserved than cell surface molecules within members of a genus. Thus, on the basis of the reactivity of the four monoclonal antibodies, Gmür and Wyss (35) were able to distinguish among the three proposed genotypes of *B. intermedius*.

According to results obtained from competitive ELISA experiments, it was suggested that serum antibody from patients with chronic periodontitis recognized the same epitopes as the monoclonal antibodies prepared against *B. intermedius* (35). The competitive-inhibition titers of the sera from diseased patients were low; but more importantly, there appeared to be a significant inhibition (20–60%) of the monoclonal antibody binding with the control human sera when assayed at a 1:10 dilution. The results of these experiments would seem to limit the usefulness of the monoclonal antibodies as reagents in immunodiagnosis.

The four monoclonal antibodies against *B. intermedius* were also used in an attempt to identify their corresponding antigens (35). Based on differential extraction procedures and immunoblotting, it was suggested that two of the antibodies (37BI6.1 and 39BI1.1) may recognize carbohydrate determinants in the lipopolysaccharide, while the other two antibodies (38BI1 and 40BI3.2) may bind to a complex, proteinaceous molecule and a protein with an apparent molecular weight of 150,000, respectively. Antigen (Ag) 38 was apparently distributed among the former *B. melaninogenicus* subsp. *melaninogenicus* strains. These experiments were preliminary in nature, and more detailed analyses are required to validate the true identity of the antigens.

The periodontopathic bacterium *A. actinomycetemcomitans* has attracted considerable attention in terms of its antigenic character and multitude of virulence factors. Important probes, in the form of monoclonal antibodies, are currently being developed for the analysis of these antigens and factors. Earlier studies used whole bacteria or cell sonicates as antigen preparations for the generation of hybridomas. The main emphasis was on the identification and speciation of clinical oral isolates of these bacteria, as in the case of the studies in which monoclonal antibodies were developed against *Bacteroides* species. Indirect immunofluorescence microscopy, employing both polyclonal antibodies prepared in rabbits and monoclonal antibody, provided sensitivities ranging from 82 to 100%, when compared to calculating colony-forming units (CFU) on selective medium plates, for the detection of *A. actinomycetemcomitans* in subgingival plaque samples (4). As these authors point out, monoclonal antibodies have select advantages over polyclonal antiserum due to their specificity for individual determinants, and thus reduce the problems of false-positive reactions and high backgrounds. However, the specific monoclonal antibody must be chosen carefully, since all bacterial cell surface antigens and virulence factors are not equally expressed in all strains encountered in clinical samples. For example, as discussed earlier in this chapter (Section II,C), the leukotoxin of *A. actinomycetem-comitans* is found only in serotype a and b strains. This may be overcome by using mixtures of monoclonal antibodies which recognize different serospecific antigens and virulence factors as the diagnostic reagent; however, choosing the right antibodies still requires careful consideration. In view of these considerations, diagnosis and taxonomy at the serotype or strain level necessitates the high degree of specificity characteristic of monoclonal antibodies; therefore, this approach is justified. In similar studies the immunofluorescent-labeling method was also employed with monoclonal antibody, but it was coupled with the technique of flow cytometry to identify and quantitate cells of *A. actinomycetem-comitans* (3,7). These monoclonal antibodies were prepared against different serotypes of *A. actinomycetemcomitans* by immunizing mice with whole or sonicated bacteria (53,69). More recent evidence suggests that these antibodies may recognize lipopolysaccharide or capsular polysaccharide (70). It is difficult to evaluate the results of these studies because, at the time of this writing, they have been published only in abstract form.

The primary approach used in the studies just discussed was to obtain monoclonal antibodies against *A. actinomycetemcomitans* that could be used for the diagnosis and quantitation of this microorganism in subgingival plaque samples from patients with periodontal disease. In a separate study, a different approach was used to obtain monoclonal antibodies that recognized a specific virulence factor of *A. actinomycetemcomitans*. These antibodies were then used as probes to identify, characterize, and isolate the specific factor. This type of approach will be discussed in more detail in Section III,B of this review.

3. Monoclonal Antibodies against Other Orally Relevant Antigens

Lipoteichoic acids represent major cell surface antigens in most gram-positive cells (55,134). Several laboratories have produced hybridomas which make monoclonal antibodies against lipoteichoic acids. In one such study BALB/c mice were immunized with lipoteichoic acids extracted from *S. mutans* BHT or *S. mutans* Ingbritt and *S. faecium* (45). One class of hybridomas that were obtained using the *S. mutans* lipoteichoic acids produced antibodies which recognized the polyglycerol phosphate backbone which is common to all lipoteichoic acids. Those hybridomas that were recovered when *S. faecium* lipoteichoic acid was used as the immunogen were thought to be specific for the kojibiosyl moieties (glucose α-1$\rightarrow$2 glucose) present on the lipoteichoic acid of group D streptococci. In a separate study, lipoteichoic acid backbone-specific monoclonal antibodies of the IgM class were obtained using lipoteichoic acid from *Lactobacillus fermentum* (E. T. Lally *et al.*, unpublished observations).

In both of the studies just discussed an interesting approach was used to select for IgM-secreting hybridomas by applying a modification of the Jerne plaque assay. In this classical hemolytic assay, immunoglobulin-secreting cells, from the spleen of a mouse injected with sheep erythrocytes (SRBC), were mixed with SRBC in agar (46,74). Following a preincubation, to allow the cells to continue secreting and/or synthesizing immunoglobulins, complement is added. The secreted antibodies bind to the erythrocytes, complement is fixed, and lysis occurs with the formation of clear plaques in a background of unlysed cells. A single molecule of IgM in the presence of complement is sufficient to induce the lysis of a single erythrocyte; however, IgG is considerably less efficient in this assay (26). The sensitivity of the method has been increased and it has been adapted for cell micromanipulation (22,86). Thus, plaque-forming cells could be selected for further study. In the approach used by Jackson and co-workers (45) and E. T. Lally *et al.* (unpublished observations), hybridomas which produced lipoteichoic acid-specific IgM antibodies were detected by directly sensitizing SRBC with lipoteichoic acid. Cell culture supernatants were assayed for hemolytic activity in the presence of complement. As a modification of this assay, it seems feasible that clones could be examined directly by incorporating sensitized erythrocytes and complement in the soft agar and simply examining the plates for plaque formation.

Monoclonal antibodies against lipoteichoic acid will prove to be useful for the purification and localization of the molecule in the oral streptococci. *Streptococcus sanguis,* one of the predominant microorganisms in developing human dental plaque, coaggregates with various species of gram-positive and gram-negative oral bacteria (12). In several of these intergeneric coaggregation systems, between *S. sanguis* and *Fusobacterium nucleatum* (60) and *S. sanguis* and *Bacterionema matruchotii* (59), morphologically distinct structures, designated corncobs, are formed. The results from recent experiments suggest that lipoteichoic acid may be one of the *S. sanguis* cell surface molecules that participates, either directly or indirectly, in cell–cell binding (23). In this study the biochemical separation and antigenic purity of the lipoteichoic acid preparation was monitored by use of a backbone-specific monoclonal antibody. The monoclonal antibody, in conjunction with heterologous anti-*S. sanguis* serum, was used in immunoelectrophoresis to establish that the lipoteichoic acid preparation was free from contaminating streptococcal cell surface antigens. Attempts were made to inhibit cell–cell aggregation in both the *F. nucleatum* and *B. matruchotii* corncob systems with the lipoteichoic acid-specific monoclonal antibody. The antibody repeatedly failed to inhibit the coaggregation. These results were reminiscent of those reported for the type 1 fimbria-mediated binding of *A. viscosus* to saliva-treated hydroxyapatite (see Section III,A) (16,17). Conversely, other investigators have been able to inhibit the binding of *S. sanguis* to saliva-coated hydroxyapatite using monoclonal antibodies which were believed to recognize fimbriae located on these cells (27). However, the initial report on this monoclonal antibody was vague and additional information concerning its characterization will be required to evaluate the data fully. Future applications of the monoclonal antibody include the localization of lipoteichoic acid on the cell surface of corncob-forming strains of *S. sanguis* by immunostaining of electron microscopic preparations.

B. Production of Monoclonal Antibodies Which Neutralize the Leukotoxin of *Actinobacillus actinomycetemcomitans*

The potential significance of the leukotoxin to the pathogenicity of *A. actinomycetemcomitans* and the suggestion that it may represent a reliable indicator of juvenile periodontitis prompted the development of monoclonal antibodies specific for this molecule. Details covering the preparation and selection of the hybridomas will be presented especially for those not familiar with these techniques.

1. Hybridoma Procedures

BALB/cJ female mice, 12–16 weeks old, were immunized with 10 μg of polymyxin-extracted protein from *A. actinomycetemcomitans* JP2. This strain was selected because extracts routinely yielded the highest activity in the leukotoxin assay. The protein preparation was emulsified in complete Freund adjuvant. The mice were boosted on days 10, 20, and 30 with protein in incomplete Freund adjuvant and bled via the retroorbital plexus on day 37. Sera were tested for the presence of antileukotoxin antibody by the biological assay described below. Mice whose sera showed inhibition of leukotoxin in the biological assay were segregated and allowed to rest for 60 days. Three days before fusion, the animals received 10 μg of polymyxin-extracted protein intravenously. On the day of the fusion, spleens were removed aseptically, and a single-cell suspension was made with a loose-fitting tissue homogenizer. The cells were washed once in Dulbecco minimal essential medium (10% fetal calf serum), and the erythrocytes were lysed with 0.17 M ammonium chloride–Tris buffer. Spleen cells recovered in this manner had a viability of more than 95% as assessed by trypan blue exclusion.

The fusion protocol was a modification of the method of Gefter *et al.* (31). Sp2/0-Ag14 myeloma cells (107) were mixed with spleen cells (1:10) and centrifuged. A 50% polyethylene glycol solution was slowly added to the cell pellet. The pellet was gently stirred, allowed to set for 1 min, and then dispersed by the addition of Dulbecco minimal essential medium. After centrifugation, the cells were suspended in medium, and portions were placed in 96-well tissue culture plates. The next day, medium containing aminopterin (0.04 μM) was added to each well, after which the cells were fed every 3–4 days. Clones were visible 7–9 days after the fusion, and when they covered approximately one-half of the bottom of the well, they were screened for the presence of antileukotoxin antibody by inhibition in the biological assay and for recognition on Western blots. Cultures which inhibited leukotoxin activity and recognized the leukotoxin on the nitrocellulose blots were cloned according to a modification of the method of Sato *et al.* (98). Immunoglobulin subclass and light-chain determinations were achieved using monospecific antisera that had been prescreened for cross-reactivity according to the method of Slack *et al.* (109).

2. Selection Methods

A dual-screening procedure was used to select hybridomas. Spent culture medium from each clone was examined first for its ability to inhibit the cytotoxicity of the leukotoxin and second to recognize this molecule on nitrocellulose blots. This approach ensured that functional antibodies would be obtained.

The first step in the screening protocol was a biological assay previously developed and routinely used to quantitate the activity of leukotoxin preparations. This assay is based on the release of preloaded ^{51}Cr from human neutrophils (124). Briefly, human peripheral blood neutrophils were isolated from donors by dextran sedimentation and centrifugation on Ficoll-Hypaque and suspended in Hanks balanced salt solution supplemented with 0.1% gelatin (127). Inhibition of cytotoxicity was measured by a modification of the ^{51}Cr-release assay (128). To test the inhibitory activity of the monoclonal antibodies, 50 μl of polymyxin-extracted leukotoxin preparation (3.6 μg of protein) and various dilutions of the spent medium from the cloned cells were added to the ^{51}Cr-labeled neutrophils in 96-well microtiter plates. The second step was to take those culture supernatants that were positive in the biological assay and to react them with leukotoxin on Western blots. At the time that these experiments were performed, purified leukotoxin was not available. In fact, information concerning the physical properties, such as molecular size, of the molecule was lacking. Therefore, the crude polymyxin preparation that was used to immunize the mice was employed as the antigen on Western blots. The polypeptides in the polymyxin extract were separated by sodium dodecyl sulfate–polyacrylamide gel electrophoresis (SDS–PAGE) on 17.5% slab gels (24). The separated polypeptides were then electrophoretically transferred to nitrocellulose sheets by the method of Towbin and co-workers (126).

The decision to use Western blotting, in place of the ELISA, to screen cloned hybridomas for the production of leukotoxin-specific antibody was based on several factors: (i) the antigen preparation that was to be used for screening was a crude heterogeneous mixture of proteins; (ii) there was indirect preliminary evidence that the concentration of leukotoxin, on a molar basis, in these preparations was relatively low; and (iii) it has been reported that the sensitivity of the ELISA is limited by the competition of antigens, in crude mixtures, for sites on the plastic plates (8,51). Most proteins bind equally well to nitrocellulose.

3. Identification of the Leukotoxin Polypeptide

Prior to the cell fusion, sera collected from mice which had been immunized with the crude antigen preparation were examined for the presence of toxin-neutralizing antibodies. Sera that demonstrated inhibitory activity were then screened on nitrocellulose blots and compared to sera obtained from juvenile periodontitis patients. Both the mouse sera and the human sera contained antibodies which recognized a polypeptide (apparent MW 115,000–135,000), which could be observed in the antigen preparation on stained SDS–polyacrylamide gels (25). Following the fusion and cloning of the hybridomas, the spent culture medium obtained from seven clones recognized the same polypeptide (Fig. 1). Several lines of evidence established that the monoclonal antibodies were directed against the leukotoxin: (i) the antibodies inhibited the cytotoxicity of the leukotoxin as measured in the ^{51}Cr-release assay; (ii) all tested juvenile periodontitis sera which inhibited the biological activity of the leukotoxin also recognized the same polypeptide as that recognized by the monoclonal antibodies; and (iii) the proposed leukotoxin polypeptide was detected with the monoclonal antibodies only in strains of *A. actinomycetemcomitans* previously shown to be leukotoxic in the ^{51}Cr-release assay (25,124).

4. Characterization of the Leukotoxin-Specific Monoclonal Antibodies

Following subcloning of the hybridomas, three monoclonal antibodies were analyzed in more detail. As illustrated in Table II, these three antibodies were all of the IgG class and showed minor differences in inhibition titers. However,

TABLE II

Comparison of Inhibitory Activity of Monoclonal Antibodies against the Leukotoxin of *Actinobacillus actinomycetemcomitans*

Monoclonal antibody designation	Subclass and L-chain type	Neutralization titer (ng IgG protein)[a]
46A3C2	$IgG_{2,\kappa}$	170
83A4A3	$IgG_{1,\kappa}$	45
107A3A3	$IgG_{1,\kappa}$	110

[a] Expressed as amount of IgG protein that inhibited the release of 50% of the total ^{51}Cr from preloaded neutrophils; 3.6 μg of crude leukotoxin was added to 5×10^5 cells (6814 ± 243 cpm). Ascites fluids were subjected to ammonium sulfate precipitation and DEAE chromatography to isolate IgG.

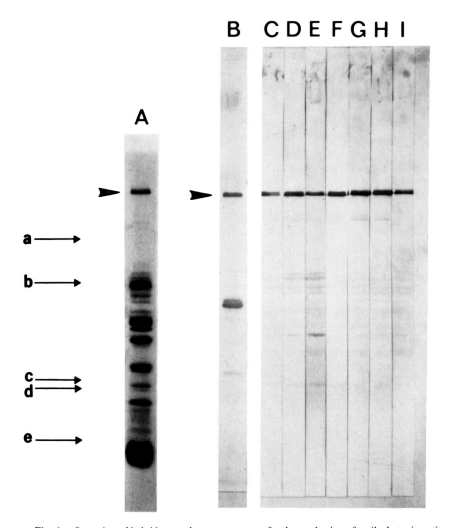

Fig. 1. Screening of hybridoma culture supernatants for the production of antileukotoxin antibodies. Crude polymyxin B-extracted proteins from strain JP2 were separated by SDS–PAGE and transferred to nitrocellulose by electroblotting. Replicate nitrocellulose blots were then incubated with the spent tissue culture medium, from cloned hybridomas that inhibited leukotoxin activity in the biological assay, followed by peroxidase-conjugated second antibody. Lane A, stained SDS–polyacrylamide gel of polymyxin B extract (42 μg of protein); lane B, nitrocellulose blot incubated with serum (1:50 dilution) from a mouse immunized with polymyxin B-extracted protein and peroxidase-conjugated sheep anti-mouse immunoglobulin (1:2000 dilution); lanes C–I, nitrocellulose blots incubated with various hybridoma culture supernatants (1:30 dilution) followed by second antibody. The arrows indicate the position of the proposed leukotoxin polypeptides. Molecular weight standards are as follows: a, bovine serum albumin (68,000); b, ovalbumin (43,000); c, lysozyme (14,300); d, cytochrome c (11,700); e, insulin (6000).

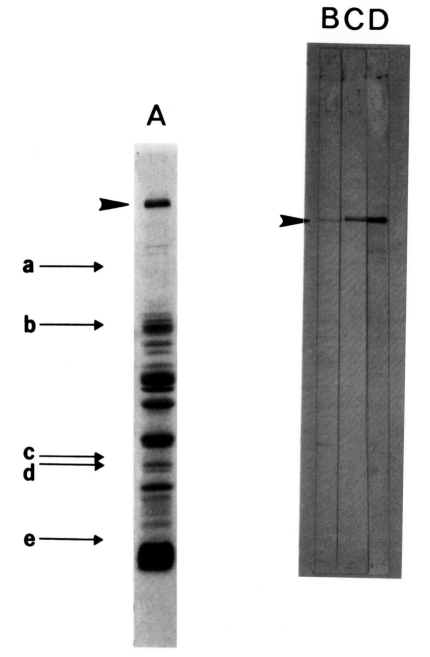

Fig. 2. Characterization of three antileukotoxin monoclonal antibodies. Spent culture medium from the three hybridomas was reacted with electroblotted polymyxin B-extracted protein (42 µg).

there appeared to be some degree of variability in binding to the leukotoxin on Western blots (Fig. 2). The results obtained from these data may suggest that monoclonal antibodies 46A3C2 and 83A4A3 may be conformational antibodies, since they had inhibition titers comparable to 107A3A3 but bound less efficiently to the leukotoxin on the Western blot. It must be kept in mind that the leukotoxin was subjected to heat (50°C for 20 min) and detergent (SDS) denaturization prior to blotting. The inhibition assay was performed using nondenatured toxin.

C. Partial Characterization of the Leukotoxin

The availability of monoclonal antibodies which recognized the leukotoxin provided invaluable probes for analyzing the physicochemical properties of the protein as well as localizing the protein in the bacterial cell. These studies are currently under way and early findings will be discussed. The monoclonal antibodies were also used to isolate the leukotoxin, and this application, along with associated problems that arose during the course of the experiments, will be discussed further below.

1. Cellular Localization

Subcellular fractions of *A. actinomycetemcomitans* were prepared. The cytoplasmic protein and cell envelope (membrane) fractions were obtained by sonication and differential centrifugation (24). The cells were also subjected to osmotic shock employing a standard procedure designed to release periplasmic enzymes gently from *Escherichia coli* (85). The cell fractions were then analyzed with monoclonal antibody on Western blots. Monoclonal reactive leukotoxin polypeptide was found primarily in the osmotic shock extract, while trace amounts of leukotoxin could infrequently be found in the cytoplasmic fraction. The osmotic shock-extracted toxin was found to be cytotoxic in the ^{51}Cr-release assay. Monoclonal reactive leukotoxin could not be found under the conditions employed in this experiment, either in the cell envelope fraction or extracellularly in the spent growth medium. These results suggest that the leukotoxin may be localized primarily in the periplasmic space or at least on the inner surface of the outer membrane. A previous study showed that the leukotoxin could be extracted from whole cells by treatment with the membrane-perturbing antibiotic polymyxin B (128). Polymyxin B acts like a detergent, intercalating in the lipid bilayer of the membrane. The release of leukotoxin from whole cells by osmotic shock was consistent with those results obtained with polymyxin. There

---

All culture supernatants were obtained after 4 days of growth (2×10^5 cells plated) and were used at a 1:30 dilution with each nitrocellulose strip. Lane A, stained SDS–polyacrylamide gel of polymyxin B extract; lanes B–D, nitrocellulose blots of crude antigen, shown in lane A, incubated with spent culture medium from hybridomas 46A3C2, 83A4A3, and 107A3A3, respectively. Reprinted with permission from DiRienzo *et al.* (25).

is a precedent for the periplasmic location of bacterial toxins, since Hirst *et al.* (41) demonstrated that both the A and B subunits of the heat-labile enterotoxin of *E. coli* are located in the periplasmic space.

2. Distribution in Oral Strains of Actinobacillus actinomycetemcomitans

The simplicity of extracting leukotoxin from small quantities of cells by the osmotic shock procedure, coupled with the ease of detection using monoclonal antibody, permitted the rapid screening of bacterial strains for the presence of leukotoxin. Various strains of *A. actinomycetemcomitans* as well as strains representing species of several related oral bacteria were subjected to osmotic shock and the extracted polypeptides were separated by SDS–PAGE. Western blots were then prepared and treated with monoclonal antibody and peroxidase-conjugated anti-mouse immunoglobulin. The results are summarized in Table III. Several points should be noted concerning the results. First, the various strains of *A. actinomycetemcomitans* could be divided into three groups based on the number of polypeptides that were recognized by the monoclonal antibody. Group

TABLE III

Leukotoxin Expression in *Actinobacillus actinomycetemcomitans* as Detected with Monoclonal Antibody

		Expression of leukotoxin	
Species or strain	Serotype[a]	135K Polypeptide	130K Polypeptide
A. actinomycetemcomitans			
Y4	b	+	−
JP2	b	+	−
650	b	+	−
651	b	+	−
ATCC 29522	b	+	+
ATCC 29523	a	+	+
ATCC 29524	b	+	+
511	—[b]	−	+
627	c	−	−
652	a	−	−
Haemophilus aphrophilus			
80		−	−
81		−	−
Capnocytophaga ochracea			
25		−	−

[a] Serotyping scheme is that of Zambon and co-workers (137).

[b] Strain 511 does not fit any of the three proposed serotypes (124).

I contained a single monoclonal-reactive polypeptide species having an apparent molecular weight of 135,000. Group II strains contained the 135K polypeptide and a second polypeptide having an apparent molecular weight of 130,000. Group III lacked monoclonal-reactive polypeptides. Second, no apparent correlation existed between the conventional serotypes and the presence or absence of monoclonal-reactive leukotoxin species. If any correlation exists, it may be that serotype c strains lack leukotoxin. This observation has been noted previously on the basis of results obtained with the ^{51}Cr-release assay (124). Since only a single serotype c strain was analyzed in this study, it is premature to make the generalization that all serotype c strains lack both the 135K and 130K polypeptides. The use of monoclonal antibody in these experiments provided the first indication that the leukotoxin was heterogeneous in nature.

3. Molecular Size Heterogeneity

Attempts were made to determine the molecular basis of the heterogeneity observed in various leukotoxin preparations. Since the experiments on the strain distribution of the leukotoxin indicated that some preparations contained at least two monoclonal antibody-reactive species, the heterogeneity of the leukotoxin was examined following various separation conditions. Initially, a crude polymyxin preparation of the leukotoxin, from A. actinomycetemcomitans, was separated by two-dimensional PAGE (1) and detected by Western blotting (126). The leukotoxin separated as a major spot which comigrated with the leukotoxin polypeptide found in the single-dimension SDS gel (Fig. 3) (25). The isoelectric point of this major polypeptide was in the range of 8.2 to 8.5. Only minor additional spots could be detected. These additional spots did not appear to correlate with the polypeptides observed in the strain heterogeneity experiments and appeared to represent degradation products. Minor, lower molecular weight species appear on the Western blots when leukotoxin preparations are heavily concentrated.

Interestingly, leukotoxin preparations that were extracted with polymyxin contained predominantly a 115K species. Osmotic shock extracts were usually enriched for the higher molecular weight 135K and 130K species. These two polypeptides could be easily separated on conventional single-dimension SDS gels. Separation on 17.5% and 10% SDS–polacrylamide gels is shown in Fig. 4. The 10% acrylamide gels gave somewhat increased separation; however, some sacrifice was made for resolution or band sharpness. The 17.5% and 10% acrylamide gels were subsequently used interchangeably. At the present time the nature of the heterogeneity of the A. actinomycetemcomitans leukotoxin remains unknown. However, preliminary examinations using the monoclonal antibody and several leukotoxin mutants may shed some light on this question (see Section III,D).

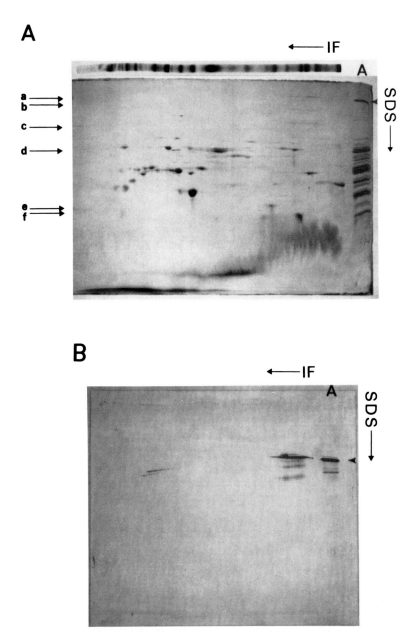

Fig. 3. Two-dimensional gel electrophoresis of polymyxin B-extracted leukotoxin fraction. Protein (100 μg) was applied to isoelectric focusing (IF) gels. One gel was stained and two gels were each overlaid on a 17.5% SDS–polyacrylamide slab gel. Polymyxin B-extracted protein was applied to a well at one end of the slab gels (lane A), and molecular weight standards were applied at the other end. One gel was then stained (panel A) and the second gel was blotted (panel B). Leukotoxin was detected by incubating the blot with monoclonal antibody 107A3A3 (in ascites fluid, 1:200 dilution). The small arrows in panels A and B indicate the position of the leukotoxin. Molecular weight standards are as follows: a, β-galactosidase (130,000); b, phosphorylase *a* (94,000); c, bovine serum albumin; d, ovalbumin; e, lysozyme; f, cytochrome *c*. Reprinted with permission from DiRienzo *et al.* (25).

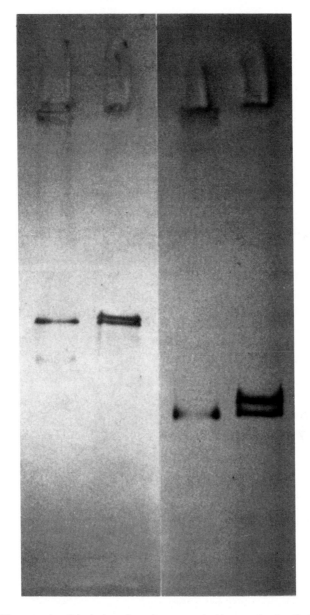

Fig. 4. Heterogeneity of the leukotoxin as demonstrated with monoclonal antibody on Western blots. Osmotic shock extracts of *Actinobacillus actinomycetemcomitans* 511 and ATCC 29524 were prepared and electrophoresed on 17.5% and 10% SDS–polyacrylamide gels. Following electrophoresis the polypeptides were transferred to nitrocellulose and detected using monoclonal antibody and peroxidase conjugated anti-mouse immunoglobulin. Lanes A and C, osmotic shock extract from strain 511; lanes B and D, osmotic shock extract from strain ATCC 29524. Lanes A and B are from a 17.5% acrylamide gel and lanes C and D are from a 10% gel.

4. Purification

The monoclonal antibodies that were produced against the leukotoxin provided a convenient means of purifying the leukotoxin by immunoaffinity chromatography. Monoclonal antibody 107A3A3 was selected for the construction of an affinity column because, of the three characterized antibodies, 107A3A3 appeared to bind leukotoxin most effectively on Western blots. Ascites fluid was subjected to ammonium sulfate precipitation. The 50% saturated precipitate was dialyzed and applied to a protein A–Sepharose CL-4B column to isolate IgG. The monoclonal antibody eluted at a pH of 6.3 and its reactivity was checked on Western blots. The purified antibody was then coupled to cyanogen bromide-activated Sepharose 4B. An osmotic shock preparation from *A. actinomycetemcomitans* Y4 was applied to the antibody column and attempts were made to elute the bound leukotoxin with various buffers. Both 0.1 *M* sodium acetate (pH 4.0) in 1 *M* sodium chloride and 0.2 *M* glycine–hydrochloric acid (pH 2.3) failed to elute the leukotoxin. Of the buffers tested, only 3.5 *M* potassium thiocyanate in 0.1 *M* sodium phosphate–0.15 *M* sodium chloride (pH 7.2) eluted the leukotoxin. The results of the immunoaffinity purification are shown in Fig. 5. Following the elution of the leukotoxin from the affinity column, there was a substantial loss of biological activity. The reason for this is not clear at the present time and experiments are in progress to solve this problem.

D. Reaction of Monoclonal Antibodies with Leukotoxin-Deficient Mutants

Prior to the production of monoclonal antibodies, several antibiotic resistance markers were introduced into *A. actinomycetemcomitans* Y4. When the monoclonal antibodies became available the antibiotic-resistant mutants were screened for their reaction with the antibodies on Western blots.

1. Phenotypic Characterization of Mutants

Table IV lists the mutants, along with their phenotypes, that were produced in this study. Originally, the double-resistance mutant strains UPA 5 and UPA 5-23 were obtained as spontaneous mutants of the wild-type parental strain UPA 1 (strain Y4). These mutants were resistant to 100 μg/ml each of nalidixic acid and streptomycin. When osmotic shock extracts of these two mutants were examined on Western blots with monoclonal antibody against the leukotoxin, it was found that UPA 5 contained a monoclonal antibody-reactive leukotoxin enriched for the lower molecular weight 130K polypeptide, while UPA 5-23 was significantly deficient in both the 135K and 130K polypeptides. Therefore, since there appeared to be either a direct or indirect correlation between antibiotic resistance and alteration of leukotoxin expression, the first step was to separate the two mutations, which resulted in the antibiotic resistances, and then reexamine the

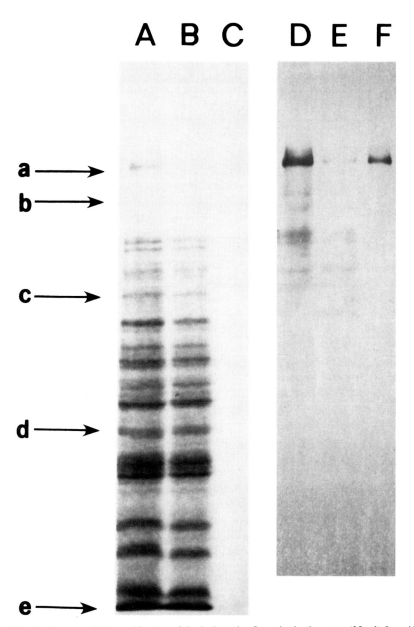

Fig. 5. Immunoaffinity purification of the leukotoxin. Osmotic shock extract (25 ml) from 10 liters of *Actinobacillus actinomycetemcomitans* Y4 culture was applied to a column containing monoclonal antibody 107A3A3 cyanogen bromide coupled to Sephadex CL-4B. The column was extensively washed with borate-buffered saline and the bound material was then eluted with 3.5 *M* potassium thiocyanate in 0.1 *M* sodium phosphate–0.15 *M* sodium chloride (pH 7.2). The unbound and bound material was then subjected to SDS–PAGE and Western blotting to assay for the leukotoxin. Lanes A–C show the stained gel and lanes D–F show the nitrocellulose blot. Lanes A and D, osmotic shock-extracted material that was applied to the column; lanes B and E, unbound material eluted from the column; lanes C and F, bound material eluted from the column. Molecular weight standards are the same as in Fig. 3.

TABLE IV

Leukotoxin Mutants of *Actinobacillus actinomycetemcomitans*

Strain designation	Phenotype[a]	Parental strain and derivation
UPA 1	$Nal^SStr^SLkt^+Env1^+$	*A. actinomycetemcomitans* Y4
UPA 5	$Nal^RStr^RLkt^AEnv1^-$	Spontaneous resistant mutant derived from UPA 1
UPA 5-23	$Nal^RStr^RLkt^DEnv1^-$	Single-colony isolate of UPA 5
UPA 1-11	$Nal^RStr^SLkt^+Env1^+$	Spontaneous resistant mutant derived from UPA 1
UPA 1-20	$Nal^RStr^SLkt^AEnv1^-$	Spontaneous resistant mutant derived from UPA 1-11

[a] Nal, Nalidixic acid; Str, streptomycin; Lkt, leukotoxin; Env1, major cell envelope protein (see reference 24); S, sensitive; R, resistant; A, altered; D, deficient; +, present; −, absent.

cells for expression of the leukotoxin. Since resistance to nalidixic acid can be caused by an alteration in either subunit A (high-level resistance) or subunit B (low-level resistance) of the DNA gyrase enzyme (73), spontaneous mutants of UPA 1 were selected for resistance up to 10 μg/ml (UPA 1–11) and 100 μg/ml (UPA 1-20) of the antibiotic. When these mutants were screened for the presence of the leukotoxin, it was discovered that expression in UPA 1-11 was identical to that of the wild-type cells, while UPA 1-20 contained an altered leukotoxin. The results obtained from Western blot analysis of osmotic shock fractions from each of the mutants are shown in Fig. 6. The samples were heavily overloaded on this blot in an attempt to detect minor variations in the leukotoxin. It should be noted that when osmotic shock extract from strain Y4 (UPA 1) was heavily concentrated, the 130K leukotoxin polypeptide was detected. Also, minor lower molecular weight bands were present and presumably resulted from the physical degradation of the leukotoxin. These results suggest that the leukotoxin heterogeneity previously observed in the various *A. actinomycetemcomitans* strains may be due to a concentration effect. That is, the level of expression of the 135K and 130K polypeptides may be equivalent in some strains, such as in ATCC 29522, or may be increased in favor of one polypeptide or the other (e.g., strains Y4 and 511; see Table III). Strains 511 may be analogous to mutant strain UPA 5. Minimally leukotoxic strains (e.g., 627 and 652) may express leukotoxin at a level similar to that in mutant UPA 5-23. Although preliminary, the data that were obtained from the analysis of the mutants would suggest that the 135K and 130K polypeptides are located on different genes which may be subject to differential regulation. However, this is speculation at the present time, and more detailed genetic analyses need to be performed. Closer examination revealed that those mutants that displayed altered leukotoxin on the blots also lacked a major cell envelope protein, previously designated Env1 (24). The loss of the Env1

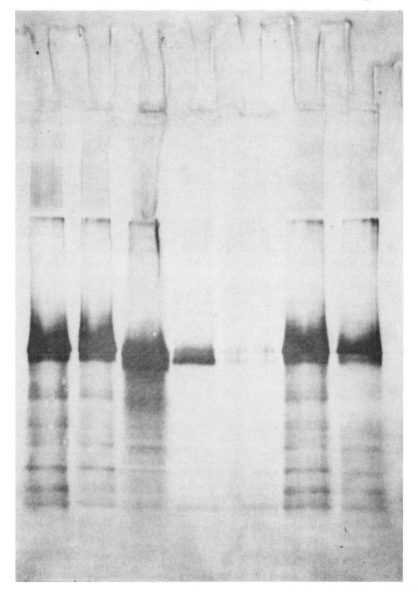

Fig. 6. The analysis of leukotoxin-deficient mutants using monoclonal antibody. Osmotic shock extracts (100 ml of culture at A_{660} 0.8 of the various antibiotic-resistant mutants were concentrated by lyophilization, the proteins were electrophoresed on SDS–polyacrylamide gels and transferred to nitrocellulose. The blot was incubated with monoclonal antibody 107A3A3 (ascites, 1:200 dilution) and peroxidase-conjugated anti-mouse immunoglobulin (1:2000 dilution). Lane A, UPA 1 (wild type, strain Y4); B, UPA 1-11; C, UPA 1-20; D, UPA 5; E, UPA 5–23; F, UPA 1: G, UPA 1 (cells grown in chemically defined medium).

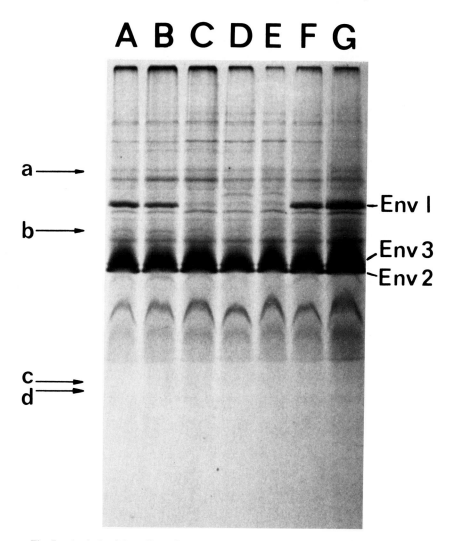

Fig. 7. Analysis of the cell envelope protein composition of the leukotoxin-deficient mutants. The cell envelope fractions from the various antibiotic-resistant mutants were prepared by sonication of the cells followed by differential centrifugation (24). These membrane preparations were then applied to a 17.5% SDS gel and stained with Coomassie Blue. Lanes A–G are the same as in Fig. 6 and the molecular weight standards are the same as in Fig. 1.

protein is shown in Coomassie Blue-stained SDS–polyacrylamide gels of cell envelope fractions isolated from the various mutants (Fig. 7). Those mutants (UPA 5, UPA 5-23, and UPA 1-20) that were resistant to high levels of nalidixic acid (100 μg/ml) lacked the Env1 protein. The relationship between the leukotoxin and the Env1 protein is not known. In subsequent experiments, presented below, the loss of the Env1 protein in these mutants appeared to be an independent event related to the acquisition of nalidixic acid resistance.

Analysis of leukotoxin mutants with the monoclonal antibodies on Western blots provided distinct advantages over the sole use of other analytical methods, such as a biologically functional assay. The primary advantage was that the actual gene product could be directly observed, so that structural changes in the protein that did not necessarily affect activity could be detected. Alternatively, mutations that affected the biological activity of the molecule could be correlated with structural changes. Along these lines the mutants were assayed for cytotoxicity in the ^{51}Cr-release assay. The results of the biological assay were in excellent agreement with those of the Western blot analysis. Mutant strains UPA 5 and UPA 5-23 demonstrated minimal if any leukotoxic activity (Fig. 8). The leukotoxic activity of strain UPA 1-11, the low-level nalidixic acid-resistant mutant, was comparable to the activity expressed by the wild-type cells. Unexpectedly, mutant UPA 1-20, which contained altered leukotoxin, also expressed wild-type

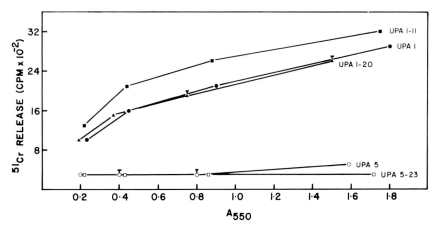

Fig. 8. Expression of leukotoxin activity by the various mutants: (■) UPA 1-11; (●) UPA 1; (▲) UPA 1-20; (○) UPA 5; (□) UPA 5-23. The bacteria were harvested, washed, and added, in increasing concentrations, to ^{51}Cr-labeled human neutrophils as described in the text. Normal human serum was added to all samples to enhance the cytotoxicity of the leukotoxin. Maximum release of label from the neutrophils, determined by lysis of the cells with Triton X-100, was 8217 ± 291 cpm per well. The buffer controls were 302 ± 20 cpm per well.

levels of leukotoxic activity. However, in this experiment the cells were grown in the absence of antibiotics. These findings suggested that (i) UPA 5 and UPA 5-23 represented mutants that were altered in either the structural or regulatory genes; and (ii) UPA 1-20 did not contain a mutation in the leukotoxin gene. Rather, high levels of nalidixic acid appeared to alter leukotoxin expression.

2. Effect of Nalidixic Acid on Leukotoxin Expression

It thus was apparent that nalidixic acid affected the expression of the leukotoxin. To test this hypothesis the mutant strains UPA 1-20 and UPA 5-23 were grown in the presence and absence of 100 μg/ml of the antibiotic, and leukotoxin expression was examined on Western blots (Fig. 9). As can be observed following Western blot analysis, nalidixic acid significantly reduced the amount of leukotoxin that was synthesized by the cells and appeared to inhibit the expression of the 135K polypeptide to a greater extent than that of the 130K polypeptide. As a control, when UPA 5-23 was grown in the absence of either nalidixic acid or streptomycin, leukotoxin still was not expressed. These results substantiated the initial observation that UPA 5-23 was mutated in the leukotoxin gene. The effect of nalidixic acid on leukotoxin expression was examined more critically by employing the monoclonal antibody in semiquantitative studies. The advantage of having the high-level nalidixic acid-resistant mutant, UPA 1-20, was that the effect of increasing levels of the antibiotic on the expression of the leukotoxin could be examined without altering cell growth. The mutant strain UPA 1-20 was grown in concentrations of nalidixic acid ranging from 0 to 100 μg/ml of culture. As shown in Fig. 10, concentrations of the antibiotic up to 100 μg/ml had no effect on cell growth of UPA 1-20 compared to the parental strain UPA 1. Growth of the wild-type cells was clearly inhibited by low concentrations of the antibiotic (Fig. 10A). Cells were removed following 9 hr of growth in the various concentrations of nalidixic acid, and osmotic shock extracts were prepared and electrophoresed on a SDS–polyacrylamide gel and blotted to nitrocellulose. The leukotoxin was then detected using monoclonal antibody. The results are shown in Fig. 11. There appeared to be a direct correlation between the concentration of nalidixic acid in the culture and the expression of the leukotoxin.

Based on the mechanism of action of nalidixic acid, its effect on the expression of the leukotoxin most likely occurs at the level of transcription. It is not clear at present why the synthesis of leukotoxin should be selectively inhibited by this antibiotic. One possible explanation is that the leukotoxin gene is located on an extrachromosomal element, such as a plasmid. The replication of a plasmic may be more sensitive to nalidixic acid than that of the bacterial chromosome. Attempts to find a plasmid in A. actinomycetemcomitans Y4 have failed. In addition, when UPA 1 was treated with acridine orange in an attempt to cure the cells of a possible plasmid, no measurable effect on the expression of the leuko-

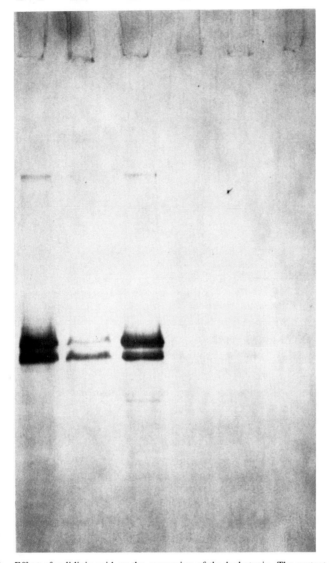

Fig. 9.   Effect of nalidixic acid on the expression of the leukotoxin. The mutant strains UPA 1-20 and UPA 5-23 were cultured in the presence and absence of 100 μg/ml of nalidixic acid or streptomycin. The osmotic shock fractions were then prepared and examined for leukotoxin expression on a Western blot using monoclonal antibody 107A3A3. Lane A, UPA 1 (no antibiotics); lane B, UPA 1-20 (nalidixic acid); lane C, UPA 1-20 (no antibiotics); lane D, UPA 5-23 (nalidixic acid and streptomycin); lane E, UPA 5-23 (streptomycin); lane F, UPA 5-23 (no antibiotics).

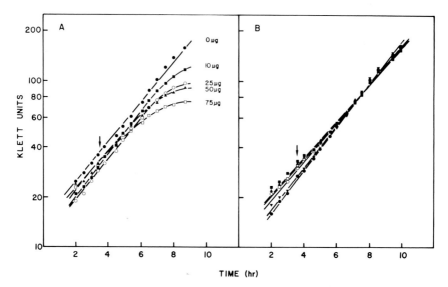

Fig. 10. Effect of nalidixic acid on the growth of *Actinobacillus actinomycetemcomitans* UPA 1 and UPA 1-20. The bacteria were grown in a peptone–yeast extract–glucose medium for approximately 3 hr, at which time the cultures were divided. Each culture then received either 0 (●), 10 (■), 25 (○), 50 (▲), 75 (□), or 100 (▼) μg/ml of nalidixic acid and growth was continued. Growth was followed with a Klett–Summerson colorimeter using a red filter. The arrows indicate the time of addition of the antibiotic. (A) UPA 1; (B) UPA 1-20.

toxin was measured. A bacteriophage has been found in one strain of *A. actinomycetemcomitans;* however, there did not appear to be any correlation between the presence or absence of the bacteriophage and level of leukotoxin expression (122).

IV. CONCLUSIONS

The studies presented in this chapter have employed monoclonal antibodies for (i) the taxonomic identification and diagnosis of specific bacteria in clinical samples; (ii) immunodiagnosis of diseased patients; (iii) identification, characterization, and isolation of specific antigens and virulence factors from these bacteria; and (iv) isolation of mutants deficient in a specific virulence factor. At the present time, species-specific or serotype-specific monoclonal antibody collections have not been developed to the extent where monoclonal antibodies can replace conventional rabbit antisera for use in the serotyping of oral bacteria and the diagnosis of diseased patients. Much of the monoclonal antibody work is in the early stages of development, as evidenced by the fact that many of these

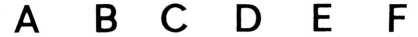

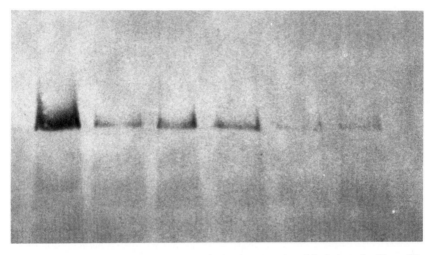

Fig. 11. Effect of nalidixic acid concentration on the expression of the leukotoxin. The antibiotic-treated cultures of UPA 1-20 from the experiment shown in Fig. 10 were centrifuged, after 9 hr of growth, to harvest and wash the cells. Osmotic shock fractions were then prepared from each culture and the proteins were separated by SDS–PAGE and transferred to nitrocellulose. The Western blot was treated with monoclonal antibody 107A3A3 and peroxidase-conjugated second antibody to detect leukotoxin. Lane A, 0 μg/ml nalidixic acid; lane B, 10 μg/ml; lane C, 25 μg/ml; lane D, 50 μg/ml; lane E, 75 μg/ml; lane F, 100 μg/ml. Only a portion of the blot is shown.

studies stress the characterization rather than the application of the antibodies. This is not meant to be a criticism of the published studies, because these preliminary characterizations of monoclonal antibodies must precede any viable application. However, it is doubtful that monoclonal antibodies will provide major advantages over currently used rabbit antisera as serotyping reagents in all situations. For example, the present serotyping scheme for strains of *S. mutans* appears to be more than adequate, showing fewer discrepancies than either biochemical or genetic typing systems. The use of monoclonal antibodies may add a minor improvement to this serotyping assay by providing highly standardized reagents which would allow for consistency from one laboratory to another. This approach would necessitate the production of monoclonal antibodies which recognized each of the serospecific carbohydrate determinants of *S. mutans*, since the antibodies already produced against the major antigens I–III demonstrate some degree of serotype cross-reactivity. Alternatively, monoclonal antibodies should supply the specificity required of a serotyping scheme for *Bacteroides* species. Several of the monoclonal antibodies which have been produced against *B. intermedius* apparently show a correlation with previously established genotypes; however, a more extensive collection of hybridomas is required to assemble a complete serotyping scheme which will be completely compatible with the DNA homology data. A total of only eight hybridomas have been characterized for *B. intermedius* and *B. gingivalis*. One of the *B. gingivalis* monoclonal antibodies cross-reacted with *B. intermedius,* and one of the *B. intermedius* antibodies also recognized *B. loescheii, B. melaninogenicus,* and *B. corporis.* Some of these problems associated with cross-reactivity along species lines may be alleviated by using cell fractions or purified components as the immunogen. A partial serotype-specific collection of monoclonal antibodies was reported in the case of *A. actinomycetemcomitans,* but the data were too preliminary to evaluate adequately the usefulness of the collection.

Another preliminary application of monoclonal antibodies in oral microbiology was in immunodiagnosis. The monoclonal antibodies were used in a competitive ELISA to measure serum antibody levels and specificity for the monoclonal antibody-defined epitopes. It would seem dangerous to conclude, solely on the basis of competition studies, that the antibodies from human sera recognized the same epitopes as those recognized by the monoclonal antibodies. Factors such as steric hindrance, a high degree of cross-linking, and conformational changes in the antigen—all possibly induced changes in the antigen resulting from the binding of the first antibody—could account for indirect inhibition of the binding of the monoclonal antibody. This inhibition could occur even if the first antibody does not recognize the same epitope.

Some of the most definitive applications of monoclonal antibodies pertained to specific antigen identification, characterization, and isolation. Here the approaches varied as to the extent of available information about the bacterial antigen or component. In the case of *B. intermedius,* a species about which little information is available concerning its antigenic composition, monoclonal antibodies were made against intact bacteria and Western blotting was used to determine the identity of the reacting antigens. In other studies involving the *S. mutans* antigens I, II, I/II, and III, glucosyltransferase, and lipoteichoic acid, and the fimbriae of *A. viscosus,* the antigen(s) had been previously identified and well characterized. The monoclonal antibodies against the antigens I, II, I/II, III were useful in determining the strain distribution and relatedness among these heterogeneous proteins. This type of approach will also help delineate the functions and interrelationships of heterogeneous forms of glucosyltransferase. Other monoclonal antibodies were produced against specific antigens as a method of isolating them in pure form. Lipoteichoic acid has routinely proved difficult to purify due to its amphiphilic nature. The role of lipoteichoic acid as a cell surface adherence receptor exemplifies the importance of the availability of this molecule, free from contaminating activities. Similarly, it was established that the fimbriae of *A. viscosus* also function as important adherence receptors. The functional specificity of the two types of fimbriae were not clearly established until monoclonal antibodies were used to purify each type. Additional supporting evidence was obtained when mutants lacking both types or a single type of fimbriae were isolated by screening with the monoclonal antibodies.

The application of monoclonal antibodies to the study of the leukotoxin of *A. actinomycetemcomitans* represented a special case. Prior to hybridoma production a great deal was known about the leukotoxin, but this information pertained to the biological activity of the molecule. Since at that time only crude toxin extracts were available, a method was required to visualize the specific molecule on analytical separation systems such as SDS–polyacrylamide gels. Monoclonal antibodies provided the best solution to the problem. By using monoclonal antibodies as immunoprobes on Western blots, the physical characteristics such as molecular size, isoelectric point, and heterogeneity of the leukotoxin were discerned, even though the molecule had not heen purified. The physicochemical characterization of the leukotoxin is far from complete and a more extensive use of the available as well as new monoclonal antibodies need to be applied to this characterization. These studies will most assuredly be enhanced by the availability of highly purified leukotoxin prepared by immunoaffinity chromatography.

One application of the leukotoxin monoclonal antibodies that has the potential to yield significant information concerning the contribution of this molecule to the pathogenicity of the bacterium was the isolation of leukotoxin-deficient mutants. It is hoped that these mutants provide as much insight into the structure and role of the leukotoxin as the fimbriae-deficient mutants of *A. viscosus*. Information already obtained from the analysis of these mutants suggests that the leukotoxin may consist of two polypeptides, both recognized by the monoclonal antibodies, which are differentially expressed, and that nalidixic acid inhibits the expression of the molecule, presumably at the level of transcription.

V. PROSPECTS FOR THE FUTURE

As stated at the outset of this chapter, the application of monoclonal antibodies in oral microbiology is still in the earliest stages of development. This means that there is substantial room for growth, especially the expansion of those studies discussed here. An impressive collection of monoclonal antibodies which recognize what are considered some of the predominant oral microbial pathogens has already been compiled. Perhaps the first future goal should be to supplement this collection with additional monoclonal antibodies, especially against those bacterial species that exhibit the greatest degree of antigenic diversity. This would include members within the genera *Bacteroides* and *Fusobacterium*. In addition, little information concerning the antigenic composition of the oral spirochetes is available. Monoclonal antibodies against the spirochetes would certainly facilitate the analysis of these bacteria.

Consequently, emphasis has previously been placed on the use of monoclonal antibodies in the identification and classification of bacteria in clinical plaque samples and in the isolation and characterization of specific antigens and virulence factors. However, there are various other applications of monoclonal antibodies which have not been approached and which may provide examples to be considered for future development. The most exciting application of monoclonal antibodies in oral microbiology (a direct reflection of this author's own bias) is the use of these specific antibodies as probes in genetic systems. Immunoprobes have great potential in the screening of mutants and genetic clones produced by recombinant DNA methods. Monoclonal antibodies readily bind to bacteria on filters and can be detected by any number of procedures including peroxidase-conjugated or ^{125}I-labeled mouse immunoglobulin and ^{125}I-labeled staphylococcal protein A. Other applications include the use of monoclonal antibodies as immunostaining reagents in electron microscopy. This approach can be used to localize antigens and virulence factors on the bacterial cell surface. Virulent and avirulent strains of bacteria can be compared by this technique to examine cells for the presence of virulence factors such as capsules, fimbriae/pili, and exoenzymes. Finally, monoclonal antibodies can be used as highly specific immunohistochemical reagents to examine tissue sections for the presence of specific bacteria and their products. The question of tissue invasion has become a significant consideration in the study of mechanisms of host–cell interactions in periodontal disease. Thus, all of these applications point toward the promising use of monoclonal antibodies as highly specific probes in the study of oral bacteria.

VI. SUMMARY

Hybridoma cell lines which secrete monoclonal antibodies were prepared against cell surface antigens from two gram-positive bacteria, *Streptococcus mutans* and *Actinomyces viscosus,* associated with dental caries formation. The monoclonal antibodies against *S. mutans* recognized the previously characterized secreted antigens I, II, I/II, and III, as well as a glucosyltransferase enzyme which catalyzes the synthesis of extracellular glucans, and lipoteichoic acid. The *A. viscosus* monoclonal antibodies were prepared against fimbriae found on the surface of virulent strains of this bacterium. The antibodies were specific for the type 1 fimbriae which mediate binding of the cells to the tooth surface and type 2 fimbriae which promote the cell–cell binding of this bacterium to oral streptococci. In other studies, monoclonal antibodies were prepared against *Bac-*

teroides gingivalis and *Bacteroides intermedius,* two bacterial species which contribute to the progression of chronic periodontitis. These antibodies apparently recognized cell surface antigens, the identities of which remain to be established. Hybridoma cell lines which make monoclonal antibodies to species-specific and serospecific antigens of *Actinobacillus actinomycetemcomitans,* the primary etiological agent in localized juvenile periodontitis, were also produced. Preliminary data indicated that these antibodies may recognize cell surface polysaccharide and carbohydrate determinants in the lipopolysaccharide. Other monoclonal antibodies were specifically made against a leukotoxin synthesized by some strains of this bacterium. The antileukotoxin monoclonal antibodies were used as immunoprobes in Western blot analyses to identify and characterize the toxin. The analyses revealed the presence of two monoclonal antibody-reactive polypeptides having apparent molecular weights of 130,000 and 135,000, as well as the differential expression of these two polypeptides in various strains and leukotoxin-deficient mutants of *A. actinomycetemcomitans.* The monoclonal antibodies produced against these bacteria and their virulence factors have made substantial contributions to our understanding of the roles of oral bacteria in disease.

ACKNOWLEDGMENTS

I would especially like to thank Joanne Haller for excellent technical assistance and help in the preparation of this manuscript. I also thank my colleagues E. T. Lally and N. S. Taichman, without whom much of this work would not have been possible, for critical discussions. I am grateful to W. A. Falkler, Jr., R. Gmür, I. L. Shklair, and I. Takazoe for providing data prior to publication. This work was supported by Public Health Service grants DE-06555, DE-07118, and DE-02623 from the National Institute of Dental Research.

REFERENCES

1. Ames, G. F. L., and Nikaido, K. (1976). Two dimensional gel electrophoresis of membrane proteins. *Biochemistry* **15,** 616–623.
2. Baehni, P. C., Tsai, C.-C., McArthur, W. P., Hammond, B. F., and Taichman, N. S. (1979). Interaction of inflammatory cells and oral microorganisms. VIII. Detection of leukotoxic activity of a plaque-derived gram-negative microorganism. *Infect. Immun.* **24,** 233–243.
3. Barnett, J. M., Buchanan, W., Cuchens, M., and McArthur, W. P. (1984). Flow cytometry and immunofiltration techniques to quantitate bacterial immunofluorescent labeling. *J. Dent. Res.* **63,** 306. (Abstr.)
4. Bonta, Y., Zambon, J. J., Genco, R. J., and Neiders, M. E. (1985). Rapid identification of periodontal pathogens in subgingival plaque: Comparison of indirect immunofluorescence microscopy with bacterial culture for detection of *Actinobacillus actinomycetemcomitans. J. Dent. Res.* **64,** 793–798.

5. Bratthall, D. (1969). Immunodiffusion studies on the serologic specificity of streptococci resembling *Streptococcus mutans*. *Odontol. Revy* **20**, 231–243.

6. Bratthall, D. (1970). Demonstration of five serological groups of streptococal strains resembling *Streptococcus mutans*. *Odontol. Revy* **21**, 143–152.

7. Buchanan, W., Barnett, J. M., and McArthur, W. P. (1984). Flow cytometry quantitation of bacteria labeled with indirect fluorescent monoclonal antibodies. *J. Dent. Res.* **63**, 307. (Abstr.)

8. Cantarero, L. A., Butler, J. E., and Osborne, J. W. (1980). The adsorptive characteristics of proteins for polystyrene and their significance in solid-phase immunoassays. *Anal. Biochem.* **105**, 375–382.

9. Chludzinski, A. M., Germaine, G. R., and Schachtele, C. F. (1974). Purification and properties of dextransucrase from *Streptococcus mutans*. *J. Bacteriol.* **118**, 1–7.

10. Ciardi, J. E., Beaman, A. J., and Wittenberger, C. L. (1977). Purification, resolution, and interaction of the glucosyltransferases of *Streptococcus mutans* 6715. *Infect. Immun.* **18**, 237–246.

11. Ciardi, J. E., Rolla, G., Bowen, W. H., and Reilly, J. A. (1977). Adsorption of *Streptococcus mutans* lipoteichoic acid to hydroxyapatite. *Scand. J. Dent. Res.* **85**, 387–391.

12. Cisar, J. O. (1982). Coaggregation reactions between oral bacteria: Studies of specific cell-to-cell adherence mediated by microbial lectins. *In* "Host–Parasite Interactions in Periodontal Diseases" (R. J. Genco and S. E. Mergenhagen, eds.), pp. 121–131. Am. Soc. Microbiol., Washington, D.C.

13. Cisar, J. O., Barsumian, E. L., Curl, S. H., Vatter, A. E., Sandberg, A. L., and Siraganian, R. P. (1980). The use of monoclonal antibodies in the study of lactose-sensitive adherence of *Actinomyces viscosus* T14V. *Res, J. Reticuloendothel. Soc.* **28**, Suppl., 73–79.

14. Cisar, J. O., Barsumian, E. L., Curl, S. H., Vatter, A. E., Sandberg, A. L., and Siraganian, R. P. (1981). Detection and location of a lectin of *Actinomyces viscosus* T14V by monoclonal antibodies. *J. Immunol.* **127**, 1318–1322.

15. Cisar, J. O., Curl, S. H., Kolenbrander, P. E., and Vatter, A. E. (1983). Specific absence of type 2 fimbriae on a coaggregation-defective mutant of *Actinomyces viscosus* T14V. *Infect. Immun.* **40**, 759–765.

16. Clark, W. B. (1985). *Actinomyces* fimbriae and adherence to hydroxyapatite. *In* "Molecular Basis of Oral Microbial Adhesion" (S. E. Mergenhagen and B. Rosan, eds.), pp. 103–108. Am. Soc. Microbiol., Washington, D.C.

17. Clark, W. B., Wheeler, T. T., and Cisar, J. O. (1984). Specific inhibition of adsorption of *Actinomyces viscosus* T14V to saliva-treated hydroxyapatite by antibody against type 1 fimbriae. *Infect. Immun.* **43**, 497–501.

18. Cohn, V., Neiders, M. E., Hammond, P., and Genco, R. J. (1983). Production of monoclonal antibodies to *Actinobacillus actinomycetemcomitans*. *J. Dent. Res.* **62**, 208. (Abstr.)

19. Coley, J., Duckworth, M., and Baddiley, J. (1972). The occurrence of lipoteichoic acid in the membranes of gram-positive bacteria. *J. Gen. Microbiol.* **73**, 587–591.

20. Coykendall, A. L. (1977). Proposal to elevate the subspecies of *Streptococcus mutans* to species stature, based on their molecular composition. *Int. J. Syst. Bacteriol.* **27**, 26–30.

21. Coykendall, A. L., and Munzenmaier, A. J. (1979). Deoxyribonucleic acid hybridization among strains of *Actinomyces viscosus* and *Actinomyces naeslundii*. *Int. J. Syst. Bacteriol.* **29**, 236–240.

22. Cunningham, A. J., and Szenberg, A. (1968). Further improvements in the plaque techniques for detecting single antibody-forming cells. *Immunology* **14**, 599.

23. DiRienzo, J. M., Porter-Kaufman, J., Haller, J., and Rosan, B. (1985). Corncob formation: A morphological model for molecular studies of bacterial interactions. *In* "Molecular Basis of Oral Microbial Adhesion" (S. E. Mergenhagen and B. Rosan, eds.), pp. 172–176. Am. Soc. Microbiol., Washington, D.C.

24. DiRienzo, J. M., and Speiler, E. L. (1983). Identification and characterization of the major cell envelope proteins of oral strains of *Actinobacillus actinomycetemcomitans*. *Infect. Immun.* **39**, 253–261.

25. DiRienzo, J. M., Tsai, C.-C., Shenker, B. J., Taichman, N. S., and Lally, E. T. (1985). Monoclonal antibodies to the leukotoxin of *Actinobacillus actinomycetemcomitans*. *Infect. Immun.* **47**, 31–36.

26. Dresser, D. W., and Greaves, M. F. (1973). Assays for antibody-producing cells. *In* "Handbook of Experimental Immunology" (D. M. Weir, ed.), 2nd Ed., Chap. 27. Blackwell, Oxford.

27. Fachon-Kalweit, S., Elder, B. L., and Fives-Taylor, P. (1985). Antibodies that bind to fimbriae block adhesion of *Streptococcus sanguis* to saliva-coated hydroxyapatite. *Infect. Immun.* **48**, 617–624.

28. Fillery, E. D., Bowden, G. H., and Hardie, J. M. (1978). A comparison of strains of bacteria designated *Actinomyces viscosus* and *Actinomyces naeslundii*. *Caries Res.* **12**, 299–312.

29. Fukui, K., Fukui, Y., and Moriyama, T. (1974). Purification and properties of dextransucrase and invertase from *Streptococcus mutans* HS6. *J. Bacteriol.* **118**, 796–804.

30. Furuta, T., Nisizawa, T., Chiba, J., and Hamada, S. (1983). Production of monoclonal antibody against a glucosyltransferase of *Streptococcus mutans* 6715. *Infect. Immun.* **41**, 872–875.

31. Gefter, M., Margulies, D., and Scharff, M. (1977). A simple method for polyethylene glycol-promoted hybridization of mouse myeloma cells. *Somatic Cell Genet.* **3**, 231–236.

32. Gibbons, R. J., Berman, K. S., Knoettner, P., and Kapsimalis, B. (1966). Dental caries and alveolar bone loss in gnotobiotic rats infected with capsule forming streptococci of human origin. *Arch. Oral Biol.* **11**, 549–560.

33. Gibbons, R. J., and MacDonald, J. B. (1961). Degradation of collagenous substrates by *Bacteroides melaninogenicus*. *J. Bacteriol.* **81**, 614–621.

34. Gmür, R., and Guggenheim, B. (1983). Antigenic heterogeneity of *Bacteroides intermedius* as recognized by monoclonal antibodies. *Infect. Immun.* **42**, 459–470.

35. Gmür, R., and Wyss, C. (1985). Monoclonal antibodies to characterize the antigenic heterogeneity of *Bacteroides intermedius*. *In* "Monoclonal Antibodies against Bacteria" (A. J. L. Macario and E. Conway de Macario, eds.), Vol. I, pp. 91–119. Academic Press, Orlando, Florida.

36. Guggenheim, B., and Newbrun, E. (1969). Extracellular glucosyltransferase activity of an HS strain of *Streptococcus mutans*. *Helv. Odontol. Acta* **13**, 84–97.

37. Hamada, S., Gill, K., and Slade, H. D. (1976). Chemical and immunological properties of the type f polysaccharide antigen of *Streptococcus mutans*. *Infect. Immun.* **14**, 203–211.

38. Hamada, S., Ooshima, T., Torii, M., Imanishi, H., Masuda, N., Sobue, S., and Kotani, S. (1978). Dental caries induction in experimental animals by clinical strains of *Streptococcus mutans* isolated from Japanese children. *Microbiol. Immunol.* **22**, 301–314.

39. Hamada, S., and Slade, H. D. (1980). Biology, immunology, and cariogenicity of *Streptococcus mutans*. *Microbiol. Rev.* **44**, 331–384.

40. Hanazawa, S., Saitoh, K., Ohmori, Y., Nishihara, H., Fujiwara, S., and Kitano, S. (1984). Production of monoclonal antibodies that recognize specific and cross-reactive antigens of *Bacteroides gingivalis*. *Infect. Immun.* **46**, 285–287.

41. Hirst, T. R., Randall, L. L., and Hardy, S. J. S. (1984). Cellular location of heat-labile enterotoxin in *Escherichia coli*. *J. Bacteriol.* **157**, 637–642.

42. Hofstad, T. (1970). Biological activities of endotoxins from *Bacteroides melaninogenicus*. *Arch. Oral Biol.* **15**, 343–348.

43. Hughes, M., MacHardy, S. M., Sheppard, A. J., Davies, P., and Ivanyi, J. (1982). Use of monoclonal antibody for the preparation of a dental caries vaccine. *J. Dent. Res.* **61**, 546. (Abstr.)

44. Iacono, V. J., Taubman, M. A., Smith, D. J., and Levine, M. J. (1975). Isolation and immunochemical characterization of the group-specific antigen of *Streptococcus mutans* 6715. *Infect. Immun.* **11**, 117–128.

45. Jackson, D. E., Wong, W., Largen, M. T., and Shockman, G. D. (1984). Monoclonal antibodies to immunodeterminants of lipoteichoic acids. *Infect. Immun.* **43**, 800–803.

46. Jerne, N. K., Nordin, A. A., and Henry, C. (1963). The agar plaque technique for recognizing antibody-producing cells. *In* "Cell-Bound Antibodies" (B. Amos and H. Koprowski, eds.), pp. 109–125. Wistar Inst. Press, Philadelphia, Pennsylvania.

47. Johnson, J. L., and Holdeman, L. V. (1983). *Bacteroides intermedius* comb. nov. and descriptions of *Bacteroides corporis* sp. nov. and *Bacteroides levii* sp. nov. *Int. J. Syst. Bacteriol.* **33**, 15–25.

48. Jordan, H. V., and Keyes, P. H. (1964). Aerobic, gram-positive, filamentous bacteria as etiological agents of experimnal periodontal disease in hamsters. *Arch. Oral Biol.* **9**, 401–414.

49. Jordan, H. V., Keyes, P. H., and Bellack, S. (1972). Periodontal lesions in hamsters and gnotobiotic rats infected with *Actinomyces* of human origin. *J. Periodont. Res.* **7**, 21–28.

50. Kamen, P. R. (1983). Inhibition of keratinocyte proliferation by extracts of *Actinobacillus actinomycetemcomitans. Infect. Immun.* **42**, 1191–1194.

51. Kenny, G. E., and Dunsmoor, C. L. (1983). Principles, problems, and strategies in the use of antigenic mixtures for the enzyme-linked immunosorbent assay. *J. Clin. Microbiol.* **17**, 655–665.

52. Kiley, P., and Holt, S. C. (1980). Characterization of the lipopolysaccharide from *Actinobacillus actinomycetemcomitans* Y4 and N27. *Infect. Immun.* **30**, 862–873.

53. Klass, J., Berthold, P., and McArthur, W. (1982). Monoclonal antibodies against *Actinobacillus actinomycetemcomitans. J. Dent. Res.* **61**, 333. (Abstr.)

54. Knox, K. W., Markham, J. L., and Wicken, J. A. (1976). Formation of cross-reacting antibodies against cellular and extracellular lipoteichoic acid of *Streptococcus mutans* BHT. *Infect. Immun.* **13**, 647–652.

55. Knox, K. W., and Wicken, A. J. (1973). Immunological properties of lipoteichoic acids. *Bacteriol. Rev.* **37**, 215–257.

56. Krasse, B., and Carlsson, J. (1970). Various types of streptococci and experimental caries in hamsters. *Arch. Oral Biol.* **15**, 25–32.

57. Kuramitsu, H. K. (1975). Characterization of extracellular glucosyltransferase activity of *Streptococcus mutans. Infect. Immun.* **12**, 738–749.

58. Lambe, D. W., Jr. (1974). Determination of *Bacteroides melaninogenicus* serogroups by fluorescent antibody staining. *Appl. Microbiol.* **28**, 561–567.

59. Lancy, P., Jr., Appelbaum, B., Holt, S. C., and Rosan, B. (1980). Quantitative *in vitro* assay for "corncob" formation. *Infect. Immun.* **29**, 663–670.

60. Lancy, P., Jr., DiRienzo, J. M., Appelbaum, B., Rosan, B., and Holt, S. C. (1983). Corncob formation between *Fusobacterium nucleatum* and *Streptococcus sanguis. Infect. Immun.* **40**, 303–309.

61. Lehner, T., Russell, M. W., Caldwell, J., and Smith, R. (1982). Immunization with purified protein antigens from *Streptococcus mutans* against dental caries in Rhesus monkeys. *Infect. Immun.* **34**, 407–415.

62. Lehner, T., Wilton, J. M. A., Ivanyi, L., and Manson, J. D. (1975). Immunological aspects of juvenile periodontitis (periodontosis). *J. Periodont. Res.* **9**, 261–272.

63. Linzer, R., Gill, K., and Slade, H. D. (1976). Chemical composition of *Streptococcus mutans* type c antigen: Comparison to type a, b, and d antigens. *J. Dent. Res.* **55**, 109A–115A.

64. Linzer, R., and Slade, H. D. (1974). Purification and characterization of *Streptococcus mutans* group d cell wall polysaccharide antigen. *Infect. Immun.* **10**, 361–368.

65. Listgarten, M. A., Lai, C.-H., and Evian, C. I. (1981). Comparative antibody titers to *Ac-*

tinobacillus actinomycetemcomitans in juvenile periodontitis, chronic periodontitis and periodontally healthy subjects. *J. Clin. Periodontol.* **8**, 155–164.

66. Mandell, R. L., and Socransky, S. S. (1981). A selective medium for *Actinobacillus actinomycetemcomitans* and the incidence of the organism in juvenile periodontitis. *J. Periodontol.* **52**, 593–598.

67. Markham, J. L., Knox, K. W., Wicken, A. J., and Hewett, M. J. (1975). Formation of extracellular lipoteichoic acid by oral streptococci and lactobacilli. *Infect. Immun.* **12**, 378–386.

68. Marx, A., Petcovici, M., Bittner, J., Antohi, M., and Ardeleanu, J. (1982). Isolation and characterization of a cross-reacting antigen in strains of Bacteroidaceae. Infect. Immun. **36**, 943–948.

69. McArthur, W., and Klass, J. (1983). Monoclonal antibody analysis of *Actinobacillus actinomycetemcomitans*. *J. Dent. Res.* **62**, 657. (Abstr.)

70. McArthur, W. P., Stroup, S., and Scidmore, N. (1985). Identification and partial characterization of *Actinobacillus actinomycetemcomitans* serotype antigens. *J. Dent. Res.* **64**, 371. (Abstr.)

71. Melvaer, K. L., Helgeland, K., and Rolla, G. (1974). A charged component in purified polysaccharide preparations from *Streptococcus mutans* and *Streptococcus sanquis*. *Arch. Oral Biol.* **19**, 589–595.

72. Michalek, S. M., McGhee, J. R., and Navia, J. M. (1975). Virulence of *Streptococcus mutans:* A sensitive method for evaluating cariogenicity in young, gnotobiotic rats. *Infect. Immun.* **12**, 69–75.

73. Miller, J. H. (1972). "Experiments in Molecular Genetics." Cold Spring Harbor Lab., Cold Spring Harbor, New York.

74. Mishell, R. I., and Dutton, R. W. (1967). Immunization of dissociated spleen cell cultures from normal mice. *J. Exp. Med.* **126**, 423.

75. Mohan, S. B., Newman, B. M., and Cole, J. A. (1979). The interconversion of dextranase and mutansucrase activities from cariogenic strains of *Streptococcus mutans*. *FEMS Microbiol. Lett.* **5**, 69–72.

76. Moore, W. E. C., Holdeman, L. V., Cato, E. P., Smibert, R. M., Burmeister, J. A., Palcanis, K. G., and Ranney, R. R. (1985). Comparative bacteriology of juvenile periodontitis. *Infect. Immun.* **48**, 507–519.

77. Moore, W. E. C., Holdeman, L. V., Smibert, R. M., Hash, D. E., Burmeister, J. A., and Ranney, R. R. (1982). Bacteriology of severe periodontitis in young adult humans. *Infect. Immun.* **38**, 1137–1148.

78. Moore, W. E. C., Ranney, R. R., and Holdeman, L. V. (1982). Subgingival microflora in periodontal disease: Cultural studies. *In* "Host–Parasite Interactions in Periodontal Diseases" (R. J. Genco and S. E. Mergenhagen, eds.), pp. 13–26. Am. Soc. Microbiol., Washington, D.C.

79. Mouton, C., Hammond, P. G., Slots, J., Reed, M. J., and Genco, R. J. (1981). Identification of *Bacteroides gingivalis* by fluorescent antibody staining. *Ann. Microbiol. (Paris)* **132B**, 69–83.

80. Mukasa, H., and Slade, H. D. (1973). Structure and immunological specificity of the *Streptococcus mutans* group b cell wall antigen. *Infect. Immun.* **7**, 578–585.

81. Mukasa, H., and Slade, H. D. (1973). Extraction, purification, and chemical and immunological properties of the *Streptococcus mutans* group "a" polysaccharide cell wall antigen. *Infect. Immun.* **8**, 190–198.

82. Mukasa, H., and Slade, H. D. (1973). Mechanism of adherence of *Streptococcus mutans* to smooth surfaces. I. Roles of insoluble dextran-levan synthetase enzymes and cell wall polysaccharide antigen in plaque formation. *Infect. Immun.* **8**, 555–562.

83. Musaka, H., and Slade, H. D. (1974). Mechanism of adherence of *Streptococcus mutans*

smooth surfaces. III. Purification and properties of the enzyme complex responsible for adherence. *Infect. Immun.* **10**, 1135–1145.

83a. Naito, Y., Okuda, K., Kato, T., and Takazoe, I. (1985). Monoclonal antibodies against surface antigens of *Bacteroides gingivalis*. *Infect. Immun.* **50**, 231–235.

84. Nakamura, T., Suginaka, Y., and Takazoe, I. (1976). Heparinase activity in lesion of periodontal diseases. *Bull. Tokyo Dent. Coll.* **17**, 147–155.

85. Neu, H. C., and Heppel, L. A. (1965). The release of enzymes from *Escherichia coli* by osmotic shock and during the formation of spheroplasts. *J. Biol. Chem.* **240**, 3685–3692.

86. Nossal, G. J. V., Lewis, H., and Warner, N. L. (1971). Differential sensitivity of haemolytic plaque methods at various stages of the immune response. *Cell. Immunol.* **2**, 13.

87. Nowotny, A., Behling, U. H., Hammond, B., Lai, C.-H., Listgarten, M., Pham, P. H., and Sanavi, F. (1982). Release of toxic microvesicles by *Actinobacillus actinomycetemcomitans*. *Infect. Immun.* **37**, 151–154.

88. Okuda, K., and Takazoe, I. (1973). Antiphagocytic effects of the capsular structure of a pathogenic strain of *Bacteroides melaninogenicus*. *Bull. Tokyo Dent. Coll.* **14**, 99–104.

89. Perch, B., Kjems, E., and Ravn, T. (1974). Biochemical and serological properties of *Streptococcus mutans* from various human and naimal sources. *Acta Pathol. Microbiol. Scand.* **82**, 357–370.

90. Pulverer, G., Ko, H. L., Wegrzynowicz, Z., and Jeljaszewicz, J. (1977). Clotting and fibrinolytic activities of *Bacteroides melaninogenicus*. *Zentralbl. Bakteriol. Parsitenkd. Infektionskr. Hyg., Abt. 1: Orig.. Reihe A* **239**, 510–513.

91. Ranney, R. R., Yanni, N. R., Burmeister, J. A., and Tew, J. G. (1982). Relationship between attachment loss and pr-cipitating antibody to *Actinobacillus actinomycetemcomitans* in adolescents and young adults having severe periodontal destruction. *J. Periodontol.* **53**, 1–7.

92. Reed, M. J., Slots, J., Mouton, C., and Genco, R. J. (1980). Antigenic studies of oral and nonoral black-pigmented *Bacteroides* strains. *Infect. Immun.* **29**, 564–574.

93. Robertson, P. B., Lantz, M., Marucha, P. T., Kornman, K. S., Trummel, C. L., and Holt, S. C. (1982). Collagenolytic activity associated with *Bacteroides* species and *Actinobacillus actinomycetemcomitans*. *J. Periodont. Res.* **17**, 275–283.

94. Russell, M. W. (1979). Purification and properties of a protein surface antigen of *Streptococcus mutans*. *Microbios* **25**, 7–18.

95. Russell, M. W., Bergmeier, L. A., Zanders, E. D., and Lehner, T. (1980). Protein antigens of *Streptococcus mutans:* Purification and properties of a double antigen and its protease-resistant component. *Infect. Immun.* **28**, 486–493.

96. Russell, M. W., and Lehner, T. (1978). Characterization of antigens extracted from cells and culture fluids of *Streptococcus mutans* serotype c. *Arch. Oral Biol.* **23**, 7–15.

97. Russell, M. W., Zanders, E. D., Bergmeier, L. A., and Lehner, T. (1980). Affinity purification and characterization of protease-susceptible antigen I of *Streptococcus mutans*. *Infect. Immun.* **29**, 999–1006.

98. Sato, K., Slesinski, R., and Littlefield, J. (1972). Chemical mutagenesis at the phosphoribosyl transferase locus in cultured human lymphoblasts. *Proc. Natl. Acad. Sci. U.S.A.* **69**, 1244–1248.

99. Scales, W. R., Long, L. W., and Edwards, J. R. (1975). Purification and characterization of a glycosyltransferase complex from the culture broth of *Streptococcus mutans* FA1. *Carbohydr. Res.* **42**, 325–338.

100. Scherp, H. W. (1971). Dental caries: Prospects for prevention. *Science* **173**, 1199–1205.

101. Sharpe, M. E., Brock, J. H., Knox, K. W., and Wicken, A. J. (1973). Glycerol teichoic acid as a common antigenic factor in lactobacilli and some other gram-positive organisms. *J. Gen. Microbiol.* **74**, 119–126.

102. Shenker, B. J., Kushner, M. E. and Tsai, C.-C. (1982). Inhibition of fibroblast proliferation by *Actinobacillus actinomycetemcomitans*. *Infect. Immun.* **38**, 986–992.
103. Shenker, B. J., McArthur, W. P., and Tsai, C.-C. (1982). Immune suppression induced by *Actinobacillus actinomycetemcomitans*. I. Effects on human peripheral blood lymphocyte responses to mitogens and antigens. *J. Immunol.* **128**, 148–154.
104. Shklair, I. L., and Keene, H. J. (1974). A biochemical scheme for the separation of the five varieties of *Streptococcus mutans*. *Arch. Oral Biol.* **19**, 1079–1081.
105. Shklair, I. L., and Keene, H. J. (1976). Biochemical characterization and distribution of *Streptococcus mutans* in three diverse populations. *In* "Proceedings: Microbial Aspects of Dental Caries" (H. M. Stiles, W. J. Loesche, and T. C. O'Brien, eds.), Microbiology Abstracts, Vol. 3, Spec. Suppl., pp. 201–210. Inf. Retrieval, Washington, D.C.
106. Shklair, I. L., Simonson, L. G., Bial, J. J., and Quiring, R. C. (1985). Diagnostic value of a coagglutination procedure using monoclonal antibodies to *B. gingivalis*. *J. Dent. Res.* **64**, 354. (Abstr.)
107. Shulman, M., Wilde, C. D., and Kohler, G. (1978). A better cell line for making hybridomas secreting specific antibodies. *Nature (London)* **276**, 269–271.
108. Simonson, L. G., Merrell, B., Rouse, R., and Shklair, I. L. (1985). Production and characterization of monoclonal antibodies to *Bacteroides gingivalis*. *J. Dent. Res.* **64**, 354. (Abstr.)
108a. Simonson, L. G., Merrell, B. R., Rouse, R. F., and Shklair, I. L. (1986). Production and characterization of monoclonal antibodies to *Bacteroides gingivalis*. *J. Dent. Res.* **65**, 95–97.
109. Slack, J., der Balian, G. P., Nahm, M., and Davie, J. M. (1980). Subclass restriction of murine antibodies. II. The IgG plaque-forming cell response to thymus-independent Type 1 and Type 2 antigens in normal mice and mice expressing an x-linked immunodeficiency. *J. Exp. Med.* **151**, 853–862.
110. Slack, J. M., and Gerencser, M. A. (1975). "Actinomyces Filamentous Bacteria: Biology and Pathogenicity." Burgess, Minneapolis, Minnesota.
111. Slots, J. (1976). The predominant cultivable organisms in juvenile periodontitis. *Scand. J. Dent. Res.* **84**, 1–10.
112. Slots, J. (1979). Subgingival microflora and periodontal disease. *J. Clin. Periodontol.* **6**, 351–382.
113. Slots, J. (1981). Enzymatic characterization of some oral and nonoral gram-negative bacteria with the API ZYM system. *J. Clin. Microbiol.* **14**, 288–294.
114. Slots, J., Evans, R. T., Lobbins, P. M., and Genco, R. J. (1980). *In vitro* antimicrobial susceptibility of *Actinobacillus actinomycetemcomitans*. *Antimicrob. Agents Chemother.* **18**, 9–12.
115. Slots, J., Reynolds, H. S., and Genco, R. J. (1980). *Actinobacillus actinomycetemcomitans* in human periodontal disease: A cross-sectional microbiological investigation. *Infect. Immun.* **29**, 1013–1020.
116. Slots, J., Rosling, B., and Genco, R. J. (1983). Suppression of penicillin-resistant oral *Actinobacillus actinomycetemcomitans* with tetracycline: Considerations in endocarditis prophylaxis. *J. Periodontol.* **54**, 193–196.
117. Slots, J., Zambon, J. J., Rosling, B. G., Reynolds, H. S., Christersson, L. A., and Genco, R. J. (1982). *Actinobacillus actinomycetemcomitans* in human periodontal disease. Association, serology, leukotoxicity and treatment. *J. Periodontal Res.* **17**, 447–448.
118. Smith, R., Lehner, T., and Beverley, P. C. L. (1984). Characterization of monoclonal antibodies to *Streptococcus mutans* antigenic determinants I/II, I, II, and III and their serotype specificities. *Infect. Immun.* **46**, 168–175.
119. Socransky, S. S. (1970). Relationship of bacteria to the etiology of periodontal disease. *J. Dent. Res.* **49**, 203–222.
120. Socransky, S. S., Hubersak, C., and Propas, D. (1970). Induction of periodontal destruction in

gnotobiotic rats by a human oral strain of *Actinomyces naeslundii. Arch. Oral Biol.* **15,** 993–995.

121. Socransky, S. S., Tanner, A. C. R., Haffajee, A. D., Hillman, J. D., and Goodson, J. M. (1982). Present status of studies on the microbial etiology of periodontal diseases. *In* "Host–Parasite Interactions in Periodontal Diseases" (R. J. Genco and S. E. Mergenhagen, eds.), pp. 1–12. Am. Soc. Microbiol., Washington, D.C.

122. Stevens, R. H., Hammond, B. F., and Lai, C. H. (1982). Characterization of an inducible bacteriophage from a leukotoxic strain of *Actinobacillus actinomycetemcomitans. Infect. Immun.* **35,** 343–349.

123. Syed, S. A., Loesche, W. J., Pape, H. L., and Grenier, E. (1975). Predominant cultivable flora isolated from human root surface plaque. *Infect. Immun.* **11,** 727–731.

124. Taichman, N. S., McArthur, W. P., Tsai, C.-C., Baehni, P. C., Shenker, B. J., Berthold, P., Evian, C., and Stevens, R. (1982). Leukocidal mechanisms of *Actinobacillus actinomycetemcomitans. In* "Host—Parasite Interactions in Periodontal Diseases" (R. J. Genco and S. E. Mergenhagen, eds.), pp. 261–269. Am. Soc. Microbiol., Washington, D.C.

125. Taichman, N. S., Shenker, B. J., Tsai, C.-C., Glickman, L. T., Baehni, P. C., Stevens, R., and Hammond, B. F. (1984). Cytopathic effects of *Actinobacillus actinomycetemcomitans* on monkey blood leukocytes. *J. Periodont. Res.* **19,** 133–145.

126. Towbin, H., Staehelin, T., and Gordon, J. (1979). Electrophoretic transfer of proteins from polyacrylamide gels to nitrocellulose sheets: Procedure and some applications. *Proc. Natl. Acad. Sci. U.S.A.* **76,** 4350–4354.

127. Tsai, C.-C., McArthur, W. P., Baehni, P. C., Evian, C., Genco, R. J., and Taichman, N. S. (1981). Serum neutralizing activity against *Actinobacillus actinomycetemcomitans* leukotoxin in juvenile periodontitis. *J. Clin. Periodontol.* **8,** 338–348.

128. Tsai, C.-C., Shenker, B. J., DiRienzo, J. M., Malamud, D., and Taichman, N. S. (1984). Extraction and isolation of a leukotoxin from *Actinobacillus actinomycetemcomitans* with polymyxin B. *Infect. Immun.* **43,** 700–705.

129. van Palenstein-Helderman, W. H. (1981). Microbial etiology of periodontal disease. *J. Clin. Periodontol.* **8,** 261–280.

130. van Steenbergen, T. J. M., Vlaanderen, C. A., and de Graaff, J. (1982). Deoxyribonucleic acid homologies among strains of *Bacteroides melaninogenicus* and related species. *J. Appl. Bacteriol.* **53,** 269–276.

131. Wetherell, J. R., Jr., and Bleiweis, A. S. (1975). Antigens of *Streptococcus mutans:* Characterization of a polysaccharide antigen from walls of strain GS-5. *Infect. Immun.* **12,** 1341–1348.

132. Wetherell, J. R., and Bleiweis, A. S. (1978). Antigens of *Streptococcus mutans:* Isolation of a serotype-specific and a cross-reactive antigen from walls of strain V-100 (serotype e). *Infect. Immun.* **19,** 160–169.

133. Wheeler, T. T., and Clark, W. B. (1980). Fibril-mediated adherence of *Actinomyces viscosus* to saliva-treated hydroxyapatite. *Infect. Immun.* **28,** 577–584.

134. Wicken, A. J., and Knox, K. W. (1974). Lipoteichoic acids—a new class of baterial antigens. *Science* **187,** 1161–1167.

135. Zambon, J. J. (1985). *Actinobacillus actinomycetemcomitans* in human periodontal disease. *J. Clin. Periodontol.* **12,** 1–20.

136. Zambon, J. J., DeLuca, C., Slots, J., and Genco, R. J. (1983). Studies of leukotoxin from *Actinobacillus actinomycetemcomitans* using the promyelocytic HL-60 cell line. *Infect. Immun.* **40,** 205–212.

137. Zambon, J. J., Slots, J., and Genco, R. J. (1983). Serology of oral *Actinobacillus actinomycetemcomitans* and serotype distribution in human periodontal disease. *Infect. Immun.* **41,** 19–27.

138. Zambon, J. J., Slots, J., Miyasaki, K., Linzer, R., Cohen, R., Levine, M., and Genco, R. J. (1984). Purification and characterization of theserotype c antigen from *Actinobacillus actinomycetemcomitans*. *Infect. Immun.* **44**, 22–27.
139. Zanders, E. D., and Lehner, T. (1981). Separation and characterization of a protein antigen from cells of *Streptococcus mutans*. *J. Gen. Microbiol.* **122**, 217–225.

12

Current and Future Applications of Monoclonal Antibodies against Bacteria in Veterinary Medicine

DAVID M. SHERMAN AND R. J. F. MARKHAM[1]
Department of Large Animal Clinical Sciences
College of Veterinary Medicine
University of Minnesota
St. Paul, Minnesota

I. INTRODUCTION

Since Kohler and Milstein first reported the development of hybridoma technology in 1975, a revolution has taken place in biomedical research and clinical medicine. In the area of infectious diseases, monoclonal antibodies have been used as powerful probes for defining the antigenic structure, virulence mechanisms, and host responses to a broad range of pathogens including bacteria (72), viruses (164), and parasites (89). Numerous advances in immunodiagnosis, pro-

[1]Present address: Department of Pathology and Microbiology, Faculty of Veterinary Medicine, University of Prince Edward Island, Charlottetown, Prince Edward Island, Canada C1A 4P3.

295

phylaxis, and therapy have resulted, and future applications are forthcoming, at an ever-accelerating rate (26).

A general introduction to hybridoma technology and potential applications of monoclonal antibodies in veterinary medicine first appeared in the veterinary literature in 1982 (5). As is often the case, new knowledge leads to increased specialization, as evidenced by this present volume focusing on monoclonal antibodies solely against bacteria. This particular chapter is further specialized, and deals specifically with a discussion of current and future applications for monoclonal antibodies against bacteria in clinical veterinary medicine.

II. BACKGROUND

Researchers and clinicians in veterinary medicine are cognizant of the tremendous impact that monoclonal antibodies are having in the areas of biomedical research and clinical application in human medicine, and reports of research involving monoclonal antibodies have begun to appear in the veterinary literature. Relatively little research activity however, is directed toward the study of bacteria. The cumulative Index Veterinarius for 1982 had no entries under monoclonal antibodies, while the 1983 edition had 69. Most entries dealt with viral antigens and identifiction of eukaryotic cell surface markers. Only three papers dealt specifically with bacterial antigens. In the 1984 edition, 7 of 71 monoclonal antibody citations involved bacteria, while in 1985, 22 of 102 entries dealt specifically with bacteria. In view of the scarcity of published material, the emphasis in this chapter on current and future applications of monoclonal antibodies in veterinary medicine will out of necessity deal largely with future uses.

Understanding and controlling infectious disease continues to be a major challenge in veterinary medicine, and bacterial pathogens are still a major concern. In 1984, $6 million in research funds were available for veterinary research from the United States Department of Agriculture, Science and Education Administration, on a competitive basis to study all animal diseases (31). Sixty-six percent of these funds were awarded to researchers studying infectious disease problems, and 44% of this portion went specifically to the study of bacterial diseases. It is reasonable to assume that an increasing number of bacterial disease investigations will include the use of monoclonal antibodies in the future.

Four major uses for monoclonal antibodies against bacteria in veterinary medicine are readily identifiable: characterization of bacterial antigens and virulence factors, elucidation of the pathogenesis of bacterial infections, improvements in immunodiagnosis, and clinical applications in treatment and prophylaxis. The focus of this presentation will be primarily on diagnostic and clinical applications, acknowledging from the outset that advances in these areas depend critically on advances in basic research on the structure and function of bacterial pathogens. The recent development of a monoclonal antibody to the K99 pilus of enteropathogenic *E. coli* for passive immunization of calves against enteric colibacillosis (127) was only possible because the development of hybridoma technology was preceded by years of basic research by numerous workers on the identification of adherence factors on enteric bacteria and their role in the pathogenesis of diarrhea (34). The antigenic structures, virulence attributes, and pathogenic mechanisms of many important bacterial pathogens in veterinary medicine are still uncharacterized. Now that hybridoma technology is readily available as a research tool, monoclonal antibodies will undoubtedly aid in first defining these unknowns and then providing new diagnostic and clinical applications.

There are certain limitations in the practice of veterinary medicine which make the potential diagnostic and clinical uses of monoclonal antibodies very attractive. The food animal practitioner must often carry out a thorough clinical examination and diagnostic workup in the isolation of a barn or feedlot, arrive at a specific diagnosis, and institute a therapeutic plan, all in a single farm visit. When an entire herd or flock is threatened with the spread of a rapidly disseminated infectious disease, this process takes on some urgency and the accuracy of the diagnosis becomes extremely important. Submission of samples to a distant diagnostic laboratory can be impractical. The development of rapid, reliable immunodiagnostic test kits for use on the farm is a recognized need. Certain immunodiagnostic procedures, such as enzyme-linked immunosorbent assays (ELISA), are adaptable for on-farm or in-practice use, and the inclusion of monoclonal antibodies as reagents in these kits will greatly enhance their practicality. The specificity of monoclonal antibodies would allow diagnostic tests to be performed directly on crude specimens such as feces, pus, mastitic milk, and tracheal lavage fluid without the intermediate step of bacterial culture (26). Furthermore, these monospecific reagents virtually eliminate the problems of cross-reactivity which can occur with conventionally derived polyclonal reagents. Specific diseases in which such diagnostic capability would be advantageous to the practitioner will be discussed.

A clinical application with tremendous potential in veterinary medicine is disease prevention by passive immunization, particularly when a newly initiated infection threatens to spread rapidly through a susceptible herd or flock. In many situations, numerous extrinsic factors play a role in the initiation and spread of bacterial disease. These factors include weather conditions, concurrent viral infections, sanitation, nutritional status, stress factors, stocking rates, ventilation, and recent transport (12). Disease outbreaks are often explosive and unpredictable. In many cases, active immunization with vaccines has not been undertaken because disease outbreaks were unexpected, efficacious vaccines are not available, or the cost–benefit ratio of prophylaxis was not considered. In situations such as these, the practitioner currently must intervene with antibiotic therapy in an effort to reduce morbidity and mortality. However, the use of antibiotic therapy in food-producing animals is coming under increasing scrutiny due to concern about transfer of drug resistance from animal to human pathogens (55). Intervention with parenteral administration of monoclonal antibodies directed against specific virulence factors of the pathogens involved in order to reduce morbidity offers an attractive alternative to antibiotic therapy. As the knowledge of virulence factors in bacterial pathogens increases, more disease outbreaks will undoubtedly be handled in this way. Specific disease entities where this approach is currently being employed as well as diseases in which such intervention is likely to be successful will be discussed in detail.

III. RESULTS AND DISCUSSION

Practical applications of monoclonal antibodies in clinical veterinary medicine must be preceded by a firm basic knowledge of the structural character, virulence factors, and pathogenic mechanisms of disease-producing bacteria. The structure of this chapter is based on the structure of bacteria. It should become readily apparent that as more is known about the role of a particular structural component in the causation of disease, the more firmly based is speculation about the applications of monoclonal antibodies against that bacterial component.

The limitations of space prohibit extensive discussions of the disease conditions presented in this chapter. Although an attempt is made to provide sufficient background material on each disease, readers not familiar with clinical veterinary medicine are referred to a standard textbook of veterinary medicine for further clarification (12).

A. Bacterial Pilus Antigens

Pili are proteinaceous, filamentous appendages on the cell surface of certain bacteria (34) (Fig. 1). They are also known as fimbriae, adhesins, adherence factors, or colonizing factors. The role of pili in enabling certain pathogens to colonize epithelial surfaces successfully is well established. In human medicine, pili have been recognized as virulence factors in infections with *Neisseria gonorrhoeae* (107), enteropathogenic Escherichia coli (EPEC) (27), and *Pseudomonas aeruginosa* (161), among others. In veterinary medicine, the importance of pilus-mediated adherence has also been identified in EPEC infections causing neonatal enteric colibacillosis of calves, lambs, and pigs (12,34), *Moraxella bovis* infections causing infectious bovine keratoconjunctivitis (IBK; pinkeye) (113), and *Bacteroides nodosus* infections causing foot rot of sheep (145). A role for pilus-mediated adherence is being investigated for a number of other important veterinary pathogens including various *Salmonella* (88), *Pasteurella* (40),

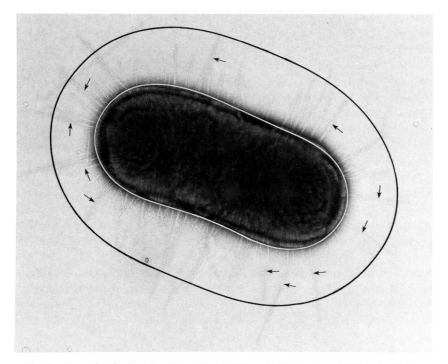

Fig. 1. Example of a heavily piliated *Escherichia coli*. This is *E. coli* O78 isolated from a turkey. (Photograph courtesy of Dr. L. H. Arp, Department of Veterinary Pathology, Iowa State University, Ames, Iowa.)

and *Bordetella* (41) species. This knowledge has led to the development of pilus-enriched vaccines for active immunization against some of these pathogens (2,61,91,94,99,100,121,145,160). In the case of the enteropathogenic *E. coli,* monoclonal antibodies have been developed for diagnostic use as well as for passive immunization of newborn calves and pigs (122,127,159). These developments as well as potential applications of monoclonal antibodies for control of pinkeye, foot rot, and other pilus-mediated infections in veterinary medicine will be discussed.

1. Pili of Enteropathogenic Escherichia coli

a. The K99 Pilus

i. Passive Immunization. The development of a monoclonal antibody against the K99 pilus of EPEC for passive protection of newborn calves against fatal enteric colibacillosis (127) is illustrative of how firm knowledge of the pathogenesis and epidemiology of a specific disease can lead to innovative methods of disease control. Strains of noninvasive *E. coli* capable of producing diarrhea in neonates must possess two virulence factors, both of which are plasmid mediated (44,93). First, they must be enterotoxigenic, possessing either heat-stable or heat-labile enterotoxin capable of inducing hypersecretion by villous epithelial cells. Second, they must possess pili to colonize the gut successfully by adherence to the villous epithelium. The physical proximity of the bacteria to the villous surface, facilitated by pilus adherence, maximizes the deleterious effects of the enterotoxin. Nonpiliated enterotoxigenic strains and piliated nonenterotoxigenic strains cannot produce disease of equal magnitude to the enteropathogenic strains which possess both pilus and toxin.

The K99 pilus is found on EPEC infecting calves, lambs, and pigs (92,104). It was first reported in 1972 and was identified at that time as Kco, the common K antigen (139). In 1975 it was designated as K99 (104). Isolation of the pilus can be accomplished with either a salt extraction procedure, ultrasonication, or mechanically, by heating and shaking of a cell suspension. Early reports on the structure of the K99 pilus suggested that it was composed of two protein subunits, a major component of MW 22,500 and a minor subunit of MW 29,500 (59). More recent work indicates that the pilus is composed of only a single subunit of MW 18,400 (19). Electron microscopic examination of K99 reveals it to be a fimbria of helical configuration with a diameter of 4.8 nm. Purified pili are strongly immunogenic.

The susceptibility of calves and lambs to colonization by K99-positive EPEC is age dependent. These species become resistant to experimental challenge after 2 days of age, as has been demonstrated both *in vivo* and *in vitro* (117,136). Although the nature of this natural resistance is not well understood, the clinical significance of this observation was profound. It led to the hypothesis that if susceptibility to enteric colibacillosis occurs only in the first few days of life, the presence of K99-specific antibody in the gut lumen during that time might successfully block intestinal adherence by K99-positive EPEC, thus inhibiting colonization until such time that the calf possessed natural resistance to infection (2). In livestock species, maternal antibodies are derived from colostral ingestion rather than by transplacental transfer (83). Experiments were undertaken to demonstrate whether cows vaccinated prepartum with killed bacterins containing either K99-positive strains of *E. coli* or purified K99 pili would produce and concentrate K99-specific antibodies in their colostrum. Calves ingesting this colostrum at birth would then be protected from enteric colibacillosis. This hypothesis was proven repeatedly to be accurate in experimental challenge studies (2,47,99). As a result, numerous vaccines have become commercially available for active immunization of the cow for passive protection of the calf. The history of vaccine development in enteric colibacillosis of calves has recently been reviewed (46).

Although these vaccines have been used with apparent success, some practical disadvantages to maternal vaccination have been recognized. Pregnant cows must be handled for vaccination twice during the first year and once during each subsequent year of the vaccination program (48). Some livestock owners are reluctant to accept the cost and inconvenience of preventative vaccination unless they have recently experienced an outbreak of enteric colibacillosis in their herds. Such outbreaks are difficult to predict, since the epizootiology of neonatal calf diarrhea includes a variety of management and environmental factors. When outbreaks do occur suddenly in unvaccinated herds, it is too late to immunize actively those pregnant cows that are close to parturition. These concerns prompted investigation of an alternative method of passive immunization of newborn calves, namely, the oral administration of K99-specific hybridoma-derived monoclonal antibody shortly after birth. The development of this K99-specific monoclonal antibody and its effacacy in protecting calves against fatal enteric colibacillosis in challenge trials has been reported (127). It represents the first known application of a monoclonal antibody for passive immunization against an important bacterial disease. The details of this work will be briefly reviewed.

The source of antigen was the K99 pilus of strain B41 EPEC, isolated and purified according to the method of Isaacson (59). The antigen, in complete Freund's adjuvant was injected into BALB/c mice. Spleens were removed after a series of three antigen injections and hybridomas were produced by polyethylene glycol-mediated fusion of mouse spleen cells with mouse plasmacytoma cell line P3-NS-1-Ag 4/1. Resulting hybridomas were grown in selective medium containing hypoxanthine, aminopterin, and thymidine in 24-well tissue culture plates. Supernatants from wells with hybridoma clones were screened for K99-reactive antibody using an ELISA technique with purified K99 as the antigen. Hybridoma monoclones producing K99-specific monoclonal antibody were isolated by limiting dilution. A single clone (2BD4E4) was selected and injected intraperitoneally into specific pathogen-free BALB/c mice, preconditioned with pristane. Mice were killed 10–60 days later and ascitic fluid aspirated. The fluid was clarified by centrifugation and stored at $-20°C$.

Characterization of the K99-specific monoclonal antibody was accomplished using several techniques including ELISA, bacterial agglutination, and immunoprecipitation of radiolabeled EPEC strain B44. The monoclonal antibody from clone 2BD4E4 was shown to be IgG_1 by ELISA with rabbit anti-mouse IgG_1 antibody. A pool of ascitic fluid from this clone exhibited a titer of 10^{-5} in the K99–ELISA system. Immunoglobulin constituted 45–50% of the protein in the ascites fluid as determined by sodium dodecyl sulfate–polyacrylamide gel electrophoresis (SDS–PAGE) (Fig. 2). The antibody was found to be reactive only with K99 antigen in radioimmunoprecipitation of L-[^{35}S]methionine-labeled *E. coli* lysates followed by SDS–PAGE. This immunoglobulin at an initial concentration of 10 mg/ml agglutinated EPEC strains B44 and B41 grown at 37°C

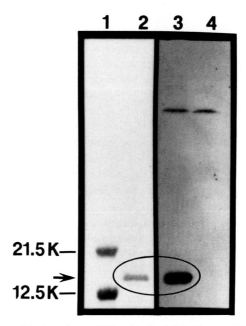

Fig. 2. Immunoprecipitation of an L-[^{35}S]methionine-labeled lysate of EPEC strain B44 with the K99-specific monoclonal antibody orally administered to calves. Immunoprecipitates were subjected to electrophoresis in a 12.5% acrylamide slab gel. Proteins in lanes 1 and 2 were detected by Coomassie Blue staining prior to salicylation of the gel. Molecular weight markers (in thousands, K) are indicated in lane 1. The K99 antigen used subsequently for production of the K99-specific monoclonal antibody is indicated by the arrow in lane 2. Lane 3 represents the radioactive antigen precipitated from EPEC strain B44 by the K99-specific monoclonal antibody. Lane 4 represents a similar precipitate by fibronectin-specific monoclonal antibody. Reprinted from reference 127 by permission of the American Society of Microbiology, Copyright © 1983, from *Infection and Immunity,* 1983, **42,** 653–658.

(K99 pilus expressed) to a dilution of 10^{-4}, but did not agglutinate cells grown at 18°C (K99 pilus not expressed), even when used at 10^{-1}.

Three separate challenge trials were conducted to evaluate the efficacy of orally administered K99-specific monoclonal antibody in protecting neonatal calves against enteric colibacillosis. In the first trial newborn calves were fed colostrum at birth and challenged orally with 2.6×10^{10} organisms of EPEC strain B44 (O9:K30;K99;F41:H−) at 12 hr of age. At 10 hours of age, treated calves received 1 ml of clarified mouse ascites fluid containing K99-specific monoclonal antibody with a titer of 1:12,000 as determined by passive hemagglutination. Control calves received no placebo. In the second and third trials, newborn calves were colostrum deprived at birth. These calves were challenged with an average of 5×10^9 organisms of EPEC strain B44 at 12 hr of age. Treated calves received the same oral dose of mouse ascites fluid at 10 hr of age.

Control calves received a placebo of 1 ml mouse ascites fluid containing monoclonal antibody specific for fibronectin. The only difference between trials 2 and 3 was that in trial 2, calves receiving treatment were known to the investigator while trial 3 was performed as a double blind. In all trials calves were examined every 12 hr and their clinical status was scored based on an assessment of state of dehydration, fecal consistency, and mental attitude, up to 72 hr postchallenge.

Treatment with the K99-specific monoclonal antibody did not affect the incidence of diarrhea after challenge with EPEC strain B44. There was no difference in the proportion of treated and control calves that developed diarrhea in any of the three trials (Table I), nor was there any significant difference in the average score of fecal consistency between treated and control groups in any of the three trials (Table II). As calculated in trial 1 only, there was also no significant difference in the time of onset of diarrhea after challenge between the control and treated calves.

In contrast to the above results, there was a significant difference in the incidence of severe dehydration as measured by estimated loss of skin elasticity between control and treated calves (Table I). The proportion of calves that became severely dehydrated after challenge was significantly lower in calves receiving the K99-specific monoclonal antibody as compared with control calves in all three trials. This reduction was highly significant ($p < 0.001$) when the results of the three trials were combined. There was also a significant reduction

TABLE I

Clinical Response of Calves after Challenge with EPEC Strain B44[a]

Trial	K99-Specific monoclonal antibody-treated calves			Controls		
	Diarrhea[b]	Clinical dehydration[c]	Death	Diarrhea	Clinical dehydration	Death
1	4/7	1/7[d]	1/7[d]	5/7	5/7	5/7
2	5/5	1/5[d]	1/5[d]	4/4	4/4	4/4
3	12/16	6/16[d]	6/16[d]	5/6	5/6	5/6
TOTAL	21/28	8/28[e]	8/28[e]	14/17	14/17	14/17
	(75%)	(29%)	(29%)	(82%)	(82%)	(82%)

[a] Adapted and reprinted from reference 127 by permission of the American Society of Microbiology, Copyright © 1983, from *Infection and Immunity*, 1983, **42**, 653–658.

[b] Expressed as the proportion of calves in the group that developed a fecal consistency score of 3 after challenge. A score of 3 represented severe, watery diarrhea.

[c] Expressed as the proportion of calves in the group that developed a clinical dehydration score of 2, representing severe dehydration.

[d] $p < .05$ versus control by one-tailed χ^2 test.

[e] $p < .001$ versus control by one-tailed χ^2 test.

TABLE II

Mean Clinical Scores of Calves after Challenge with EPEC Strain B44[a,b]

Trial	Calves	MCS (0–8)	DEP (0–3)	DEHY (0–2)	FC (0–3)	Weight loss (kg)	Duration of diarrhea (hr)	Onset of diarrhea after challenge (hr)
1	T	2.9 ± 2.7 (<.05)	0.4 ± 1.1 (<.025)	0.4 ± 0.8 (<.0125)	2.0 ± 1.4 (NS)	ND	22.5 ± 3.0 (<.025)	31.0 ± 24.9 (NS)
	C	6.1 ± 3.3	2.1 ± 1.5	1.6 ± 0.8	2.4 ± 1.1	ND	58.8 ± 42.5	14.8 ± 3.7
2	T	4.2 ± 2.2 (<.005)	0.8 ± 1.3 (<.005)	0.4 ± 0.9 (<.005)	3.0 ± 0 (NS)	3.2 ± 2.8 (<.025)	ND	ND
	C	8.0 ± 0	3.0 ± 0	2.0 ± 0	3.0 ± 0	7.6 ± 2.3	ND	ND
3	T	4.7 ± 2.7 (<.0125)	1.3 ± 1.2 (<.0025)	0.9 ± 1.0 (<.0025)	2.6 ± 0.9 (NS)	3.1 ± 3.0 (<.05)	ND	ND
	C	7.3 ± 1.6	2.7 ± 0.8	1.8 ± 0.4	2.8 ± 0.4	5.9 ± 3.3	ND	ND
Combined	T	4.1 ± 2.4 (<.001)	1.0 ± 1.2 (<.001)	0.7 ± 0.9 (<.001)	2.5 ± 1.0 (NS)	3.1 ± 2.9 (<.0025)	ND	ND
	C	7.0 ± 3.8	2.5 ± 1.1	1.8 ± 0.6	2.7 ± 0.8	6.6 ± 3.0	ND	ND

[a] Adapted and reprinted from reference 127 by permission of the American Society of Microbiology, Copyright © 1983, *Infection and Immunity*, 1983, **42**, 653–658.

[b] All data are expressed as mean ± SD; numbers within parentheses are *p* values versus control, using the one-tailed *t*-test. Abbreviations: T, treated group; C, control group; MCS, maximum clinical score; DEP, degree of depression; DEHY, degree of dehydration; FC, fecal consistency; NS, not significant; ND, not done.

in the severity of systemic illness between treatment and control groups in all three trials as measured by comparison of mean scores earned for degree of clinical dehydration, degree of clinical depression, and maximum clinical score (Table II). In addition, a significant difference was noted in the duration of diarrhea after challenge when measured in trial 1, and a significant difference was observed in the degree of weight loss between treated and control calves when measured in trials 2 and 3 (Table II).

Most importantly, treatment with the K99-specific monoclonal antibody significantly reduced mortality in challenged calves in all three trials (Table I). When the results of all three trials were considered together, the mortality rate in the calves receiving the K99-specific monoclonal antibody was only 29% as compared with 82% in the control calves. This difference was highly significant ($p < 0.001$).

It was concluded that treatment with 1 ml of mouse ascitic fluid containing K99-specific monoclonal antibody reduced the severity of diarrhea and the mortality rate after challenge with EPEC strain B44. This finding supported the earlier work (2) which indicated that immunization of cows with purified K99 antigen before calving stimulated their production of K99-specific antibodies which were passively transferred to their calves and which prevented fatal diarrhea. In this study, antibody directed only against the K99 pilus of EPEC significantly reduced the severity of diarrhea caused by strain B44, which carries two adherence pili (K99 and F41), as well as the K30 capsular antigen, which is also believed to mediate adherence (98). This suggests that the degree of colonization and, hence, the clinical severity of disease, was reduced by the K99-specific monoclonal antibody. The fact that diarrhea was not eliminated completely was attributed to the possibility that either performed enterotoxin was present in the challenge inoculum, that the dose of monoclonal antibody was not sufficient to block adherence by K99 pili completely, or that F41-mediated adherence with some colonization of the gut may have occurred. The fact that 29% of treated calves died was attributed to several factors, including the deprivation of colostrum in trials 2 and 3, and the presence of concurrent infections. Postmortem examination in some treated calves revealed the presence of concurrent rotavirus and/or coronavirus in the intestine.

This work has led to the development and use of a commercially available K99-specific monoclonal antibody preparation for oral administration in newborn calves to prevent fatal enteric colibacillosis.[2] The application of hybridoma technology for the development of a K99-specific antibody which could be prepared by conventional means has been perceived by some as a case of technologic overkill. In fact, a conventionally raised K99-specific antibody product for oral administration directly to calves has been developed and marketed in

---

[2]Genecol™99, Molecular Genetics, Inc., Minnetonka, Minnesota.

Israel (151). However, hybridoma technology has advanced so dramatically since the first published report in 1975, that the cost of producing hybridoma-derived monoclonal antibody compares favorably to the production of conventional antisera (C. C. Muscoplat, Molecular Genetics, Inc., Minnetonka, Minnesota, personal communication). The superiority to conventionally produced antisera is obvious when the specificity, concentration, and uniformity of hybridoma-derived antibody is considered.

ii. Immunodiagnosis. The development of a monoclonal antibody to the K99 pilus should have a considerable impact on the diagnosis of enteric colibacillosis. Rapid diagnosis of enteropathogenic *E. coli* as a cause of neonatal diarrhea is important for several reasons. The disease tends to spread rapidly among newborn calves, particularly when cattle are maintained in close quarters (12). Numerous etiologic agents may produce diarrhea in young calves. Although EPEC account for the majority of these infections, rotavirus, coronavirus, *Salmonella* sp., *Clostridium perfringens,* cryptosporidia, and other less common pathogens may also occur (12,16,152). A specific diagnosis of K99-positive EPEC allows the practitioner to choose an appropriate therapy, initiate a preventative program, and offer a more accurate prognosis.

The conventional diagnostic procedure has been the collection of a fecal swab from the live calf or an ileal swab from necropsy, with subsequent culture on bacteriologic medium favoring pilus expression such as Minca-Is (45). After overnight incubation, several colonies are selected and slide agglutination tests are performed using conventionally raised antisera to K99. Alternately, colonies are smeared on a slide and examined using fluorescent-antibody techniques with K99-specific antisera conjugated to fluorescein. Several limitations exist with these methods. With both techniques, overnight culture is required for isolation of EPEC before a diagnosis can be made. Practitioners may not be equipped to perform either test. Since many nonpathogenic *E. coli* may be present in fecal swabs, inappropriate selection of colonies from the initial culture may lead to false-negative results.

In 1979, Ellens *et al.* (24) reported on the development of an ELISA technique which allowed detection of the K99 antigen directly from calf feces. In a comparison with the conventional culture and agglutination technique, the diagnostic sensitivity of the ELISA was equivalent to the standard test. However, overnight culture was eliminated and test results were available in 6 hr. The ELISA employed a rabbit-derived K99-specific antisera purified by adsorption of the hyperimmune serum with a K99-negative variant of the parent strain from which the pilus was first derived. To perform the ELISA, extensive processing of the fecal specimen was first required. Samples were diluted in phosphate-buffered saline, homogenized by ultrasonication, and then centrifuged for clarification. Some cross-reactivity occurred when bovine coronavirus was present in the fecal specimens and required blocking with bovine anticoronavirus serum.

Mills and Tietze (86) have reported on the use of K99-specific monoclonal antibody (2BD4E4) in a sandwich ELISA for detection of K99 pilus on *E. coli* isolates after bacterial culture of fecal samples. More recently, a sandwich ELISA technique utilizing a K99-specific monoclonal antibody for detection of the K99 antigen directly from fecal samples has been developed (D. E. Reed, Molecular Genetics, Inc., Minnetonka, Minnesota, personal communication). The technique requires no preparation of the fecal sample, yields results in less than an hour, and is designed as a test kit for use in the veterinary practice. The source of the monoclonal antibody is again clone 2BD4E4. A fecal swab or a 0.2-g sample of feces is suspended ina tube of diluent buffer by shaking. The K99-specific monoclonal antibody linked to horseradish peroxidase is added to the tube. A polystyrene wand coated with the K99-specific monoclonal antibody is then placed in the sample tube and incubated for 15 min. The wand is then washed in cold water and placed in a second tube containing the enzyme substrate. After 15 min, the color change is visually observed. A positive control is run with each sample as a color standard. Results are based on the concentration of pilus antigen in the sample and are read as negative (< 0.1 µg of K99 antigen), low positive ($0.1-1.0$ µg), or high positive (< 1 µg of K99 antigen). Due to the consistent concentration and avidity of the monoclonal reagents, the sensitivity of the test can be easily titrated to a desired level of sensitivity.

The specificity of this test system has been demonstrated by testing fecal samples from gnotobiotic calves infected with various enteric viruses as well as by testing bacterial cultures of numerous species and strains of enteric bacteria known to be K99 negative. Two variations of this test system using monoclonal antibody reagents have been reported: a competitive ELISA test and a three-step sandwich ELISA system (159). The latter has since been marketed commercially to practicing veterinarians.[3]

b. The K88 Pilus. The K88 pilus is found only on EPEC isolated from porcine enteric colibacillosis. Presence of the pilus is plasmid mediated, and there appears to be a strong association with certain O serotypes of EPEC, most notably O8, O45, O138, O141, O147, O149, and O157 (34). Strains carrying the K88 pilus may produce either heat-stable or heat-labile enterotoxin, or both (135). Pili on K88-positive strains are visible with electron microscopy and have a diameter of 2.1 nm (34). The molecular weight range is 23,500–26,000 (90). Three immunologically distinct K88 pilus structures are recognized (K88ab, K88ac, and K88ad), with the ''a'' fraction representing a common antigenic determinant (43,106). Partial amino acid sequences of the three K88 antigens have been characterized (34). The plasmid genes responsible for their production have been isolated by molecular cloning (34).

The progress in understanding the role of the K88 adhesin in porcine enteric

---

[3]Coli-Tect[TM]99, *E. coli* K-99 Antigen Test Kit, Molecular Genetics, Inc., Minnetonka, Minnesota.

colibacillosis, and the development of vaccines to prevent clinical disease is analogous to that described above for the K99 pilus. The K88 antigen was first described in 1961 as a serologically distinct antigen associated with *E. coli* strains isolated from pigs with edema disease and neonatal enteritis (105). It was later demonstrated that the K88 antigen was an adherence factor which facilitated colonization of the small intestine (6,65,158). This was confirmed by several *in vivo* and *in vitro* studies wherein adherence of K88-positive EPEC to intestinal villous epithelium was blocked by antisera against the K88 antigen (65,134,138,158). Based on these findings, vaccine trials were carried out and demonstrated that sows vaccinated with K88-positive EPEC would produce high levels of colostral K88-specific antibody which would passively protect newborn suckling pigs from enteric disease produced by K88-positive EPEC (119,120). Numerous commercial vaccines are now available for immunization of sows to control K88-positive EPEC-induced enteritis in their offspring (157).

As was described in the case of enteric colibacillosis of calves due to K99-positive EPEC, numerous epidemiologic factors contribute to the development of clinical disease, and in swine herds managed in confinement systems, neonatal colibacillosis can be unpredictable in onset and severe in nature (3). Analogous to the situation in calves, in swine herds where active immunization of sows has not been carried out prior to an outbreak of piglet enteritis, morbidity and mortality might be reduced through passive immunization of newborn pigs by direct oral administration of K88-specific antibody. P. L. Sadowski (Molecular Genetics, Inc., Minnetonka, Minnesota, personal communication) has produced K88-specific monoclonal antibodies using techniques similar to those described earlier for the production of the K99-specific monoclonal antibody. Three distinct monoclonal antibodies have been produced, showing specificity for the a, b, and c antigenic determinants of the K88 antigen. The protective effects of both the a and c antibodies when administered orally to newborn pigs have been demonstrated in challenge trials using a K88ac-positive EPEC strain (122).

It is interesting to note that in Europe, where active immunization of sows using vaccines containing K88ab and K88ac-positive strains of EPEC has been carried out for a number of years, EPEC isolates obtained from the intestines of pigs dying of colibacillosis in field outbreaks are increasingly of the K88ad variety and less frequently of the K88ab variety (43). It appears that vaccination is exerting some selection pressure on EPEC, and that the organisms are responding with variation in their adherence structures (34). Passive immunization of piglets with monoclonal antibodies could also potentially contribute to this selection pressure. Alternatively, the avidity of a K88a-specific monoclonal antibody might be capable of blocking adherence by all K88-positive EPEC, despite variations in their secondary structure.

One potential limitation of passive immunization by oral administration of K88-specific monoclonal antibody arises from the fact that, unlike K99-positive

EPEC infections in the calf, which are restricted to the first few days of life, K88-positive EPEC infections in pigs can occur throughout the suckling and weaning periods (157). Continuous administration of monoclonal antibody would be impractical, and passive immunization would have to be employed only in the face of outbreaks, or at known peak periods of susceptibility, namely during the first few days of life and again, just after weaning.

The conventional diagnostic procedures for confirming K88-positive EPEC infection in pigs are similar to those described above for K99-positive EPEC infection. A sandwich ELISA has been described for identification of the K88 pilus from bacterial suspensions of *E. coli* cultured from clinical specimens (87). It is reasonable to assume that K88-specific monoclonal antibody will facilitate the development of ELISA test kits which allow rapid detection of the K88 antigen directly from fecal specimens or swabs.

c. The 987P Pilus. The 987P pilus is also restricted to porcine isolates of EPEC (34). It is most often associated with EPEC strains O9, O20, and O141, and always is found with heat-stable enterotoxin only (34). Structurally, 987P is a glycoprotein of MW 20,000 (60). It is a rigid fimbria with a diameter of 7 nm. Unlike the other host-specific adhesins described, 987P does not demonstrate mannose-resistant hemagglutination of erythrocytes, and is coded on the bacterial chromosome rather than by a plasmid (137).

The role of 987P as an adherence factor facilitating colonization of the porcine intestine has been well established. Purified 987P pilus and Fab fragments of antibody specific for 987P have been shown to block adherence of 987P-positive EPEC strains to porcine small intestine epithelial cells *in vitro* (62). Numerous challenge trials have demonstrated that antibody to the 987P pilus will protect piglets from enteric colibacillosis with 987P-positive EPEC. Vaccination of sows with 987P-positive EPEC will increase 987P-specific antibody levels in colostrum and protect suckling pigs from clinical disease (61,91,94).

P. L. Sadowski (Molecular Genetics, Inc., Minnetonka, Minnesota, personal communication) has produced a monoclonal antibody to the 987P pilus using techniques similar to those described above for the production of the K99-specific monoclonal antibody, and protection studies have been carried out. Orally administered 987P-specific monoclonal antibody was shown to protect colostrum-deprived newborn piglets from challenge with EPEC strain 987. Significant reductions in the clinical severity of disease and in mortality rates were demonstrated as compared to challenged control pigs not receiving the monoclonal antibody.

Outbreaks of enteric colibacillosis in young pigs may be due to either K99-positive, K88-positive, or 987P-positive strains of EPEC (28). Although there is a tendency for K88-positive strains to produce diarrhea in pigs over 2 weeks of age and K99-positive and 987P-positive strains to occur more frequently in younger pigs, there is much overlap in these infections (33). This observation suggests that for prevention of enteric colibacillosis in piglets by oral administration of monoclonal antibody, the specificity of the monoclonal antibody is actually a handicap. The practical solution to this problem would be the administration of a trivalent mixture of monoclonal antibodies to the three known porcine EPEC adherence pili. A commercial product containing monoclonal antibodies against the K99, K88, and 987P adhesins is currently being evaluated for use in controlling outbreaks of enteric colibacillosis in young pigs (C. C. Muscoplat, Molecular Genetics, Inc., Minnetonka, Minnesota, personal communication).

d. The F41 Pilus. The F41 pilus is the most recently characterized adhesin of EPEC important in veterinary medicine (20). At present, F41 has been identified only in bovine strains of EPEC and can be found in conjunction with the K99 pilus in certain EPEC strains, most notably B41 (20,95). The presence of F41 is plasmid mediated. It occurs in the O9 and O101 serogroups of EPEC, and is associated exclusively with heat-stable enterotoxin (34). It has a fimbrial structure with a diameter of 3.2 nm (20). Chemical characterization reveals the F41 pilus to be a protein of MW 29,500 whose amino acid sequence has been identified (20). The role of the F41 pilus in the production of bovine enteric colibacillosis is not yet as firmly established as is the role of the K99 pilus. However, there are several observations which suggest that the F41 pilus is a virulence factor. A K99-negative, F41-positive, mutant strain of B41 (B41M) was shown to adhere to calf enterocytes *in vitro* and to produce diarrhea in newborn germfree piglets (95).

No vaccine trials have been reported to date. It is reasonable to assume, however, that once the role of F41 is clarified in bovine neonatal diarrhea, active immunization of the dam to produce F41 specific colostral antibody will be practiced. In turn, the development of an F41-specific monoclonal antibody for direct, oral passive immunization of the calf, is likely to follow.

2. Pili of Other Veterinary Bacterial Pathogens

a. Moraxella bovis. Infectious bovine keratoconjunctivitis (IBK) is a common cattle disease of major economic significance. A comprehensive review of IBK has recently been published (113). It is generally accepted that *Moraxella bovis* is the primary initiator and mediator of this disease, although a role for numerous other pathogens, including viruses, mycoplasma, and chlaymdia, have been suggested. Infection of the conjunctiva with *M. bovis* produces severe inflammation resulting in lacrimation, blepharospasm, photophobia, corneal edema, temporary blindness, and residual scarring. Ocular pain and impaired vision lead to reduced feed intake and decreased milk production with substantial economic loss to both beef and dairy cattle producers.

Numerous factors appear to contribute to the initiation of clinical disease. Outbreaks of IBK occur most commonly in the summer and autumn. This is attributed to the increased population of face flies acting as mechanical vectors for *M. bovis* and to the seasonal increase in solar radiation which predisposes the cornea to infection. This has been substantiated in experimental infection where controlled exposure to ultraviolet light prior to challenge with *M. bovis* increases the rate and severity of infection. Lack of skin pigmentation in the eyelids of certain cattle breeds also predisposes to infection. Other corneal irritants such as dust can also increase susceptibility. When multiple predisposing factors are present, severe outbreaks of IBK can occur suddenly and spread rapidly, with the morbidity rate reported as high as 80%.

Although *M. bovis* has been linked to IBK since 1945 (10), considerable doubt existed concerning its role as a primary pathogen, largely due to the difficulties encountered in consistently reproducing experimental infection. In 1972, Pedersen *et al.* (108) demonstrated that only piliated strains of *M. bovis* were capable of colonizing the conjunctiva of calves and reproducing the disease. The presence of pili in virulent strains was associated with a distinctive flat, agar-corroding, colony morphology, and was confirmed by electron microscopy. Since that time, virtually all investigations into the pathogenesis of IBK have utilized piliated strains of *M. bovis,* and, as discussed below, advances in disease control are based on manipulating the immunological response of the host to the pilus. Pili, however, are not the only recognized virulence factors of *M. bovis.* It has been reported that production of hemolysin is also a characteristic of all strains capable of producing ocular disease (110). A role for several other toxins and proteases has also been suggested (113). However, as with the enteropathogenic *E. coli,* the pilus is of major importance as the prime mediator of colonization. If colonization is blocked, the deleterious effects of additional virulence factors may be minimized.

Several lines of investigation suggest that a systemic humoral immune response may prevent infection with *M. bovis.* In field outbreaks of IBK, young cattle are more susceptible than adults, suggesting the development of a natural acquired immunity (57). Pugh *et al.* (112) have demonstrated that calves receiving colostrum from cows vaccinated with *M. bovis* are more resistant to experimental challenge than calves receiving colostrum from unvaccinated dams, when challenged with a homologous strain. It has also been demonstrated by Kopecky *et al.* (68) that calves experimentally infected in one eye subsequently develop less severe clinical disease when challenged in the other eye 21 days later. The conclusion drawn was that systemic rather than local immune responses were responsible for limiting disease. Several investigators have measured antibody responses in the serum and lacrimal secretions of infected calves. Killinger *et al.* (66) reported that in lacrimal secretion the highest and most persistent antibody titers specific for *M. bovis* were of the IgG class despite the fact that, in normal calves, IgA is the predominant antibody class in lacrimal secretion. Weech and Renshaw (156) demonstrated that the *M. bovis*-specific antibody in lacrimal secretions was directed primarily against protein antigens, including pilus, rather than carbohydrate antigens. These investigators, however, were unable to detect a serum antibody response to infection. Bishop *et al.* (11) identified an *M. bovis*-specific IgG response in the serum of challenged calves but primarily an IgA response in lacrimal secretion. Despite the somewhat contradictory findings of these investigators, it is likely that a systemic humoral immune response is an important defense against infection with *M. bovis*. The apparent efficacy of parenteral vaccination supports this conclusion.

Pugh *et al.* (111) demonstrated the importance of including pilus antigen in parenteral vaccines against *M. bovis* in 1977. Protection was demonstrated against homologous challenge strains. Recently a piliated *M. bovis* vaccine has become commercially available.[4] This vaccine is a formalin-killed, aluminum hydroxide-adjuvanted, whole-cell bacterin containing two highly piliated strains of *M. bovis,* EPP63 and FLA64. In experimental challenge trials (160) the vaccine given subcutaneously at a 28-day interval produced high circulating antibody titers to the pili of both strains, as measured by ELISA, and substantially reduced the rate of infection in vaccinated calves as compared to challenged, unvaccinated controls. This vaccine is now being used widely in the field with apparent success, although the vaccine's ability to induce protection against heterologous field strains of *M. bovis* has not been reported.

Interestingly, little published data exist regarding the characterization of *M. bovis* pilus in terms of chemical and physical structure, genetic derivation, and antigenic homology. Since IBK occurs worldwide and a variety of *M. bovis* strains are isolated from field outbreaks in different geographic areas (39), vaccine failures can be expected to occur unless vaccines are designed to induce strong antibody responses to widely shared pilus antigens. Identificâtion of common epitopes should be considered an important prerequisite for development of efficacious vaccines. Current investigations directed toward development of a pilus vaccine for gonorrhea are instructive.

Schoolnik *et al.* (124) have examined the chemical structure and antigenic diversity of gonococcal pili. Cyanogen bromide fragments of pili from different gonococcal strains were prepared and evaluated. One fragment, designated as CNBr-2 was found to encompass a highly conserved antigenic region that mediates receptor cell site binding function and is immunorecessive. Fragment CNBr-3 was identified as immunodominant and to include a variable antigenic region that confers type specificity to the pilus but is functionally inert. Virji *et al.* (153) have utilized monoclonal antibodies to gonococcal pili to demonstrate a common antigenic region and a type-specific region, both of which contain more than one epitope.

---

[4]Piliguard™ Pinkeye, Schering Corporation, Kenilworth, New Jersey.

It has been reported that pili from the genera *Neisseria, Pseudomonas,* and *Moraxella* show homologous N-terminal amino acid sequences, suggesting that these proteins may be derived from a common ancestral gene (124). This region may show little structural variation because of the necessity of conserving receptor cell site binding specificity for successful colonization of the host. Preliminary work by G. K. Schoolnik (Stanford University, School of Medicine, Stanford, California, personal communication) has begun to clarify the pilus structure of *M. bovis.* Two distinct pili have been identified on *M. bovis* strain EPP63. They are provisionally designated as heavy and light with molecular weights of 18,000 and 17,000, respectively. The amino acid sequence of both proteins has been determined. The coding for these pili is chromosomal and not plasmid mediated, and the DNA sequence coding for the light pilus has been defined. Both the heavy and light pili share a common antigenic region of approximately 40 amino acids at the N-terminus. Serologic studies show this antigenic region to be immunorecessive. The remainders of both pili are antigenically heterologous, and this variable region is immunodominant. Several field isolates of *M. bovis* have also been demonstrated to possess pili of 18,000 and 17,000 MW, but identification of a common epitope has not yet been carried out.

Clearly monoclonal antibodies could be instrumental in identifying common epitopes on *M. bovis* pili. Furthermore, monoclonal antibodies directed against common pilus epitopes might be used effectively for passive immunization of unvaccinated cattle at risk in outbreaks of IBK. The immunologic studies of host response to infection cited above suggest that parenteral injection of pilus-specific monoclonal antibody may protect against colonization of the conjunctiva, as serum IgG appears to reach the lacrimal fluid. Alternatively, monoclonal antibody could be instilled directly into the eye, injected into the subconjunctival space as is currently done with antibiotic therpay (113), or delivered over time by a sustained-release biodegradable ocular insert which has recently been developed (146). Passive immunization could provide the veterinarian with great flexibility in managing IBK, particularly in situations such as feedlots where cattle are assembled from multiple sources and may develop IBK before active immunization has had adequate time to induce a protective antibody response.

b. *Bacteroides nodosus.* Infectious foot rot of sheep is an inflammation of the skin and horny tissues of the foot. When infection progresses to the soft tissue underneath the hoof wall, severe lameness occurs. The pain and impaired mobility, which results in affected pastured sheep, leads to decreased feed intake, reduced weight gains, decreased wool production, increased susceptibility to predation, and, occasionally, starvation. It is a recognized problem in all nonarid intensive sheep-producing areas of the world. Warm temperatures, wet weather, and lush pastures are important triggers of clinical disease, and sudden outbreaks of high morbidity result when climatic conditions are optimal (12).

Bacteroides nodosus is the primary etiologic agent of infectious foot rot of sheep. It is an obligate parasite of the hoof epidermis in sheep and cattle, and is spread during clinical outbreaks by contamination of pasture by purulent discharges from infected feet (13). The pathogenic mechanisms of *B. nodosus* are not clearly defined. Virulent strains are characterized by a distinctive papillate or beaded-colony morphology (B type), a high level of proteolytic elastase activity, and abundant surface pili (29,133). It is widely held that the pilus is an important protective immunogen and has served as the basis for much vaccine research (144,149,155). However, a recent report on antibody responses of naturally infected sheep suggests that pilus may not be the predominant immunogen. Using an electroblot radioimmunoassay, antibody responses to 10 to 15 antigens were identified, with the greatest response being directed against an unidentified nonpilus antigen of 75,000 MW (102). In a comparative electron microscopic study of virulent and nonvirulent strains, Every and Skerman (30) confirmed the presence of abundant pili in virulent strains but also identified the presence of an additional outer membrane layer and aggregates of diffuse polar material which might contribute to virulence.

Beginning around 1970, reports of vaccine efficacy using piliated strains of *B. nodosus* in oil adjuvants were reported from Australia (22), New Zealand (132), and England (116). A protective effect was observed, and the level of protection roughly correlated to serum pilus antibody titers. In virtually all these studies, protection was demonstrated primarily against homologous challenge strains. However, two vaccine trials carried out in the United States using an Australian-produced vaccine demonstrated poor protection (82,140). These failures prompted investigation into serotypic heterogeneity of virulent field strains (123). It appears that pilus (K) antigens of *B. nodosus* are extremely variable. Several studies of K antigen diversity have been reported, and the number of identifiable serogroups has ranged from 3 in Australia (21) to 14 in the United States (123). Using pilus antiserum produced in rabbits, strong agglutination titers to homologous pili are consistently produced, and minor cross-reactions among heterologous pili are widespread (123).

To date, the minor cross-reactions observed in agglutination tests have not been carefully scrutinized. It is conceivable that these cross-reactions represent weak immunologic responses to common epitopes on *B. nodosus* pili but that these epitopes are immunorecessive, a situation analogous to that described for *Neisseria gonorrhoeae* and possibly *Moraxella bovis,* as previously discussed. Clearly, hybridoma-derived monoclonal antibodies to pilus fragments would be far superior to conventionally prepared rabbit antibodies for the purpose of establishing the existence of common epitopes. Identification of a common immunogenic region is critical for the further development of a broadly efficacious pilus vaccine. In addition, the specificity of monoclonal antibodies could facilitate definition of the immunogenic and pathogenic role of other *B. nodosus* surface structures implicated as virulence factors. Once common immunogens are defined on virulent strains, passive immunization by parenteral injection of monoclonal antibodies might be useful in reducing morbidity in sporadic outbreaks of infectious foot rot in unvaccinated sheep.

c. Additional Pili of Importance. As evidenced by the above discussions, attachment to epithelial cell surfaces is a critical first step in the pathogenesis of bacterial infection of mucosal surfaces, particularly when mechanical defenses such as peristalsis or ciliary activity resist colonization. Recognition of this fact has led researchers to a more careful evaluation of both fimbrial and nonfimbrial adherence factors as mediators of infectious disease in both human and veterinary medicine. This is particularly true in the study of respiratory pathogens. Respiratory tract disease continues to be one of the costliest disease entities encountered in veterinary practice. Significant economic loss occurs in the cattle, swine, and poultry industries due to respiratory infections, and trends toward confinement livestock rearing in all of these industry sectors exacerbate the spread of respiratory pathogens (9,109,166).

Studies on the nature of bacterial adherence in respiratory disease have been reported with regard to *Pasteurella multocida* (40), *Bordetella bronchiseptica* (49), *Haemophilus somnus* (143), and *Mycoplasma pneumoniae* (32) infections in various species. The usefulness of monoclonal antibodies in defining the mechanism and structures of adherence by respiratory pathogens has been nicely illustrated by Feldner *et al.* (32) in their work with *Mycoplasma pneumoniae*, a human respiratory pathogen. This study is instructive to veterinary researchers.

What was known about *M. pneumoniae* was its small size, its possession of a specialized tip structure, its mobility, and the ability to adhere to animal cells and inert surfaces. Adherence was considered to be a prerequisite for survival in the host organism, but the location and structure of the mycoplasmal adhesin was unknown. To answer these questions, mice were immunized with whole-cell suspensions of *M. pneumoniae*. Splenic lymphocytes were harvested and hybridomas produced. One hundred twenty hybridoma clones were screened for the production of adherence-inhibiting antibody using a hemadsorption assay. Through limiting dilution techniques, a single clone was isolated producing the desired antibody. Utilizing this monoclonal antibody in an indirect-immunofluorescence test on whole *M. pneumoniae* cells, a localized area of fluorescence was identified on one pole of the cell. Electron microscopic examination using ferritin-labeled antimouse monoclonal antibody confirmed that the monoclonal antibody was bound specifically to the unipolar tip structure of the organism (Fig. 3).

Pretreatment of *M. pneumoniae* cells with the tip-specific monoclonal antibody prevented adherence to sheep, rabbit, guinea pig, and human erythrocytes, demonstrating that adhesive ability was localized to the tip structure. The monoclonal antibody was then radiolabeled by addition of [^{35}S]methionine to the

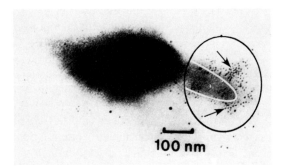

Fig. 3. Electron microscopic view of a *Mycoplasma pneumoniae* cell after incubation with adherence-inhibiting monoclonal antibody labeled with ferritin. Ferritin molecules are seen predominantly at the tip structure, confirming that the adhesive property of *M. pneumoniae* is localized to the tip structure. Adapted and reprinted from reference 32 by permission from *Nature (London)*, 1982, **298**, 765–767, Copyright © 1982, Macmillan Journals Limited.

hybridoma cell culture. *Mycoplasma pneumoniae* cultures were solubilized in SDS and the proteins separated by electrophoresis in SDS–polyacrylamide gel. The gel was then treated with the labeled monoclonal antibody. Autoradiography revealed antibody bound to a single protein in the molecular weight range 160,000–190,000. Subsequent coating of a second gel with sheep erythrocytes resulted in binding of red cells only on the same protein, indicating that the antigenic protein and the functional binding protein were identical.

Clearly hybridoma technology provides a powerful investigative tool for defining the structure and function of bacterial adhesins. The use of monoclonal antibodies in the study of veterinary respiratory pathogens will undoubtedly lead to greater understanding of host–parasite interactions and novel approaches to immunoprophylaxis by blocking the mechanisms of bacterial adherence.

B. Bacterial Toxins and Cytoplasmic Proteins

Toxin production is an important virulence mechanism, particularly for noninvasive bacteria which are able to exert profound systemic effects on the host despite localization of the infection. Clostridial infections are the classic example of this virulence mechanism. In human medicine, hybridoma technology has been applied to the study of bacterial toxins to elucidate toxin structure and pathogenic mechanisms, to improve immunodiagnostic capability, and to develop new approaches to immunotherapy. Reports of monoclonal antibodies specific for bacterial toxins include studies of diphtheria toxin (50), *Pseudomonas aeruginosa* exotoxin A (35), *Clostridium botulinum* toxins C_1 (103) and D (96), and *Clostridium tetani* tetanus toxin (154). To illustrate the potential uses of toxin-specific monoclonal antibodies in veterinary medicine, several important toxin-mediated diseases will be discussed.

1. Escherichia coli *enterotoxin*

As discussed earlier, enteropathogenic strains of *E. coli* (EPEC) possess two known important virulence factors: adherence pili to implement intestinal colonization in the face of gut peristalsis and a competing resident intestinal flora (118), and enterotoxin which stimulates intestinal epithelial cells to secrete fluid and electrolytes into the gut lumen at an accelerated rate (8). The net results of EPEC infection in the host are dehydration, acidosis, electrolyte imbalance, and death.

Two types of enterotoxin are recognized in EPEC strains isolated from livestock; heat-stable (ST) and heat-labile (LT) enterotoxins. The former stimulates villous cell hypersecretion through activation of guanylate cyclase in the epithelial cell, while the latter accomplishes the task by activation of adenylate cyclase. Transmission of both enterotoxin types is plasmid mediated. K88-Positive EPEC strains are associated with both LT and ST enterotoxins, whereas K99, F41, and 987P-positive EPEC have been found to produce only ST enterotoxin (34).

Although the value of active immunization of swine (91) and cattle (2) with piliated vaccines has been well established and passive immunization of calves with monoclonal antibody to K99 has been demonstrated to be protective (127), enterotoxin-specific monoclonal antibody could play an important future role in passive immunization of neonates. Observations that K88-positive EPEC isolates from naturally infected swine are less frequently of the K88ab type and more frequently of the K88ad type suggest that the pilus plasmid genome is responsive to selection pressure exerted by vaccination (34). This could potentially impair the long-term efficacy of highly specific monoclonal antibodies directed against variable regions of the pilus. Enterotoxin-specific monoclonal antibody offers a possible alternative for continued passive immunization. A combination of LT- and ST-specific antibodies could conceivably neutralize enterotoxins of all EPEC strains regardless of their current or future pilus specificity. The success of this strategy would depend on the inability of enterotoxin to escape immune recognition through structural variation mediated by the plasmid genome. Furthermore, if colonization is allowed to occur, the question arises of whether or not antibody can successfully bind and neutralize enterotoxins. The physically intimate association of the EPEC organism to the brush border of epithelial cells facilitated by adherence pili may present spatial constraints which limit antibody–enterotoxin interaction.

Despite these theoretical concerns, Klipstein *et al.* (67) have shown that active immunization with enterotoxin can reduce intestinal hypersecretion. Using a vaccine composed of synthetically produced ST cross-linked to the nontoxic B subunit of LT, rats and rabbits have been protected against challenge with both toxins and heterologous organisms producing these toxins. Protection was measured by a significant decrease in intestinal hypersecretion using a ligated gut loop assay. The protective effect of the vaccine was attributed to a marked increase in toxin-specific mucosal IgA in the gut.

The feasibility of producing monoclonal antibodies to *E. coli* enterotoxin has already been demonstrated. Hemelhof *et al.* (51) have reported the development of a monoclonal antibody to the heat-stable enterotoxin (STh) of a human EPEC strain. This monoclonal antibody, at a 320-fold dilution, exhibited toxin-neutralizing potency 10 times greater than that shown by conventionally raised antibody to STh. Interestingly, two other monoclonal antibodies to STh have been reported (148,165), but neither demonstrated the ability to neutralize the biologic activity of the enterotoxin. This suggests that immunogenic regions exist outside the region of functional activity in the structure of enterotoxin.

2. Cytotoxin of Pasteurella haemolytica

Pneumonic pasteurellosis is one of the costliest diseases confronting the cattle industry, particularly in the feedlot sector, where economic considerations dictate cattle management practices which predispose to outbreaks of respiratory disease. Fibrinous pneumonia due to *Pasteurella haemolytica* is considered the terminal event in a multifactorial syndrome known as the bovine respiratory disease (BRD) complex, which occurs with high frequency in North American feedlots (63).

Stress is an important predisposing factor in the development of BRD. Feeder calves entering the feedlot have often been recently weaned, unadapted to grain rations, comingled with strange cattle in sales barns, shipped long distances with inadequate feed or water, and subjected to adverse weather conditions. Comingling with cattle from multiple sources leads to the widespread transmission of respiratory tract viruses, particularly parainfluenza-3, and infectious bovine rhinotracheitis virus (58). Infections with these and other viruses are believed to predispose cattle to the development of *Pasteurella* penumonia, presumably by impairment of pulmonary clearance and/or immunosuppression. The major cause of mortality in BRD is pneumonic pasteurellosis (64).

In feedlot outbreaks of BRD, morbidity can reach 35% and mortality 10%. In addition to cattle lost, treatment costs can be staggering. Antibiotic therapy is costly and time-consuming, and antibiotic resistance in *Pasteurella* isolates is increasing (4). Efforts to reduce morbidity have traditionally included the practice of vaccinating calves against viral and bacterial pathogens as they enter the feedlot. However, many calves may already be incubating respiratory tract viruses by the time they reach the feedlot, and modified live virus vaccines have been implicated as an added stressor (77). Furthermore, *Pasteurella* bacterins may actually contribute to the severity of respiratory disease, as will be discussed later. In fact, an epidemiologic study of feedlot mortality in Canada identified vaccination of cattle upon arrival at the feedlot as one of the three most important factors contributing to increased mortality rates (78).

Although *Pasteurella multocida* is frequently isolated from outbreaks of BRD, *P. haemolytica* is considered the primary bacterial pathogen. Twelve ruminant serotypes of *P. haemolytica* are recognized, but serotype 1 is most often isolated from pneumonic lungs (115). The virulence factors and pathogenic mechanisms of *P. haemolytica* are not completely understood. While viral impairment of pulmonary clearance may promote increased bacterial entry into the distal lung, bacterial surface adhesins may facilitate continued colonization of the terminal bronchioles and alveoli. After colonization, cell wall endotoxin release is believed by some to be an initiator of the pulmonic lesions which develop (69). However, attention recently has focused on other compounds released by the organism. *Pasteurella haemolytica* has been found to produce a potent cytotoxin capable of killing polymorphonuclear leukocytes and alveolar macrophages, thus disabling the primary immunologic defense of the lung against bacterial pathogens (74,75).

The physicochemical properties of cytotoxin have been studied. Himmel *et al.* (53) have purified and partially characterized cytotoxin as a protein with a molecular weight of approximately 150,000 associated with the bacterial capsule. The protein was isolated from culture supernatant and was shown to be highly immunogenic. In immunodiffusion tests, the antigen was cross-reactive with antisera produced against all 12 serotypes of *P. haemolytica*. No reactivity was demonstrated against antisera to *P. multocida*. Toxicity against bovine alveolar macrophages was demonstrated *in vitro*. Shewen and Wilkie (128) also have reported similar immunogenic and cytotoxic findings with cytotoxin from culture supernatant.

The universal presence of cytotoxin in all serotypes of *P. haemolytica,* its immunogenicity, and its probable role as an important virulence factor make cytotoxin an ideal antigen for active immunization against pneumonic pasteurellosis. Examination of feedlot cattle submitted for necropsy and diagnosed as having respiratory disease had lower levels of serum anticytotoxic neutralizing antibodies than did animals dying of other causes, or than animals bled prior to entry into feedlots (129). Immunization with isolated cytotoxin did confer some protection against experimental challenge, although response to other (surface) antigens appeared to be required for complete protection (130). This may be an analogous situation to the EPEC, where antibodies to both the pilus and the toxin may give the best response.

Recognition of the importance of cytotoxin helps to explain the apparent negative effects of vaccination with killed whole-cell bacterins. Since cytotoxin is produced most abundantly during log-phase growth in culture (36), conventionally prepared bacterins containing bacteria from stationary-phase growth will induce much anticapsular opsonizing antibody but may produce very little cytotoxin-neutralizing antibody. This can lead to increased phagocytic activity but also may result in more efficient killing of phagocytes by cytotoxin released from ingested bacteria. The net effect of vaccination then may be an impaired immune response.

Although redesigning bacterins to promote a better anticytotoxin response would result in a better vaccine, this does not ensure the development of a better vaccination program. In fact, the realities of feedlot practice argue against the value of active immunization as a technique for controlling BRD. Most outbreaks of BRD occur within 10 to 14 days after arrival in the feedlot, when environmental stresses on the calf are at their greatest. Yet cattle vaccinated upon arrival cannot be expected to develop a strong humoral immune response within the first 2 weeks, if at all. Endogenous steroid release due to stress and concurrent viral infections may impair the animals' ability to mount an effective immune response, even with the best of vaccines. Ideally, calves should be vaccinated before marketing to the feedlot (preconditioning). However, calf raisers in general are unwilling to incur the expense of vaccination to protect the future economic interests of prospective feedlot calf buyers.

Clearly passive immunization could play an important role in controlling BRD, as it fits more logically into the epidemiologic pattern of feedlot disease and feedlot management practices. Antibody administered parenterally to cattle upon arrival at the feedlot could protect them from clinical disease during the critical adaptation period. Hybridoma technology offers a significant advantage over conventionally prepared antisera for passive immunization. It allows for the production of unlimited quantities of high-titer antibodies directed against specific virulence factors. Monoclonal antibody to cytotoxin administered alone or in conjunction with monoclonal antibodies to other antigens of *P. haemolytica* or proteins of known respiratory viral pathogens could dramatically improve current approaches to controlling respiratory disease in cattle.

3. Clostridial Toxins

A wide range of clostridial diseases affect farm animals (12), including tetanus (*Cl. tetani*), botulism (*Cl. botulinum*), blackleg (*Cl. chauvoei*), malignant edema (*Cl. septicum, Cl. novyi*), necrotic hepatitis (*Cl. novyi*), bacillary hemoglobinuria (*Cl. haemolyticum*), and enterotoxemia (*Cl. perfringens*). All of these diseases are mediated by release of potent clostridial toxins.

In general, these diseases are effectively controlled by vaccination with alum-precipitated toxoids. However, serious outbreaks continue to occur in unvaccinated animals and successful therapy depends on the administration of large doses of specific antitoxins. Commercially available, conventionally prepared antitoxins vary considerably in their cost, availability, and efficacy. The most serious limitation to treatment is the relatively high cost of administering adequate doses of antitoxin. For example, the recommended treatment regimen for an adult horse with tetanus is 300,000 units of tetanus antitoxin administered three times at 12-hr intervals (12). The current cost of this therapy is approximately $700.

It has been demonstrated that antibodies to clostridial toxins can be prepared using hybridoma technology. Oguma *et al.* (103) have reported the production of four different monoclonal antibodies against the C_1 toxin of *Cl. botulinum*, only one of which showed neutralizing activity against the biologic activity of the toxin. This suggests that in conventionally prepared antitoxins, a significant proportion of antibody which is produced may not possess neutralizing activity. Volk *et al.* (154) have produced a number of mouse monoclonal antibodies to tetanus toxoid. These antibodies bound to at least 20 different epitopes on the toxoid molecule. Mixtures of these antibodies demonstrated greater neutralizing activity than any of them alone, suggesting that efficient neutralization requires antibody binding at more than one site on the toxoid molecule.

The comparatively high titers of hybridoma-derived antibodies along with their potential for improved specificity could significantly improve the efficacy of antitoxin therapy when monoclonal antibodies are used instead of conventionally prepared antitoxin. Hybridoma technology could conceivably result in lower cost products of higher potency for therapeutic use.

4. *Protoplasmic Antigens of* Mycobacterium paratuberculosis

Paratuberculosis (Johne's disease) is a chronic granulomatous enteric infection of ruminant animals caused by the acid-fast organism *Mycobacterium paratuberculosis*. The disease occurs worldwide and is considered a major problem in the North American cattle industry. In infected herds, clinically ill animals with diarrhea shed the organism in the feces and *M. paratuberculosis* infection can be confirmed by bacterial culture techniques. This is also true of a percentage of infected animals not showing clinical signs. However, many infected animals in a herd are nonshedding carriers and cannot be identified by culture of feces (12).

Efforts at eliminating Johne's disease have been frustrated for decades by the lack of a sensitive and specific immunodiagnostic test for identification of nonshedding carrier animals. A wide range of diagnostic tests has been evaluated to detect both humoral and cellular immune responses to infection. These efforts have been reviewed (84,147). In virtually all cases diagnostic specificity was inadequate as a result of antigenic cross-reactions. *Mycobacterium paratuberculosis* shares common cell wall antigens with a variety of pathogenic and saprophytic bacteria, including other *Mycobacteria* sp., *Corynebacterium* sp., and *Nocardia* sp. (70). These historical difficulties have led to a renewed emphasis on isolation of type-specific antigens from protoplasmic extracts of *M. paratuberculosis* and the utilization of newer, more sensitive diagnostic assays such as the ELISA (85).

Abbas *et al.* (1) have reported on the isolation of an affinity-purified peptide derived from a crude protoplasmic extract of *M. paratuberculosis*. The crude extract is obtained by disruption of whole cells in a Ribi hydraulic cell press, separation of cell wall debris by centrifugation, and lyophilization of the remaining supernatant. Isolation of peptide antigens involved a complicated stepwise procedure. The crude protoplasmic extract was treated by solvent extraction and ammonium sulfate precipitation followed by gel filtration, ion exchange chromatography, and, finally, affinity chromatography. The yield of peptide antigen from crude material applied to the affinity column was 7.8%. Whereas the crude starting material demonstrated cross-reactivity to bovine antisera against *M. avium, M. phlei, M. fortuitum,* and *Nocardia asteroides* in complement fixation and ELISA tests, the purified peptide reacted only with antisera to *M. paratuberculosis* in complement fixation and ELISA with antisera diluted 1:40.

Although the purification of this antigen and its application in the ELISA system represent major advances in the immunodiagnosis of paratuberculosis, the application of hybridoma technology could eliminate the need for exhaustive purification of protoplasmic antigens. Hewitt *et al.* (52) have reported on the use of monoclonal antibodies in the serodiagnosis of human tuberculosis without the need for purification of antigen. The assay described is a competitive-inhibition assay wherein crude *M. tuberculosis* antigen (pressate) is bound to microtiter plate wells. Test sera are then incubated in coated wells, followed by the addition of ^{125}I-labeled murine monoclonal antibodies directed against type-specific antigens of *M. tuberculosis*. Plates are then washed and the amount of bound monoclonal antibody is determined by γ counting as an indirect measure of *M. tuberculosis*-specific antibody in test sera. Combinations of different antigen-specific monoclonal antibodies were employed in the assay to improve sensitivity. It was emphasized that mycobacterial infections present a wide range of antigens to the host which may be recognized or ignored to variable degrees during the host immune response. Therefore, the sensitivity of the immunoassay can be improved by utilizing monoclonal antibodies against several known type-specific antigens.

The prevalence of host recognition of the peptide antigen of *M. paratuberculosis* described by Abbas *et al.* (1) is currently unknown, although it was reported in their study that sera from 83% of the known infected animals tested were identified as positive in the ELISA assay. This antigen could be used to produce a mouse monoclonal antibody for use in the competitive-inhibition assay described, with crude protoplasmic extract of *M. paratuberculosis* serving as the test antigen. In addition, monoclonal antibodies could be used as probes to identify other protoplasmic antigens of *M. paratuberculosis* which are not cross-reactive and could therefore be used to improve the sensitivity of a competitive-inhibition test.

Morris and Ivanyi (95a) have recently reported on patterns of cross reactivity in protoplasmic antigens of various mycobacteria including *M. paratuberculosis* to a panel of ten monoclonal antibodies produced against *M. tuberculosis* and *M. leprae* antigens. A radioimmunoassay was employed to detect binding activity.

C. Bacterial Capsular Antigens

The bacterial capsule plays an important role in the pathogenesis of some bacterial infections, largely through its ability to inhibit phagocytosis. Two general mechanisms of antiphagocytic activity are recognized (56). First, abundant capsule may cover cell surface antigens such as pili and cell wall lipopolysaccharide (LPS), preventing phagocytic interaction with subcapsular determinants. Second, polysaccharide capsule does not fix complement in the absence of antibody, thus inhibiting complement-mediated opsonization. The polysaccharide capsule of many bacteria is highly immunogenic, however, and immunization with capsule-rich vaccines will promote anticapsular antibody production capable of mediating complement fixation and phagocytosis (7).

In human medicine, an exciting approach to immunotherapy is being explored using monoclonal antibodies to capsular antigens of group B *Streptococcus,* bacteria responsible for potentially fatal septicemias in newborn infants. Since these infections occur during passage through the birth canal and their occurrence is unpredictable, active immunization does not represent a practical approach to management of the problem, a situation analogous to many of the veterinary diseases already discussed. Shigeoka *et al.* (131) have reported on the development of murine monoclonal antibodies of the IgM class prepared against group B streptococcal (GBS) type III polysaccharide antigens. One of these monoclonal antibodies, when used in a rat model of infection, significantly reduced mortality in rats challenged with five different GBS type III strains. Two of these strains normally resist opsonization by human sera containing opsonizing antibody. Mortality in rats was significantly reduced even when monoclonal antibody was administered as late as 24 hr after challenge. This suggests that the antibody could be used for immunotherapy as well as immunoprophylaxis. A similar protective effect has been shown for monoclonal antibodies to capsular antigens of *Haemophilus influenzae* (37).

In veterinary medicine, the role of capsule is not well defined for many bacterial pathogens. Capsular antigens do occur widely among the Enterobacteriaceae and they have been proposed as playing a role in the adherence of enteropathogenic *E. coli* (98), in addition to the aforementioned pili. Capsular K antigens are also involved in the pathogenesis of septicemic *E. coli* infections (163). Among the gram-positive organisms, *Staphylococcus aureus,* an important mastitis pathogen, possesses numerous mechanisms for escaping phagocytosis, among them being capsule (163). Two streptococci, *S. equi* and the group E *Streptococcus* of swine, are recognized as having antiphagocytic properties.

However, this is due to possession of cell wall-associated proteins rather than polysaccharide capsule (18,162).

At present, the diagnostic, therapeutic, and prophylactic applications of monoclonal antibodies against capsular antigens of veterinary pathogens remain largely unexplored. Hybridoma technology can contribute to a better understanding of the structure, function, and importance of capsular antigens. This in turn may lead to clearer ideas for clinical applications of monoclonal antibodies.

D. Bacterial Cell Wall Antigens

Cell wall structures have received a great deal of attention both as immunogens and as virulence factors. The cell wall "O" LPS of gram-negative bacteria are strongly antigenic and serve as the basis for taxonomic classification of gram-negative organisms (42). The lipid A moiety of gram-negative bacterial LPS has been identified as a potent component of the endotoxin molecule exerting powerful, well-defined, toxic effects in infected hosts (17). The waxy cell walls of acid-fast organisms such as the mycobacteria, are instrumental in facilitating the intracellular survival of phagocytized bacteria, leading to chronic granulomatous infections (163). The peptidoglycan component of gram-positive bacterial cell wall has also been demonstrated to produce endotoxinlike activity and adjuvant activity (126). In addition, some gram-positive organisms possess cell wall-related proteins, such as protein A of *Staphylococcus aureus* and the M protein of group A streptococci, which assist the organism in avoiding phagocytosis and establishing infection (7). In this section, three potential applications for monoclonal antibodies against cell wall components of veterinary pathogens will be discussed.

1. Brucella abortus

Brucellosis, due to *Brucella abortus,* is an important zoonotic disease of ruminant animals which can cause undulant fever in humans. In the United States, a federal regulatory disease control program established in 1934, has significantly reduced, but not eliminated brucellosis in cattle. The essential elements of the control program are restriction of cattle movement, serologic identification and destruction of infected animals, and vaccination of calves with a live avirulent *B. abortus* (strain 19) vaccine. Vaccination is an important component of the program. However, the production of antibodies in vaccinated animals as well as the occurrence of other organisms which induce cross-reactive antibodies, confound the accurate serologic diagnosis of naturally occurring brucellosis infection. This is recognized as a serious obstacle to the total elimination of brucellosis from the national herd (12).

Numerous approaches to improving the strain specificity of serologic tests have been explored. Now, hybridoma technology offers the most promising solution to this long-standing problem. Identification of strain 19-specific cell wall antigens as well as type-specific antigens of *Yersinia enterocolitica*, a common cross-reacting organism, might be expedited by the use of monoclonal antibody probes. Monoclonal antibodies developed against strain-specific antigens could then be used in competitive serologic assays such as the competitive-inhibition assay described earlier for the diagnosis of tuberculosis, to discriminate natural *B. abortus* infections from both strain 19 vaccination and spontaneous infections with cross-reactive organisms. Several reports on the development of monoclonal antibodies against cell wall LPS antigens of *Brucella* strains for serodiagnostic application have already appeared (54,125,125a). The first work by Schurig (125) illustrated the use of monoclonal antibody to *Brucella* in a competitive ELISA test to discriminate antibody against *E. coli* LPS antigen from antibody to *Brucella* LPS antigen in sera from immunized animals. In another study (15), a monoclonal antibody specific for the ''O''-chain polysaccharide of *Yersinia enterocolitica* was found to agglutinate several biotypes of *B. abortus*. It was concluded that the ''A'' antigen of *B. abortus* is identical to the ''O''-chain polysaccharide of *Y. enterocolitica*.

2. Streptococcus equi

Streptococcus equi causes a severe lymphadenopathy in horses resulting in abscessation and rupture of lymph nodes primarily in the head and neck region. The condition is commonly known as strangles due to the severe respiratory impairment which can result from swelling of the pharyngeal lymph nodes. In certain management situations, *S. equi* infection can reach epidemic proportions. This is particularly true on breeding farms and in training stables where there is a continual turnover of large numbers of horses. Contamination of the environment with purulent material from draining abscesses promotes the spread of disease, and in some facilities strangles becomes an endemic problem (12). Young foals accompanying their mares to breeding farms are particularly susceptible. A commercial bacterin is available for vaccination against *S. equi*, but the degree of protection afforded by immunization is variable (25). Vaccination of susceptible foals after they have been introduced onto contaminated premises is of little value. This represents another situation in veterinary medicine where an effective product for passive immunization of populations at risk would be helpful in controlling disease.

Numerous *S. equi* antigens have been examined for their potential as protective immunogens (101), including peptidoglycans, murein–teichoic acid complex, group C carbohydrate, Lancefield extracted protein, and a cell wall protein similar to the M protein of group A streptococci. The M-like protein, first characterized by Woolcock in 1974, is of particular interest (162). It has been shown to be a potent immunogen, producing high antibody titers in both horses and rabbits. Srivastava and Barnum (142) have reported that vaccination of pony foals with purified, alum-precipitated M-like protein protected them from infection via contact exposure to a horse with active strangles. Antibody levels produced by vaccination with M-like protein were equivalent to the levels which occur after natural infection with *S. equi.*

These findings suggest that a monoclonal antibody directed against the M-like protein could be useful for passive immunization of foals against *S. equi* infection, although at this time it is unclear whether circulating serum antibody alone affords adequate protection against disease. Some evidence exists that a cellular immune response as well as a local mucosal immune response in the nasopharynx play a role in host protection (150). Nevertheless, the value of passive immunization with parenterally administered monoclonal antibody merits future evaluation.

3. Core LPS of Gram-Negative Bacterial Endotoxin

One of the most exciting potential applications of hybridoma technology in veterinary and human medicine is the development of a monoclonal antibody to the common core LPS fraction of endotoxin for uses in immunotherapy and immunoprophylaxis against a broad range of Gram-negative pathogens involved in a wide variety of specific disease entities. That such a possibility can even be theorized is a credit to the many basic and clinical researchers who have carefully studied the structure, function, and clinical effects of Gram-negative endotoxin.

Variations in "O" antigenicity of Gram-negative bacteria result from the diversity of structure of the oligosaccharide side chains of cell wall LPS. Although these "O" antigens are highly immunogenic, their structural diversity leads to serologically distinct antibody responses, with little or no cross-reactivity occurring between heterologous "O" strains. Given the staggering number of Gram-negative bacterial species and strains capable of producing serious infection, active immunization has never received serious consideration as a means of effectively controlling Gram-negative infections. However, recognition of the problem of antigenic diversity has prompted investigations into the identification of shared cell wall antigens which might serve as common immunogens in a cross-protective vaccine. McCabe *et al.* (80) have reviewed the background and developments in this area of research, and the major advances described will be briefly summarized here.

In 1966, Lüderitz *et al.* (71) reported on the structural similarities of the core portions of Gram-negative cell wall LPS in *Salmonella* sp. and other related *Enterobacteriaceae.* It was observed that, despite variations in the terminal oligosaccharide structures which confer "O" antigenicity, all species examined possessed a common core antigen composed of lipid A attached to ketodeoxyoctonate (KDO) and heptose. This core structure is immunogenic.

Mutant strains of *S. typhimurium* (14), *S. minnesota* (79), and *E. coli* (23) have been identified which fail to synthesize oligosaccharide side chains of cell wall LPS. Two stable mutants, the Re mutant of *S. minnesota* and the J5 mutant of *E. coli* O111:B$_4$, have been used in a number of immunization studies to demonstrate that antibody produced against the core LPS determinants only will significantly protect laboratory animals from challenge infection with a broad range of Gram-negative organisms including other *Salmonella* and *E. coli* species (79,167),*Klebsiella* sp. (79,167), *Pseudomonas* sp. (168), and *Haemophilus influenzae* (76).

These encouraging findings have led to investigations into the role of core LPS antibody in protecting human patients from the effects of Gram-negative septicemia. McCabe *et al.*, (81) measured naturally occurring antibody to core LPS determinants as well as antibody to type-specific antigens in 400 human patients with Gram-negative septicemia. A marked correlation was observed between antibody titer to core LPS and severity of clinical disease. Patients with high antibody titers to core LPS of 1:80 or more as measured by indirect hemagglutination were far less likely to develop shock or die than patients with low antibody titer to core LPS. This phenomenon appeared to be independent of antibody titer to type-specific antigens of infecting organisms. Ziegler *et al.* (169) immunized human volunteers with the J5 mutant of *E. coli* O111:B$_4$ and produced a human antiserum to core LPS, which was then administered to hospital patients with Gram-negative septicemia in a double-blind clinical trial. Mortality was significantly reduced in patients receiving J5 antiserum in comparison to patients receiving nonimmune serum, even among patients experiencing profound shock. These patients were infected with a broad range of unrelated Gram-negative organisms.

Mutharia *et al.* (97) have recently produced four monoclonal antibodies against the J5 mutant of *E. coli*, all of which react with purified LPS from J5 *E. coli*, the Re 595 mutant of *S. minnesota*, *Agrobacterium tumefaciens*, and *Pseudomonas aeruginosa* in addition to purified lipid A of *P. aeruginosa*. These antibodies also react in ELISA with outer membrane preparations of more than 30 strains of various Gram-negative bacteria while showing no reactivity against Gram-positive species. These results add credence to the concept of widespread conservation of single antigenic sites in the lipid A of diverse gram-negative bacteria and illustrate the power of monoclonal antibodies as investigative tools. A more recent report (87a) has shown that the cross reactivity of monoclonal antibodies against *E. coli* J5 endotoxin was even greater when the antibodies were reacted with whole heterologous organisms rather than the purified LPS extracts.

These findings have raised hopes that a vaccine containing core LPS determinants can be developed for immunization against diverse gram-negative bacterial infections. In addition, antibody against core LPS could be used for passive immunization of patients at risk, such as burn patients or immunocompromised patients on chemotherapy, as well as for immunotherapy in the early stages of

Gram-negative bacterial septicemia. Monoclonal antibody derived by hybridoma technology would be a logical method for producing therapeutic and prophylactic antibody. It obviates the problem of raising conventional antisera in human beings and would yield specific antibody in much higher concentration. The concentration of antibody administered for therapeutic purposes is probably a critical factor because, in overwhelming Gram-negative sepsis, antibody is rapidly consumed.

The potential applications of a monoclonal antibody to core LPS in veterinary medicine are numerous and the economic benefit to be derived from passive immunization and immunotherapy is enormous. Many costly clinical syndromes in livestock are known or thought to involve Gram-negative bacterial septicemia or endotoxemia (12,127a). These include, among others, colisepticemia in newborn calves, shigellosis in foals, agalactia of sows, salmonellosis of cattle and horses, postoperative endotoxemia in horses, and coliform mastitis in cattle. Many of these conditions are characterized by a high mortality rate even in the face of aggressive antibiotic therapy and supportive care. The ability to intervene in these conditions with a monoclonal antibody to core LPS would be of incalculable benefit to clinical veterinary medicine.

IV. CONCLUSIONS

Three main areas of application for monoclonal antibodies against bacterial antigens in veterinary medicine have been discussed, namely, passive immunization, improved immunodiagnostics, and immunotherapy. Although many of the proposed applications presented in this chapter are speculative, the authors have attempted to limit discussion to bacterial diseases where existing knowledge of the antigenic structure, virulence mechanisms, and host responses to infection is sufficient to make such speculation realistic. Whenever possible, these potential applications have been supported by discussion of analogous developments in human medical research to lend credence to the speculations in veterinary medicine. Only additional research involving these specific veterinary pathogens will determine whether or not the potential applications we have hypothesized can be successfully implemented in practice. It is hoped that this chapter will encourage veterinary researchers to examine critically some of our proposed applications for monoclonal antibodies. Undoubtedly many additional practical applications for hybridoma technology in veterinary medicine have eluded our imagination, and interested readers are very likely to develop additional ideas of their own. If this occurs, then the chapter has served a useful purpose.

Passive immunization using monoclonal antibodies may dramatically alter traditional approaches to disease control in veterinary medicine. Several aspects of veterinary livestock practice underscore the need for effective passive immunizing agents. Livestock producers resist the idea of active immunization against infectious diseases even when efficacious vaccines are available. Much of this resistance is due to the economic realities of livestock production where profit margins are narrow and the cost of vaccination is weighed against the risk of experiencing disease outbreaks. Unfortunately, in many cases the risks are weighed incorrectly and the veterinarian is then called in to halt the rapid spread of infectious disease through a highly susceptible population of livestock. The value of passive immunization in these situations is unquestionable, as evidenced by the apparent success of the K99-specific monoclonal antibody in controlling outbreaks of fatal diarrhea in neonatal calves due to enteropathogenic *E. coli*. In other situations, the risk of disease is recognized to be high and active immunization is carried out, but management factors preclude the value of vaccination. This is particularly true in feedlots where susceptible populations of cattle are not accessible for vaccination prior to the period of highest disease risk. Infections are established before protective antibody is produced by the host and passive immunization represents the only logical immunologic defense.

Monoclonal antibodies, because of their specificity, unlimited availability, and high titer, represent excellent passive immunizing agents. However, their potential usefulness in preventing infection must be evaluated on a case-by-case basis. When the host naturally responds to infection with a local mucosal immune response or a cellular immune response, parenteral administration of monoclonal antibody may not provide adequate protection against infection. In localized infections of mucosal surfaces, monoclonal antibody may need to be administered to specific sites when circulating antibody does not participate in immunologic control of infection. Whereas this was easily accomplished in enteric colibacillosis by oral administration of K99-specific monoclonal antibody, the logistics of administering monoclonal antibody to the terminal airways in respiratory disease are mechanically complex.

The selection of the appropriate antibody class may also be important depending on whether or not opsonization of bacteria is dependent on complement activation. It appears that in the work with antibody to the core LPS of endotoxin, antibody of the IgM class is more protective than IgG antibody. In other situations, bacteria are capable of producing proteases which degrade secretory IgA (73), and monoclonal antibodies of other classes might be more effective. The half-lives of either heterologous or homologous monoclonal antibodies must also be taken into account, especially if passive immunization or long-term therapy is anticipated.

Perhaps the most significant limitation to widespread application of monoclonal antibodies for passive immunization is the current dependency of hybridoma technology on murine cell lines. Repeated application of murine-derived monoclonal antibodies to livestock species will undoubtedly lead to the development of host antimurine antibodies which would destroy the immunologic activity of the administered monoclonal antibody, or perhaps induce allergic sensitivity. This problem requires the development of new cell lines capable of producing species-specific antibody. Recent reports of successful human–murine (38), bovine–murine (114a,141,141a), and porcine–murine (114) fusions capable of producing human, bovine, and porcine immunoglobulins, respectively, offer much hope for the future.

In the area of immunodiagnostics, monoclonal antibodies will be of particular value to veterinary medicine. As a result of their specificity, monoclonal antibodies are ideally suited for identifying specific antigens out of crude antigenic mixtures in unpurified specimens. This has been illustrated by the development of an ELISA test kit using K99-specific monoclonal antibody for detection of the K99 antigen directly from fecal samples. For the veterinarian in livestock practice who works independently and in relative isolation, the development of test kits for field use will dramatically reduce dependency on a central diagnostic laboratory and increase the availability of test results. In addition, monoclonal antibodies will undoubtedly lead to refinements in current methods of serodiagnosis, particularly in those cases where antigenic cross-reactivity leads to decreased specificity. Paratuberculosis and brucellosis are prime examples.

Immunotherapy is becoming increasingly popular in human medicine, and many potential applications exist in veterinary medicine as well. Immunotherapy is particularly attractive in veterinary medicine as an alternative to antibiotic therapy. The use of antibiotics in livestock is strictly regulated and the selection of antibiotics by practitioners often depends as much on their persistence in meat, milk, and eggs as it does on the susceptibility of the infecting organism. For example, the use of aminoglycoside antibiotics in cattle requires a 30-day withholding period before treated cattle can be marketed for meat. This inhibits the use of aminoglycosides even when their therapeutic use in indicated. Even more importantly, societal awareness and concern over adulterants in the food supply and the potential for transfer of drug resistance from animal pathogens to human pathogens, demands that the profession of veterinary medicine identify and implement effective alternatives to antibiotic use. Immunotherapy with monoclonal antibodies represents one likely alternative, and new research activity should be directed toward the development of a broad range of immunotherapeutic agents using hybridoma technology.

Although the scope of this chapter has been limited to applications of monoclonal antibodies against bacteria in veterinary medicine, equally exciting developments are occurring in the areas of veterinary virology, mycology, parasitology, and neoplastic disease. There is no doubt that hybridoma technology will accelerate the pace of basic research in veterinary medicine and lead to a broad range of diagnostic and clinical applications that will change the face of veterinary practice for years to come.

V. SUMMARY

Current and future applications of monoclonal antibodies against bacteria in veterinary medicine have been discussed. Those aspects of veterinary practice which make developments in hybridoma technology particularly attractive to veterinary medicine have been emphasized.

Existing applications of monoclonal antibodies were detailed, including the use of pilus-specific monoclonal antibodies for passive immunization of calves and piglets against enteropathogenic *E. coli* (EPEC) infections as well as the development of rapid diagnostic test kits for field diagnosis of EPEC infections.

Potential applications of monoclonal antibodies for passive immunization against a variety of veterinary pathogens were presented, including passive immunization against *Moraxella bovis* (pinkeye), *Bacteroides nodosus* (foot rot), EPEC enterotoxin (enteric colibacillosis), *Pasteurella haemolytica* (pneumonic pasteurellosis), and *Streptococcus equi* (strangles).

Potential diagnostic applications for important veterinary pathogens were discussed, including diagnosis of *Mycobacterium paratuberculosis* infection (Johne's disease) and *Brucella abortus* (brucellosis).

Potential applications for immunotherapy using monoclonal antibodies were also discussed, including therapy for clostridial infections using monoclonal antibodies against clostridial toxins, and for gram-negative bacterial infections, using monoclonal antibodies against the common core lipopolysaccharide determinants of gram-negative cell wall endotoxin.

Conclusions were presented concerning the role of hybridoma technology in the future progress of veterinary medicine.

REFERENCES

1. Abbas, B., Riemann, H. P., and Lonnerdal, B. (1983). Isolation of specific peptides from *Mycobacterium paratuberculosis* protoplasm and their use in an enzyme-linked immunosorbent assay for the detection of paratuberculosis (Johne's disease) in cattle. *Am. J. Vet. Res.* **44,** 2229–2236.
2. Acres, S. D., Isaacson, R. E., Babiuk, L. A., and Kapitany, R. A. (1979). Immunization of calves against enterotoxigenic colibacillosis by vaccinating dams with purified K99 antigen and whole cell bacterins. *Infect. Immun.* **25,** 121–126.
3. Alexander, T. J. L. (1981). Piglet diarrhoea: A guide to diagnosis and control. *Br. Vet. J.* **137,** 651–662.
4. Amstutz, H. E., Morter, R. L., and Armstrong, C. H. (1982). Antimicrobial resistance of strains of *Pasteurella hemolytica* isolated from feedlot cattle. *Bovine Practitioner* **17,** 52–55.
5. Antczak, D. F. (1982). Monoclonal antibodies: Technology and potential use. *J. Am. Vet. Med. Assoc.* **181,** 1005–1010.

6. Arbuckel, J. B. R. (1970). The location of *Escherichia coli* in the pig intestine. *J. Med. Microbiol.* **3**, 333–340.

7. Arbuthnott, J. P., Owen, P., and Russell, R. J. (1983). Bacterial antigens. *In* "Topley and Wilson's Principles of Bacteriology, Virology and Immunity" (G. Wilson and H. M. Dick, eds.), 7th Ed., Vol. 1, pp. 337–373. Williams & Wilkins, Baltimore, Maryland.

8. Argenzio, R. A., and Whipp, S. C. (1980). Pathophysiology of diarrhea. *In* "Veterinary Gastroenterology" (N. V. Anderson, ed.), pp. 220–232. Lea & Febiger, Philadelphia, Pennsylvania.

9. Bäckström, L., and Curtis, S. E. (1980). Housing and environmental influences on production. *In* "Diseases of Swine" (A. D. Leman, R. D. Glock, W. L. Mengeling, R. H. C. Penny, E. Scholl, and B. Straw, eds.), 5th Ed., pp. 737–753. Iowa State Univ. Press, Ames.

10. Baldwin, E. M. (1945). A study of bovine infectious keratitis. *Am. J. Vet. Res.* **6**, 180–187.

11. Bishop, B., Schurig, G. G., and Troutt, H. F. (1983). Enzyme-linked immunosorbent assay for measurement of anti-*Moraxella bovis* antibodies. *Am. J. Vet. Res.* **43**, 1443–1445.

12. Blood, D. C., Radostits, O. M., and Henderson, J. A. (1983). "Veterinary Medicine—A Textbook of the Diseases of Cattle, Sheep, Pigs, Goats, and Horses," 6th Ed. Baillière, London.

13. Boundy, T. (1983). Foot rot and foot conditions. *In* "Diseases of Sheep" (W. B. Martin, ed.), pp. 98–103. Blackwell, Oxford.

14. Chedid, L., Parant, M., Parant, F., and Boyer, F. (1968). A proposed mechanism for natural immunity to enterobacterial pathogens. *J. Immunol.* **100**, 292–301.

15. Cherwonogrodzky, J. W., Wright, P. F., Perry, M. B., MacLean, L., and Bundle, D. R. (1984). Identification of the *Brucella abortus* "A" antigen as the O-chain polysaccharide. *Abstr. Pap., Annu. Meet., 65th, Conf. Res. Workers Anim. Dis.* Abstr. 112.

16. Cimprich, R. E. (1981). Differential diagnosis of neonatal diarrhea in domestic animals. *Compend. Contin. Educ. Pract. Veterinarian* **3**, S26–S29.

17. Culbertson, R., and Osburn, B. I. (1980). The biologic effects of bacterial endotoxin: A short review. *Vet. Sci. Commun.* **4**, 3–14.

18. Daynes, R. A., and Armstrong, C. H. (1973). An antiphagocytic factor associated with group E *Streptococcus*. *Infect. Immun.* **7**, 298–304.

19. de Graaf, F. K., Klemm, P., and Gaastra, W. (1981). Purification, characterization and partial covalent structure of the adhesive antigen K99 of *Escherichia coli*. *Infect. Immun.* **33**, 877–883.

20. de Graaf, F. K., and Roorda, I. (1982). Production, purification and characterization of the fimbrial adhesive antigen F41 isolated from calf enteropathogenic *Escherichia coli* strain B41M. *Infect. Immun.* **36**, 751–758.

21. Egerton, J. R. (1973). Surface and somatic antigens of *Fusiformus nodosus*. *J. Comp. Pathol.* **83**, 151–159.

22. Egerton, J. R., and Burrell, D. H. (1970). Prophylactic and therapeutic vaccination against ovine foot rot. *Aust. Vet. J.* **46**, 517–522.

23. Elbein, A. D., and Heath, E. C. (1965). The biosynthesis of cell wall lipopolysaccharide in *Escherichia coli*. I. The biochemical properties of a uridine diphosphate galactose 4-epimeraseless mutant. *J. Biol. Chem.* **240**, 1919–1925.

24. Ellens, D. J., de Leeuw, P. W., and Rozemond, H. (1979). Detection of the K99 antigen of *Escherichia coli* in calf faeces by enzyme linked immunosorbent assay (ELISA). *Vet. Q.* **1**, 169–175.

25. Engelbrecht, H. (1969). Vaccination against strangles. *J. Am. Vet. Med. Assoc.* **115**, 425–427.

26. Engleberg, N. C., and Eisenstein, B. I. (1984). The impact of new cloning techniques on the diagnosis and treatment of infectious diseases. *N. Engl. J. Med.* **311**, 892–901.

27. Evans, D. G., Silver, R. P., Evans, D. J., Chase, D. G., and Gorbach, S. L. (1975). Plasmid-controlled colonization factor associated with virulence in *Escherichia coli* enterotoxigenic for humans. *Infect. Immun.* **12**, 656–667.

28. Evans, M. G., and Waxler, G. L. (1982). Piliated *Escherichia coli* and enteric disease in neonatal swine in Michigan. *Abstr. Pap., Annu. Meet., 63rd, Conf. Res. Workers Anim. Dis.*, Abstr. 238.

29. Every, D. (1979). Purification of pili from *Bacteroides nodosus* and an examination of their chemical, physical and serological properties. *J. Gen. Microbiol.* **115**, 309–316.

30. Every, D., and Skerman, T. M. (1983). Surface structure of *Bacteroides nodosus* in relation to virulence and immunoprotection in sheep. *J. Gen. Microbiol.* **129**, 225–234.

31. Federal Register (1984). Department of Agriculture: Special and alcohol fuels research grants programs for fiscal year 1984, solicitation of applications; notice. Vol. 49, p. 1160.

32. Feldner, J., Gobel, U., and Bredt, W. (1982). *Mycoplasma pneumoniae* adhesin localized to tip structure by monoclonal antibody. *Nature (London)* **298**, 765–767.

33. Francis, D. H. (1982). Prevalence of K88, K99 and 987P-positive *Escherichia coli* in piglets with colibacillosis. *Abstr. Pap., Annu. Meet., 63rd, Conf. Res. Workers Anim. Dis.* Abstr. 237.

34. Gaastra, W., and de Graaf, F. K. (1982). Host-specific fimbrial adhᵉsins of noninvasive enterotoxigenic *Escherichia coli* strains. *Microbiol. Rev.* **46**, 129–161.

35. Galloway, D. R., Hedstrom, R. C., and Pavlovskis, O. R. (1984). Production and characterization of monoclonal antibodies to exotoxin A from *Pseudomonas aeruginosa*. *Infect. Immun.* **44**, 262–267.

36. Gentry, M. J., and Confer, A. W. (1983). Serum neutralization of *Pasteurella haemolytica* cytotoxin. *Abstr. Pap., Annu. Meet., 64th, Conf. Res. Workers Anim. Dis.* Abstr. 179.

37. Gigliotti, F., and Insel, R. A. (1982). Protection from infection with *Haemophilus influenzae* type B by monoclonal antibody to the capsule. *J. Infect. Dis.* **146**, 249–254.

38. Gigliotti, F., Smith, L., and Insel, R. A. (1984). Reproducible production of protective human monoclonal antibodies by fusion of peripheral blood lymphocytes with a mouse myeloma cell line. *J. Infect. Dis.* **149**, 43–47.

39. Gil-Turnes, C., and de Araujo, F. L. (1982). Serological characterization of strains of *Moraxella bovis* using double immunodiffusion. *Can. J. Comp. Med.* **46**, 165–168.

40. Glorioso, J. C., Jones, G. W., Rush, H. G., Pentler, L. J., Darif, C. A., and Coward, J. E. (1982). Adhesion of type A *Pasteurella multocida* to rabbit pharyngeal cells and its possible role in rabbit respiratory tract infections. *Infect. Immun.* **35**, 1103–1109.

41. Goodnow, R. A. (1980). Biology of *Bordetella bronchiseptica*. *Microbiol. Rev.* **44**, 722–738.

42. Gross, R. J., and Holmes, B. (1983). The Enterobacteriaceae. *In* "Topley and Wilson's Principles of Bacteriology, Virology and Immunity" (M. T. Parker, ed.), 7th Ed., Vol. 2, pp. 272–284. Williams & Wilkins, Baltimore, Maryland.

43. Guinée, P. A. M., and Jansen, W. H. (1979). Behavior of *Escherichia coli* K antigens K88ab, K88ac, and K88ad in immunoelectrophoresis, double diffusion, and hemagglutination. *Infect. Immun.* **23**, 700–705.

44. Guinée, P. A. M., Jansen, W. H., and Agterberg, C. M. (1976). Detection of the K99 antigen by means of agglutination and immunoelectrophoresis in *Escherichia coli* isolates from calves and its correlation with enterotoxigenicity. *Infect. Immun.* **13**, 1369–1377.

45. Guinée, P. A. M., Veldkamp, J., and Jansen, W. H. (1977). Improved Minca medium for the detection of K99 antigen in calf enterotoxigenic strains of *Escherichia coli*. *Infect. Immun.* **15**, 676–678.

46. Haggard, D. L., and Sherman, D. M. (1984). Vaccine development in the prevention of bovine enteric colibacillosis. *Compend. Contin. Educ. Pract. Veterinarian* **6**, S347–S353.

47. Haggard, D. L., Johnson, D. W., Springer, J. A., Ward, G. E., and Vosdingh, R. A. (1982).

Evaluation of an *Escherichia coli* bacterin containing the K99 antigen for preventing bovine neonatal enteric colibacillosis. *Vet. Med. Small Anim. Clin.* **77**, 1391–1394.

48. Haggard, D. L., Springer, J. A., and Vosdingh, R. A. (1982). Efficacy of a single annual booster inoculation of cows with *Escherichia coli* bacterin for preventing enterotoxigenic colibacillosis in neonatal calves. *Vet. Med. Small Anim. Clin.* **77**, 1525–1527.

49. Hansen, G. A., Pedersen, K. B., and Riising, K. B. (1983). Protection against colonization of *Bordetella bronchiseptica* in the upper respiratory tract of the pig. *In* "Atrophic Rhinitis in Pigs" (K. B. Pedersen and N. C. Nielsen, eds.), pp. 89–97. Comm. Eur. Communities, Luxembourg.

50. Hayakawa, S., Tsuyoshi, U., Mekada, E., Moynihan, M. R., and Okada, Y. (1983). Monoclonal antibody against diphtheria toxin. *J. Biol. Chem.* **258**, 4311–4317.

51. Hemelhof, W., Retore, P., De Mol, P., Butzler, J. P., Takeda, T., Miwatani, T., and Yakeda, Y. (1984). Production of a monoclonal antibody against heat-stable enterotoxin produced by human strain of enterotoxigenic *Escherichia coli*. *Lancet* **1**, 1011–1012.

52. Hewitt, J., Coates, A. R. M., Mitchison, D. A., and Ivanyi, J. (1982). The use of murine monoclonal antibodies without purification of antigen in the serodiagnosis of tuberculosis. *J. Immunol. Methods* **55**, 205–211.

53. Himmel, M. E., Yates, M. D., Laverman, L. H., and Squire, P. G. (1982). Purification and partial characterization of a macrophage cytotoxin from *Pasteurella haemolytica*. *Am. J. Vet. Res.* **43**, 764–767.

54. Holman, P. J., Adams, L. G., Hunter, D. M., Heck, F. C., Nielsen, K. H., and Wagner, G. G. (1983). Derivation of monoclonal antibodies against *Brucella abortus* antigens. *Vet. Immunol. Immunopathol.* **4**, 603–614.

55. Holmberg, S. D., Osterholm, M. T., Senger, K. A., and Cohen, M. L. (1984). Drug-resistant *Salmonella* from animals fed antimicrobials. *N. Engl. J. Med.* **311**, 617–622.

56. Horwitz, M. A. (1982). Phagocytosis of microorganisms. *Rev. Infect. Dis.* **4**, 104–123.

57. Hughes, D. E., and Pugh, G. W. (1970). A five-year study of infectious bovine keratoconjunctivitis in a beef herd. *J. Am. Vet. Med. Assoc.* **157**, 443–451.

58. Irwin, M. R., McConnell, S., Coleman, J. D., and Wilcox, G. E. (1979). Bovine respiratory disease complex: A comparison of potential predisposing etiologic factors in Australia and the United States. *J. Am. Vet. Med. Assoc.* **175**, 1095–1099.

59. Isaacson, R. E. (1977). K99 surface antigen of *Escherichia coli:* purification and partial characterization. *Infect. Immun.* **15**, 272–279.

60. Isaacson, R. E., and Richter, P. (1981). *Escherichia coli* 987P pilus: Purification and partial characterization. *J. Bacteriol.* **146**, 784–789.

61. Isaacson, R. E., Dean, E. A., Morgan, R. L., and Moon, H. W. (1980). Immunization of suckling pigs against enterotoxigenic *Escherichia coli*-induced diarrheal disease by vaccinating dams with purified K99 or 987P pili: Antibody production in response to vaccination. *Infect. Immun.* **29**, 824–826.

62. Isaacson, R. E., Fusco, P. C., Brinton, C. C., and Moon, H. W. (1978). *In vitro* adhesion of *Escherichia coli* to porcine small intestinal epithelial cells: Pili as adhesive factors. *Infect. Immun.* **21**, 392–397.

63. Jensen, R., and Mackey, D. R. (1979). "Diseases of Feedlot Cattle," 3rd Ed., pp. 59–66. Lea & Febiger, Philadelphia, Pennsylvania.

64. Jensen, R., Pierson, R. E., Braddy, P. M., Saari, D. A., Lauerman, L. H., England, J. J., Keyvanfar, H., Collier, J. R., Horton, D. P., McChesney, A. E., Benitez, A., and Christie, R. M. (1976). Shipping fever pneumonia in yearling feedlot cattle. *J. Am. Vet. Med. Assoc.* **169**, 500–506.

65. Jones, G. W., and Rutter, J. M. (1972). Role of the K88 antigen in the pathogenesis of neonatal diarrhea caused by *Escherichia coli* in piglets. *Infect. Immun.* **6**, 918–927.

66. Killinger, A. H., Weisiger, R. M., Helper, L. C., and Mansfield, M. E. (1978). Detection of *Moraxella bovis* antibodies in the SIgA, IgG and IgM classes of immunoglobulin in bovine lacrimal secretions by an indirect fluorescent antibody test. *Am. J. Vet. Res.* **39**, 931–934.
67. Klipstein, F. A., Engert, R. F., and Houghten, R. A. (1983). Protection in rabbits immunized with a vaccine of *Escherichia coli* heat-stable toxin cross-linked to the heat-labile toxin B subunit. *nfect. Immun.* **40**, 888–893.
68. Kopecky, K. E., Pugh, G. W., and McDonald, T. J. (1983). Infectious bovine keratoconjunctivitis: Evidence for general immunity. *Am. J. Vet. Res.* **44**, 260–262.
69. Lillie, L. E. (1974). The bovine respiratory disease complex. *Can. Vet. J.* **15**, 233–242.
70. Lind, A. (1978). Mycobacterial antigens. *Ann. Microbiol.* **129A**, 99–107.
71. Lüderitz, O., Staub, A. M., and Westphal, O. (1966). Immunochemistry of O and R antigens of *Salmonella* and related *Enterobacteriaceae*. *Bacteriol. Rev.* **30**, 192–255.
72. Macario, A. J. L., and Conway de Macario, E. (1984). Antibacterial monoclonal antibodies and the dawn of a new era in the control of infection. *Surv. Synth. Pathol. Res.* **3**, 119–130.
73. Male, C. J. (1979). Immunoglobulin A1 protease production by *Haemophilus influenzae* and *Streptococcus pneumoniae*. *Infect. Immun.* **26**, 254–261.
74. Markham, R. J. F., and Wilkie, B. N. (1980). Interaction between *Pasteurella haemolytica* and bovine alveolar macrophages: Cytotoxic effect on macrophages and impaired phagocytosis. *Am. J. Vet. Res.* **41**, 18–22.
75. Markham, R. J. F., Ramnaraine, M. L. R., and Muscoplat, C. C. (1982). Cytotoxic effect of *Pasteurella haemolytica* on bovine polymorphonuclear leukocytes and impaired production of chemotactic factors by *Pasteurella haemolytica*-infected alveolar macrophages. *Am. J. Vet. Res.* **43**, 285–288.
76. Marks, M. I., Ziegler, E. J., Douglas, H., Corbeil, L. B., and Braude, A. I. (1982). Induction of immunity against lethal *Haemophilus influenzae* type b infection by *Escherichia coli* core lipopolysaccharide. *J. Clin. Invest.* **69**, 742–749.
77. Martin, S. W. (1983). Vaccination: Is it effective in preventing respiratory disease or influencing weight gains in feedlot calves? *Can. Vet. J.* **24**, 10–19.
78. Martin, S. W., Meek, A. H., Davis, D. G., Johnson, J. A., and Curtis, R. A. (1982). Factors associated with mortality and treatment costs in feedlot calves: The Bruce county beef project, years 1978, 1979, 1980. *Can. J. Comp. Med.* **46**, 341–349.
79. McCabe, W. R. (1972). Immunization with R mutants of *S. minnesota*. I. Protection against challenge with heterologous gram negative bacilli. *J. Immunol.* **108**, 601–610.
80. McCabe, W. R., DeMaria, A., and Johns, M. (1980). Potential use of shared antigens for immunization against gram-negative bacillary infections. *In* "New Developments with Human and Veterinary Vaccines" (A. Mizrahi, I. Hertman, M. A. Klingberg, and A. Kohn, eds.), pp. 107–117. Alan R. Liss, New York.
81. McCabe, W. R., Kreger, B. E., and Johns, M. (1972). Type specific and cross-reactive antibodies in gram-negative bacteremia. *N. Engl. J. Med.* **287**, 261–267.
82. McGowan, B. (1973). Report on the committee of diseases of sheep and goats. *Proc. Annu. Meet., 77th, U.S. Anim. Health Assoc.* p. 362.
83. McGuire, T. C., and Adams, D. S. (1982). Failure of colostral immunoglobulin transfer to calves: Prevalence and diagnosis. *Compend. Contin. Educ. Pract. Veterinarian* **4**, S35-S39.
84. Merkal, R. S. (1973). Laboratory diagnosis of bovine paratuberculosis. *J. Am. Vet. Med. Assoc.* **163**, 1100–1102.
85. Merkal, R. S. (1984). Paratuberculosis: Advances in cultural, serologic, and vaccination methods. *J. Am. Vet. Med. Assoc.* **184**, 939–943.
86. Mills, K. W., and Tietze, K. L. (1984). Monoclonal antibody enzyme-linked immunosorbent assay for identification of K99-positive *Escherichia coli* isolates from calves. *J. Clin. Microbiol.* **19**, 498–501.

87. Mills, K. W., Phillips, R. M., Kelly, B. L., and Baughman, G. L. (1982). Using enzyme-linked immunosorbent assay to detect *Escherichia coli* K88 pili antigens from clinical isolates. *Am. J. Vet. Res.* **43**, 365–367.

87a. Miner, K. M., Manyak, C. L., Williams, E., Jackson, J., Jewell, M., Gammon, M. T., Ehrenfreund, C., Hayes, E., Callahan, L. T., Zweerink, H., and Sigal, N. H. (1986). Characterization of murine monoclonal antibodies to *Escherichia coli* J5. *Infect. Immun.* **52**, 56–62.

88. Mintz, C. S., Cliver, D. O., and Deibel, R. H. (1983). Attachment of *Salmonella* to mammalian cells *in vitro*. *Can. J. Microbiol.* **29**, 1731–1735.

89. Mitchell, G. F. (1981). Hybridomas in immunoparasitology. *In* "Monoclonal Hybridoma Antibodies: Techniques and Applications" (J. G. R. Hurrell, ed.), pp. 139–149. CRC Press, Boca Raton, Florida.

90. Mooi, F. R., and de Graaf, F. K. (1979). Isolation and characterization of K88 antigens. *FEMS Microbiol. Lett.* **5**, 17–20.

91. Moon, H. W. (1981). Protection against enteric colibacillosis in pigs suckling orally vaccinated dams: Evidence for pili as protective antigens. *Am. J. Vet. Res.* **42**, 173–177.

92. Moon, H. W., Nagy, B., Isaacson, R. E., and Ørskov, I. (1977). Occurrence of K99 antigen on *Escherichia coli* isolated from pigs and colonization of pig ileum by K99$^+$ enterotoxigenic *E. coli* from calves and pigs. *Infect. Immun.* **15**, 614–620.

93. Moon, H. W., Whipp, S. C., and Skartvedt, S. M. (1976). Etiologic diagnosis of diarrheal diseases of calves: Frequency and methods for detecting enterotoxin and K99 antigen production by *Escherichia coli*. *Am. J. Vet. Res.* **37**, 1025–1029.

94. Morgan, R. L., Isaacson, R. E., Moon, H. W., Brinton, C. C., and To, C. C. (1978). Immunization of suckling pigs against enterotoxigenic *Escherichia coli*-induced diarrheal disease by vaccinating dams with purified 987P or K99 pili: Protection correlates with pilus homology of vaccine and challenge. *Infect. Immun.* **22**, 771–777.

95. Morris, J. A., Thorns, C., Scott, A. C., Sojka, W. J., and Wells, G. A. (1982). Adhesion *in vitro* and *in vivo* associated with an adhesive antigen (F41) produced by a K99 mutant of the reference strain *Escherichia coli* B41. *Infect. Immun.* **36**, 1146–1153.

95a. Morris, J. A., and Ivanyi, J. (1985). Immunoassays of field isolates of *Mycobacterium bovis* and other *Mycobacteria* by use of monoclonal antibodies. *J. Med. Microbiol.* **19**, 367–373.

96. Murayama, S. (1983). *Clostridium botulinum* type D toxin: Purification, characterization and comparison with type C_1 toxin in molecular properties. *Jpn. J. Vet. Res.* **31**, 93.

97. Mutharia, L. M., Crockford, G., Bogard, W. C., and Hanock, R. E. W. (1984). Monoclonal antibodies specific for *Escherichia coli* J5 lipopolysaccharide: Cross reaction with other gram-negative bacterial species. *Infect. Immun.* **45**, 631–636.

98. Myers, L. L. (1978). Enteric colibacillosis in calves: Immunogenicity and antigenicity of *Escherichia coli* antigens. *Am. J. Vet. Res.* **39**, 761–765.

99. Nagy, B. (1980). Vaccination of cows with a K99 extract to protect newborn calves against experimental enterotoxic colibacillosis. *Infect. Immun.* **27**, 21–24.

100. Nagy, B., Moon, H. W., Isaacson, R. E., To, C. C., and Brinton, C. C. (1978). Immunization of suckling pigs against enteric enterotoxigenic *Escherichia coli* infection by vaccinating dams with purified pili. *Infect. Immun.* **21**, 269–274.

101. Nara, P. L., Krakowka, S., Powers, T. E., and Garg, R. C. (1983). Experimental *Streptococcus equi* infection in the horse: Correlation with *in vivo* and *in vitro* immune responses. *Am. J. Vet. Res.* **44**, 529–534.

102. O'Donnell, I. J., Stewart, D. J., and Clark, B. L. (1983). Serological identification of pilus antigen and other protein antigens of *Bacteroides nodosus* using electro-blot radioimmunoassay after electrophoretic fractionation of the proteins on sodium dodecyl sulfate polyacrylamide gels. *Aust. J. Biol. Sci.* **36**, 15–20.

103. Oguma, K., Agui, T., Syuto, B., Kimura, K., Iida, H., and Kubo, S. (1982). Four different monoclonal antibodies against type C_1 toxin of *Clostridium botulinum*. *Infect. Immun.* **38**, 14–20.

104. Ørskov, I., Ørskov, F., Smith, H. W., and Sojka, W. J. (1975). The establishment of K99, a thermolabile, transmissible *Escherichia coli* K antigen, previously called "Kco", possessed by calf and lamb enteropathogenic strains. *Acta Pathol. Microbiol. Scand., Sect. B* **83**, 31–36.

105. Ørskov, I., Ørskov, F., Sojka, W. J., and Leach, J. M. (1961). Simultaneous occurrence of *E. coli* B and L antigens in strains from diseased swine. *Acta Pathol. Microbiol. Scand., Sect. B* **53**, 404–422.

106. Ørskov, I., Ørskov, F., Sojka, W. J., and Wittig, W. (1964). K antigens K88ab (L) and K88ac (L) in *E. coli*. A new O antigen: O147 and a new K antigen: K89 (B). *Acta Pathol. Microbiol. Scand., Sect. B* **62**, 439–447.

107. Pearce, W. A., and Buchanan, T. M. (1978). Attachment role of gonococcal pili. Optimum conditions and quantitation of adherence of isolated pili to human cells *in vitro*. *J. Clin. Invest.* **61**, 931–943.

108. Pedersen, K. B., Froholm, L. O., and Bovre, K. (1972). Fimbriation and colony type of *Moraxella bovis* in relation to conjunctival colonization and development of keratoconjunctivitis in cattle. *Acta Pathol. Microbiol. Scand., Sect. B* **80**, 911–918.

109. Pickard, J. R., and Woods, G. T. (1981). Weaner–stocker calf management. *In* "Current Veterinary Therapy, Food Animal Practice" (J. L. Howard, ed.), pp. 162–166. Saunders, Philadelphia, Pennsylvania.

110. Pugh, G. W., and Hughes, D. E. (1968). Experimental bovine infectious keratoconjunctivitis caused by sunlamp irradiation and *Moraxella bovis* infection: Correlation of hemolytic ability and pathogenicity. *Am. J. Vet. Res.* **29**, 835–839.

111. Pugh, G. W., Hughes, D. E., and Booth, G. D. (1977). Experimentally induced infectious bovine keratoconjunctivitis: Effectiveness of a pilus vaccine against exposure to homologous strains of *Moraxella bovis*. *Am. J. Vet. Res.* **38**, 1519–1522.

112. Pugh, G. W., McDonald, T. J., Kopecky, K. E., and Beall, C. W. (1980). Experimental infectious bovine keratoconjunctivitis: Effects of feeding colostrum from vaccinated cows on development of pinkeye in calves. *Am. J. Vet. Res.* **41**, 1611–1614.

113. Punch, P. I., and Slatter, D. H. (1984). A review of infectious bovine keratoconjunctivitis. *Vet. Bull.* **54**, 193–207.

114. Raybould, T. J. G., Willson, P. J., McDougal, L. J., and Watts, T. C. (1985). A porcine–murine hybridoma that secretes porcine monoclonal antibody of defined specificity. *Am. J. Vet. Res.* **46**, 1768–1769.

114a. Raybould, T. J. G., Crouch, C. F., McDougall, L. J., and Watts, T. C. (1985). Bovine-murine hybridoma that secretes bovine monoclonal antibody of defined specificity. *Am. J. Vet. Res.* **46**, 426–427.

115. Rehmtulla, A. J., and Thomson, R. G. (1981). A review of the lesions in shipping fever of cattle. *Can. Vet. J.* **22**, 1–8.

116. Roberts, D. S., Foster, W. H., Kerry, J. B., and McCalder, H. A. (1972). An alum-treated vaccine for the control of foot rot in sheep. *Vet. Rec.* **91**, 428–429.

117. Runnels, P. L., Moon, H. W., and Schneider, R. A. (1980). Development of resistance with host age to adhesion of K99+ *Escherichia coli* to isolated intestinal epithelial cells. *Infect. Immun.* **28**, 298–300.

118. Rutter, J. M. (1980). Bacterial colonization of the alimentary tract in neonatal diarrhoea of animals. *Proc., Int. Symp. Neonat. Diarrhea* (S. D. Acres, A. J. Forman, and H. Fast, eds.), pp. 183–195. Vet. Infect. Dis. Organ., Saskatoon, Canada.

119. Rutter, J. M., and Anderson, J. C. (1972). Experimental neonatal diarrhoea caused by an

enteropathogenic strain of *Escherichia coli* in piglets: A study of the disease and the effects of vaccinating the dam. *J. Med. Microbiol.* **5,** 197–210.

120. Rutter, J. M., and Jones, G. W. (1973). Protection against enteric disease caused by *Escherichia coli*—a model for vaccination with a virulence determinant? *Nature (London)* **242,** 531–533.

121. Rutter, J. M., Jones, G. W., Brown, G. T. H., Burrows, M. R., and Luther, P. D. (1976). Antibacterial activity in colostrum and milk associated with protection of piglets against enteric disease caused by K88 positive *Escherichia coli. Infect. Immun.* **13,** 667–676.

122. Sadowski, P. L., Hermanson, V., and Hoffsis, G. (1984). Protection of pigs from fatal colibacillosis through the use of "a" and "c" specific monoclonal antibodies to the K88 pilus. *Abstr. Pap., Annu. Meet., 65th, Conf. Res. Workers Anim. Dis.* Abstr. 281.

123. Schmitz, J. A., and Gradin, J. L. (1980). Serotypic and biochemical characterization of *Bacteroides nodosus* isolates from Oregon. *Can. J. Comp. Med.* **44,** 440–446.

124. Schoolnik, G. K., Fernandez, R., Tai, J. Y., Rothbard, J., and Gotschlich, E. C. (1984). Gonococcal pili. Primary structure and receptor binding domain. *J. Exp. Med.* **159,** 1351–1370.

125. Schurig, G. G. (1983). Use of competitive-ELISA with monoclonal antibodies to *Brucella* for diagnostic purposes: A model with cross-reactive *E. coli* antigens. *Abstr. Pap., Annu. Meet., 64th, Conf. Res. Workers Anim. Dis.* Abstr. 193.

125a. Schurig, G. G., Hammerberg, C., and Finkler, B. R. (1984). Monoclonal antibodies to *Brucella* surface antigens associated with the smooth lipopolysaccharide complex. *Am. J. Vet. Res.* **45,** 967–971.

126. Schwab, J. H. (1979). Acute and chronic inflammation induced by bacterial cell wall structures. *In* "Microbiology" (D. Schlessinger, ed.), pp. 209–214. Am. Soc. Microbiol., Washington, D.C.

127. Sherman, D. M., Acres, S. D., Sadowski, P. L., Springer, J. A., Bray, B., Raybould, T. J. G., and Muscoplat, C. C. (1983). Protection of calves against fatal enteric colibacillosis by orally administered *Escherichia coli* K99-specific monoclonal antibody. *Infect. Immun.* **42,** 653–658.

127a. Sherman, D. M. (1986). New prospects for control of endotoxin mediated diseases in veterinary medicine. *Minnesota Vet.* **26,** 33–36.

128. Shewen, P. E., and Wilkie, B. N. (1982). Cytotoxin of *Pasteurella haemolytica* acting on bovine leukocytes. *Infect. Immun.* **35,** 91–94.

129. Shewen, P. E., and Wilkie, B. N. (1983). *Pasteurella haemolytica* cytotoxin neutralizing activity in sera from Ontario beef cattle. *Can. J. Comp. Med.* **47,** 497–498.

130. Shewen, P. E., and Wilkie, B. N. (1984). Immunity to *Pasteurella haemolytica* serotype 1. *In* "Bovine Respiratory Disease: A Symposium" (R. W. Loan, ed.), pp. 480–481. Texas A&M Univ. Press, College Station.

131. Shigeoka, A. O., Pincus, S. H., Rote, N. S., and Hill, H. R. (1984). Protective efficacy of hybridoma type-specific antibody against experimental infection with group B *Streptococcus. J. Infect. Dis.* **149,** 363–372.

132. Skerman, T. M., and Cairney, I. M. (1972). Experimental observations on prophylactic and therapeutic vaccination against foot rot in sheep. *N. Z. Vet. J.* **20,** 205–211.

133. Skerman, T. M., Erasmuson, S. K., and Every, D. (1981). Differentiation of *Bacteroides nodosus* biotypes and colony variants in relation to their virulence and immunoprotective properties in sheep. *Infect. Immun.* **32,** 788–795.

134. Smith, H. W. (1972). The nature of the protective effect of antisera against *Escherichia coli* diarrhoea in piglets. *J. Med. Microbiol.* **5,** 345–353.

135. Smith, H. W., and Gyles, C. L. (1970). The relationship between two apparently different enterotoxins produced by enteropathogenic strains of *Escherichia coli* of porcine origin. *J. Med. Microbiol.* **3,** 387–401.

136. Smith, H. W., and Halls, S. (1967). Observations by the ligated intestinal segment and oral

inoculation methods on *Escherichia coli* infections in pigs, calves, lambs and rabbits. *J. Pathol. Bacteriol.* **93**, 499–529.

137. Smith, H. W., and Huggins, M. B. (1978). The influence of plasmid-determined and other characteristics of enteropathogenic *Escherichia coli* on their ability to proliferate in the alimentary tracts of piglets, calves and lambs. *J. Med. Microbiol.* **11**, 471–492.

138. Smith, H. W., and Linggood, M. A. (1971). The effect of antisera in protecting pigs against experimental *Escherichia coli* diarrhoea and oedema disease. *J. Med. Microbiol.* **4**, 487–493.

139. Smith, H. W., and Linggood, M. A. (1972). Further observations on *Escherichia coli* enterotoxins with particular regard to those produced by atypical piglet strains and by calf and lamb strains: The transmissible nature of these enterotoxins and of a K antigen possessed by calf and lamb strains. *J. Med. Microbiol.* **5**, 243–250.

140. Snyder, S. P. (1974). Foot rot research at Oregon State University, a progress report. *Ore. Agric. Exp. Stn., Spec. Rep.* No. 410, pp. 47–49.

141. Srikumaran, S., Guidry, A. J., and Goldsby, R. A. (1983). Bovine × mouse hybridomas that secrete bovine immunoglobulin G_1. *Science* **220**, 52–524.

141a. Srikumaran, S., Guidry, A. J., and Goldsby, R. A. (1984). Production and characterization of bovine immunoglobulins G_1, G_2, and M from bovine × murine hybridomas. *Vet. Immunol. Immunopathol.* **5**, 323–342.

142. Srivastava, S. K., and Barnum, D. A. (1983). Vaccination of pony foals with M-like protein of *Streptococcus equi*. *Am. J. Vet. Res.* **44**, 41–45.

143. Stephens, L. R., and Little, P. B. (1981). Ultrastructure of *Haemophilus somnus*, causative agent of bovine infectious thromboembolic meningoencephalitis. *Am. J. Vet. Res.* **42**, 1638–1640.

144. Stewart, D. J. (1978). The role of various antigenic fractions of *Bacteroides nodosus* in eliciting protection against foot rot in vaccinated sheep. *Res. Vet. Sci.* **24**, 14–19.

145. Stewart, D. J., Clark, B. L., Peterson, J. E., Griffiths, D. A., and Smith, E. F. (1982). Importance of pilus associated antigen in *Bacteroides nodosus* vaccines. *Res. Vet. Sci.* **32**, 140–147.

146. Theodorakis, M. C., Brightman, A. H., Otto, J. M., Tomes, J. E., and Whitlock, T. W. (1983). A polymer insert for treating infectious bovine keratoconjunctivitis. *Trans. Annu. Sci. Program Coll. Vet. Ophthalmol., 14th* pp. 23–37.

147. Thoen, C. O., and Muscoplat, C. C. (1979). Recent developments in diagnosis of bovine paratuberculosis (Johne's disease). *J. Am. Vet. Med. Assoc.* **174**, 838–840.

148. Thompson, M. R., Gianella, R. A., Deutsch, A., and Brandwein, H. (1983). Monoclonal antibodies directed against *E. coli* heat-stable enterotoxins (STa). *Proc. Jt. Conf. Cholera (U.S.–Jpn. Coop. Med. Sci. Program), 19th* Abstr. p. 89.

149. Thorley, C. M., and Egerton, J. R. (1981). Comparison of alum-absorbed or non-alum-absorbed oil emulsion vaccines containing either pilate or non-pilate *Bacteroides nodosus* cells in inducing and maintaining resistance of sheep to experimental foot rot. *Res. Vet. Sci.* **30**, 32–37.

150. Timoney, J. F., and Galan, J. E. (1984). The protective response of the horse to an avirulent strain of *Streptococcus equi*. *Abstr. Pap., Annu. Meet., 65th, Conf. Res. Workers Anim. Dis.* Abstr. 97.

151. Trainin, Z., Brenner, J., Kornitzer, I., Tamarin, R., Cohen, A., and Meiron, R. (1981). Oral passive immunization of newborn calves against enterotoxigenic *Escherichia coli*. *Refu. Vet.* **38**, 1–6.

152. Tzipori, S. (1981). The aetiology and diagnosis of calf diarrhoea. *Vet. Rec.* **108**, 510–514.

153. Virji, M., Heckels, J. E., and Watt, P. J. (1983). Monoclonal antibodies to gonococcal pili: Studies on antigenic determinants on pili from variants of strain P9. *J. Gen. Microbiol.* **129**, 1965–1973.

154. Volk, W. A., Bizzini, B., Snyder, R. M., Bernhard, E., and Wagner, R. R. (1984). Neu-

tralization of tetanus toxin by distinct monoclonal antibodies binding to multiple epitopes on the toxin molecular. *Infect. Immun.* **45,** 604–609.

155. Walker, P. D., Short, J., Thomson, R. O., and Roberts, D. S. (1973). The fine structure of *Fusiformis nodosus* with special reference to the location of antigens associated with immunity. *J. Gen. Microbiol.* **77,** 351–360.

156. Weech, G. M., and Renshaw, H. W. (1983). Infectious bovine keratoconjunctivitis: Bacteriologic, immunologic, and clinical responses of cattle to experimental exposure with *Moraxella bovis. Comp. Immunol. Microbiol. Infect. Dis.* **6,** 81–94.

157. Wilson, M. R. (1981). Enteric colibacillosis. *In* "Diseases of Swine," (A. D. Leman, R. D. Glock, W. L. Mengeling, R. H. C. Penny, E. Scholl, and B. Straw, eds.), 5th Ed., pp. 471–477. Iowa State Univ. Press, Ames.

158. Wilson, M. R., and Hohmann, A. W. (1974). Immunity to *Escherichia coli* in pigs: Adhesion of enteropathogenic *Escherichia coli* to isolated intestinal epithelial cells. *Infect. Immun.* **10,** 776–782.

159. Wolfe, K. H., Sadowski, P. L., Brandwein, H. J., Deutsch, A., and Reed, D. E. (1984). A diagnostic kit for the detection of the K99 *E. coli* pilus in feces. *Proc. Annu. Meet. Am. Assoc. Vet. Lab. Diagn.* pp. 205–211.

160. Wolff, T. (1984). Piliated pinkeye bacterin for the prevention of infectious bovine keratoconjunctivitis in cattle. *Agri-Practice* **5,** 34–40.

161. Woods, D. E., Straus, D. C., Johanson, W. G., Berry, V. K., and Bass, J. A. (1980). Role of pili in adherence of *Pseudomonas aeruginosa* to mammalian buccal epithelial cells. *Infect. Immun.* **29,** 1146–1151.

162. Woolcock, J. B. (1974). Purification and antigenicity of an M-like protein of *Streptococcus equi. Infect. Immun.* **10,** 116–122.

163. Woolcock, J. B. (1979). "Bacterial Infection and Immunity in Domestic Animals," pp. 35–43. Elsevier, Amsterdam.

164. Yewdell, J. W., and Gerhard, W. (1981). Antigenic characterization of viruses by monoclonal antibodies. *Annu. Rev. Microbiol.* **35,** 185–206.

165. Yokota, T., Ito, T., and Kuwahara, S. (1983). Production and characterization of monoclonal antibodies to heat-labile and heat-stable enterotoxins of *Escherichia coli. Proc. Jt. Conf. Cholera (U. S.–Jpn. Coop. Med. Sci. Program), 19th* Abstr. p. 96.

166. Zander, D. V. (1984). Principles of disease prevention: Diagnosis and control. *In* "Diseases of Poultry" (M. S. Hofstad, J. H. Barnes, B. W. Calnek, W. M. Reid, and H. W. Yoder, eds.), 8th Ed., pp. 1–37. Iowa State Univ. Press, Ames.

167. Ziegler, E. J., Douglas, H., Sherman, J. R., Davis, C. E., and Braude, A. I. (1973). Treatment of *E. coli* and *Klebsiella* bacteremia in agranulocytic animals with antiserum to a UDP-GAL epimerase-deficient mutant. *J. Immunol.* **111,** 433–438.

168. Ziegler, E. J., McCutchan, J. A., Douglas, H., and Braude, A. I. (1975). Prevention of lethal *Pseudomonas* bacteremia with epimerase deficient *E. coli* antiserum. *Trans. Assoc. Am. Physicians* **88,** 101–108.

169. Ziegler, E. J., McCutchan, J. A., Fierer, J., Glauser, M. P., Sadoff, J. C., Douglas, H., and Braude, A. I. (1982). Treatment of gram negative bacteremia and shock with human antiserum to a mutant *Escherichia coli. N. Engl. J. Med.* **307,** 1225–1230.

Index